Principles and Practices in Clinical Research

This book comprehensively reviews the fundamental principles, ethical considerations, regulatory frameworks, and emerging trends in clinical research. The introductory chapters explore the fundamentals of clinical research, its historical context, and the pivotal role of key stakeholders. The book explores regulatory frameworks in various regions, including the USA, EU countries, non-EU countries, and India. It also delves into the implementation of International Conference on Harmonization (ICH) guidelines, ensuring compliance and quality in clinical trials. It meticulously dissects ethical considerations, delving into historical breaches to underscore the paramount importance of ethical integrity. The chapters outline regulatory standards, emphasize data accuracy and confidentiality, and prepare researchers for regulatory inspections and audits. Moreover, the chapters provide a concise yet comprehensive guide to protocol development and statistical analysis in clinical research. From the inception of research protocols to the intricacies of statistical analysis, the book offers practical insights and methodologies crucial for conducting rigorous and ethically sound research. Moreover, it critically examines emerging trends, from the integration of digital health technologies to the burgeoning role of machine learning and artificial intelligence. This book is intended for researchers, healthcare professionals, and regulatory stakeholders.

Key Features:

- Provides an in-depth examination of the fundamental principles underlying clinical research
- Reviews regulatory frameworks across multiple regions, including the USA, EU, non-EU countries, and India
- Discusses the importance of ethics in clinical research, the role of ethical committees, and the informed consent process
- Covers fundamental clinical research methods, including study design, protocol development, and statistical analysis
- Addresses cutting-edge trends and innovations within clinical research, including the application of machine learning and AI tools

Principles and Practices in Clinical Research

Comprehensive Guide to Methodologies, Ethics, and Regulations

Edited by
Nidhi and Anoop Kumar

CRC Press
Taylor & Francis Group
Boca Raton London New York

CRC Press is an imprint of the
Taylor & Francis Group, an **informa** business

Designed cover image: Shutterstock

First edition published 2027
by CRC Press
2385 NW Executive Center Drive, Suite 320, Boca Raton FL 33431

and by CRC Press
4 Park Square, Milton Park, Abingdon, Oxon, OX14 4RN

CRC Press is an imprint of Taylor & Francis Group, LLC

ISBN: 978-1-032-87518-7 (hbk)
ISBN: 978-1-032-87527-9 (pbk)
ISBN: 978-1-003-53308-5 (ebk)

DOI: 10.1201/9781003533085

Typeset in Times
by Apex CoVantage, LLC

Contents

Preface

Clinical research stands at the intersection of scientific discovery, ethical responsibility, and societal trust. As medicine continues to advance at an unprecedented pace, so too does the complexity of the research that fuels it. Today's clinical investigator must navigate not only rigorous methodological demands but also an intricate landscape of ethical principles, regulatory frameworks, and stakeholder expectations. For newcomers, this landscape can appear daunting; for experienced researchers, it evolves quickly enough to require continual learning.

Principles and Practices in Clinical Research: Comprehensive Guide to Methodologies, Ethics, and Regulations was written to serve as a clear, accessible roadmap through this multifaceted terrain. Our goal is to demystify the processes that underpin high-quality clinical inquiry—from designing a sound protocol and selecting appropriate endpoints to safeguarding participant rights, managing data integrity, and meeting regulatory obligations across diverse jurisdictions.

This book does not presume deep prior expertise. Instead, it begins with foundational concepts and builds toward more advanced, practice-oriented discussions, integrating real-world examples and contemporary challenges faced by today's research community. Throughout these chapters, we emphasize a central theme: scientific excellence must be inseparable from ethical rigor. Sound methodology without ethical grounding can undermine public trust, while ethical aspirations without methodological strength fail to generate meaningful evidence.

We hope this guide benefits a wide audience: students taking their first steps into clinical investigation, clinicians seeking to contribute to the evidence base, research coordinators and administrators navigating day-to-day operations, and experienced investigators aiming to stay current with evolving standards. Regulators, ethics board members, and industry professionals may also find clarity and practical insights within these pages.

Above all, we offer this book in the spirit of strengthening the scientific enterprise that ultimately serves patients. As you explore the chapters ahead—whether sequentially or based on your immediate needs—we invite you to engage critically, reflect on the responsibilities inherent in research, and contribute thoughtfully to the future of clinical science.

About the Editors

Nidhi, Ph.D., MAMS, is an accomplished academician and clinical scientist serving as Associate Professor in the Department of Translational and Clinical Research at Jamia Hamdard, New Delhi. She obtained her Ph.D. in Pharmacology from University College of Medical Sciences & GTB Hospital (Delhi University) and previously completed her M. Pharm and B. Pharm in Pharmacology and Pharmaceutical Sciences from Jamia Hamdard.

With over 22 years of teaching and research experience, her expertise spans neuropharmacology, exploring repurposed or indigenous drugs for the treatment of epilepsy and autism, along with neuroinflammatory pathways. She has also worked on neuro-behavioral changes due to pharmacotherapeutics in diabetes and cancer patients. Dr. Nidhi has made significant contributions through her work on cognitive and psychological impairments in chronic conditions such as diabetes and cancer, leveraging standardized neuropsychological tools, depression scales, and quality-of-life instruments to generate clinically actionable insights. Her experience extends across clinical trial operations, pharmacovigilance, pharmacoepidemiology, and translational research, and she has been actively involved in both medical and pharmacy education at undergraduate and postgraduate levels. A recipient of multiple awards for her research work presented in various national and international conferences, including the Dr. Vinod Kumar Bhargava Award by the National Academy of Medical Sciences, she has also received ICMR grants for her research work.

Anoop Kumar currently works as Assistant Professor in the Department of Pharmacology, Delhi Institute of Pharmaceutical Education and Research (DIPSAR), Delhi Pharmaceutical Sciences & Research University (DPSRU), Govt of NCT of Delhi. He has more than ten years of teaching and research experience in reputed organizations like Cipla Pharmaceutical Limited, Baddi; Shanti Niketan College of Pharmacy, Mandi; Sun Pharmaceutical Industries Limited, Gurugram; Translational Health Science Institute (THSTI), Faridabad; ISF College of Pharmacy, Moga, Punjab; and the National Institute of Pharmaceutical Education and Research (NIPER), Raebareli. Recently, he has also been included in the top 2% list of scientists released by Stanford. His current h-index is 31 and i10-index is 79, with 3767 citations and more than 100 research and review articles. His lab gets funding from various government bodies like DST SERB, ICMR, NIF, and IIT-Delhi. His research interests are in the following areas: (1) drug repurposing, (2) meta-analysis of clinical trials, (3) network pharmacology, (4) pharmacoeconomic studies, (5) signal analysis in pharmacovigilance, and (6) animal experimental studies.

1 Introduction to Clinical Research

Haya Majid[1] *and Raman Sehgal*[2]
[1]Department of Translational and Clinical Research, School of Chemical and Life Sciences, Jamia Hamdard, New Delhi, India
[2]Department of Clinical Research, Medanta-The Medicity, Gurugram, Haryana, India

1.1 INTRODUCTION

Clinical research is a subfield of medicine that studies human subjects to find answers to certain health-related queries. This research can include trials of new drugs, medical devices, or interventions, as well as observational studies that look at health outcomes in different populations. The goal is to gather data that can inform medical decisions, guide policy, and improve health outcomes (Kandi and Vadakedath 2023).

1.2 HISTORY OF CLINICAL RESEARCH

Over many years, the development of clinical research has been an intriguing path, marked by significant milestones that have shaped the field into what it is today. The evolution of clinical research has been driven by the need to understand human health, improve medical treatments, and ensure patient safety. This journey has involved the development of ethical standards, the establishment of regulatory frameworks, and the advancement of scientific methodologies.

1.2.1 Ancient and Medieval Roots (Before 1500s)

The roots of clinical research can be traced back to ancient civilizations, where early forms of medical experimentation were practiced.

- **Ancient Egypt and Greece:** The Ebers Papyrus (circa 1550 BCE) from ancient Egypt is one of the earliest known medical texts, documenting various treatments and remedies. Hippocrates, the "Father of Medicine," in ancient Greece (circa 460–370 BCE), advocated for the observation and documentation of symptoms, laying the foundation for evidence-based medicine. However, systematic clinical trials as we know them today did not exist during this period.
- **Islamic Golden Age:** Medical knowledge was greatly advanced by doctors such as Ibn Sina (Avicenna) and Al-Razi (Rhazes) throughout the Islamic Golden Age (8th–14th century). Avicenna's "The Canon of Medicine" emphasized the importance of clinical observations and experimentation, influencing medical practices in Europe for centuries.

1.2.2 The Birth of Clinical Trials (1500s–1700s)

The Renaissance period marked the beginning of more systematic approaches to clinical research, though the concept of controlled trials was still in its infancy.

DOI: 10.1201/9781003533085-1

- **James Lind's Scurvy Experiment (1747):** In order to determine the most effective therapy for scurvy among sailors, Scottish physician James Lind carried out the first known controlled clinical study in 1747. Lind divided 12 sailors with scurvy into groups, giving each group different treatments, including citrus fruits, which ultimately proved to be the most effective. This trial is considered a landmark in clinical research history as it introduced the concept of control groups and comparative treatments.
- **Early Pharmacology:** During the 17th and 18th centuries, there was growing interest in the systematic testing of medicinal substances. William Withering, an English physician, conducted one of the first documented clinical studies on the use of digitalis (derived from foxglove plants) for treating heart conditions in the late 1700s. His work demonstrated the importance of dosage and careful observation in clinical trials.

1.2.3 The 19th Century: Foundations of Modern Clinical Research

The 19th century saw the establishment of principles that would form the basis of modern clinical research, including the development of more rigorous scientific methods and ethical considerations.

- **Placebo-Controlled Trials:** The concept of placebo control, where one group receives the experimental treatment and another receives an inert substance, began to take shape in the 19th century. This approach was important for distinguishing between the actual effects of a treatment and the placebo effect.
- **Advances in Medical Ethics:** The 19th century also saw the beginnings of ethical considerations in clinical research. The Nuremberg Code, established after World War II, was influenced by earlier ethical debates about the use of human subjects in medical experiments, which began to surface in this period.
- **Public Health and Epidemiology:** John Snow's work during the 1854 cholera outbreak in London laid the groundwork for modern epidemiology and public health research. Snow's systematic collection and analysis of data demonstrated the importance of observational studies in understanding and controlling disease.

1.2.4 The 20th Century: The Emergence of Ethical and Regulatory Frameworks

The 20th century was a transformative period for clinical research, characterized by the development of ethical standards, regulatory oversight, and the formalization of clinical trial methodologies.

- **The Flexner Report (1910):** Abraham Flexner's study on American health schooling highlighted the importance of scientific integrity in therapeutic investigation and practice, and ultimately led to significant improvements in medical education. This report laid the foundation for modern medical education and research standards.
- **Nuremberg Code (1947):** Following the atrocities of medical experiments conducted during World War II, the Nuremberg Code was established, setting forth ethical guidelines for human experimentation. The code emphasized voluntary consent, the right to withdraw, and the need for scientifically valid research, marking a pivotal moment in the history of clinical research ethics.
- **Thalidomide Tragedy (1960s):** The thalidomide tragedy, where a drug prescribed to pregnant women led to severe birth defects, underscored the need for stringent drug testing and regulation. As a result of this incident, the United States passed the Kefauver-Harris Amendment in 1962, requiring pharmaceutical companies to provide proof of the efficacy and safety of their goods prior to approval.
- **Declaration of Helsinki (1964):** The World Medical Association adopted the Declaration of Helsinki, which established moral guidelines for people participating in scientific

studies. It emphasized informed consent, the importance of scientifically sound research, and the need to weigh risks against potential benefits.

- **Randomized Controlled Trials:** The 20th century also saw the formalization of randomized controlled trials (RCTs) as the gold standard for clinical research. The British Medical Research Council carried out the initial significant RCT in 1948 to evaluate streptomycin's effectiveness in combating TB. RCTs, which provide solid data on the effectiveness as well as reliability of medical therapies, have emerged as the mainstay of evidence-based health care.

1.2.5 The Late 20th Century to Present: Technological and Ethical Advancements

The late 20th century to the present day has seen rapid advancements in clinical research, driven by technological innovations, globalization, and evolving ethical standards.

- **Technological Innovations:** Advances in technology, including the development of electronic health records, data analytics, and genomics, have revolutionized clinical research. These technologies enable large-scale data collection, more precise trial designs, and personalized medicine approaches.
- **Good Clinical Practice Guidelines:** A worldwide standard for the planning, execution, and documentation of clinical trials was created in the 1990s by the International Council for Harmonization of Technical Requirements for Pharmaceuticals for Human Use (ICH) via the establishment of Good Clinical Practice (GCP) standards. The reliability of clinical trial information, as well as the safety of human participants, is guaranteed by GCP rules.
- **Expansion of Global Clinical Research:** The globalization of clinical research has expanded the scope and scale of clinical trials, with studies increasingly conducted across multiple countries. This has led to greater diversity in clinical trial populations but has also raised challenges related to regulatory harmonization and ethical oversight.
- **Patient-Centered Outcomes Research:** Patient-centered outcomes research (PCOR), which aims to identify the consequences that are most important to patients, has gained popularity in recent years. This approach emphasizes the involvement of patients in the research process and the consideration of patient-reported outcomes in clinical trials.
- **Ethical Challenges in the Digital Age:** New ethical issues pertaining to data privacy, informed consent, and the use of big data in clinical research have been brought about by the growth of digital health technologies, such as wearable technology and mobile health applications. These developments have prompted ongoing discussions about how to adapt ethical frameworks to the digital age (research and 2010 2024; education and 2005 2005; Update and 2008 2024; Obs and 1999 2024; Chalmers,. . ., and 2002 2024).

1.3 CHARACTERIZATION OF CLINICAL RESEARCH

Clinical research is often categorized into several types, as shown in Figure 1.1.

1.3.1 Interventional Studies (Clinical Trials)

Interventional studies, often referred to as clinical trials, are systematic research investigations where participants are assigned specific interventions based on a detailed research protocol. Since they offer vital information on the efficacy, safety, and best practices of novel therapies or interventions, these studies are essential to expanding medical knowledge and enhancing patient care. Although clinical trials are usually organized into stages, each with specific goals and subject groups, investigators may gradually get a thorough grasp of how the treatment affects the health of participants.

Phase I Trials represent the initial step in testing a new intervention on humans. A limited number of people, usually between 20 and 100, participate in these studies; they might be healthy volunteers or patients with the illness under study. Assessing the intervention's safety is the main objective of Phase I studies. Researchers focus on determining the appropriate dosage range by gradually increasing doses and closely monitoring participants for any adverse effects. Additionally, Phase I trials help identify any potential side effects and gather preliminary data on how the intervention behaves in the body, including absorption, distribution, metabolism, and excretion. Although these trials provide essential safety data, their small size means that the findings are often limited and require further investigation in subsequent phases.

Phase II Trials are designed to expand on the safety data obtained in Phase I and to begin assessing the efficacy of the intervention. Larger numbers of people with the ailment the intervention is meant to treat—typically several hundred—participate in these studies. Phase II studies' main goals are to ascertain the efficacy of the intervention, adjust the dosage schedule, and further assess its safety profile. Researchers carefully monitor participants to assess how well the intervention works in controlling or alleviating symptoms and whether it provides a meaningful benefit compared to existing treatments. Phase II trials also continue to monitor for side effects, which may become more apparent as the sample size increases. The data collected during this phase are crucial for determining whether the intervention has sufficient potential to warrant further investigation in larger, more definitive trials.

Phase III Trials are critical in establishing the intervention's overall efficacy and safety in contrast to a placebo or currently accepted medical therapy. These studies have a huge and varied participant base, sometimes in the thousands, spread over many sites. The primary goal of Phase III trials is to confirm the intervention's effectiveness in a broader population and gather comprehensive safety data. Researchers use this phase to evaluate how well the intervention performs in real-world settings and to find any long-term or uncommon adverse effects. Phase III trials are typically randomized and controlled, with participants assigned to either the new intervention or a control group (such as a placebo or standard treatment). The results of these trials provide the robust evidence needed for regulatory approval, as they demonstrate that the intervention offers a significant benefit over existing options and can be used safely in a wide patient population.

Phase IV trials, also referred to as post-marketing surveillance studies, take place after regulatory bodies' approval of the intervention for general use. In a much wider and more diverse population than was feasible in the early stages, these studies are still tracking the intervention's long-term efficacy and safety. In order to identify any uncommon or chronic adverse effects that would not have been noticeable in the more controlled settings of previous stages, Phase IV studies are crucial. They also help identify any new risks associated with long-term use, interactions with other medications, or effectiveness in different subgroups of the population. By continuing to collect data on the intervention's performance in the general population, Phase IV trials ensure that the benefits of the treatment continue to outweigh the risks and allow for ongoing refinement of its use in clinical practice (Thiese 2014).

1.3.2 Observational Studies

Observational studies do not involve active intervention by the researchers. Instead, they observe participants in their natural settings and collect data to investigate the relationships between exposures, risk factors, and health outcomes. These studies are critical for understanding how various factors influence health and disease in real-world settings.

Cohort studies are a favored form of observational research in which a number of people who have something in common, such as a particular exposure or demographic trait, are followed over time to observe the development of specific health outcomes. Cohort studies may be retrospective, in which researchers examine historical data to evaluate outcomes based on prior exposures, or prospective, in which individuals are tracked ahead in time from the moment of exposure to the occurrence of outcomes. Prospective cohort studies are particularly valuable for establishing temporal relationships between exposure and outcome, which is crucial for inferring potential causal links. For example, a prospective cohort investigation might examine the prevalence of lung cancer in a group of smokers and non-smokers across a number of years. Conversely, retrospective cohort studies are typically faster and less expensive but may be limited by the availability and accuracy of historical data. Cohort studies are effective methods for determining risk factors for illnesses and researching the long-term impact of exposures.

Case-control studies are another essential observational study design, particularly useful for studying rare diseases or conditions. In case-control studies, researchers identify individuals with a specific condition or disease (cases) and contrast them with others who don't have the condition (controls). The primary objective is to look retrospectively at the participants' histories to identify factors that may have contributed to the development of the condition. In comparison to cohort studies, case-control studies are often more successful and economical because they focus on a smaller group of individuals and do not require long-term follow-up. For instance, a case-control study might compare the past exposure to a suspected environmental toxin in individuals with a rare cancer (cases) to those without the cancer (controls) to identify potential risk factors. However, one of the main challenges of case-control studies is the potential for recall bias, where participants may not accurately remember or report past exposures, which can affect the study's findings. Despite this limitation, case-control studies are invaluable for exploring associations between exposures and rare diseases.

Cross-sectional studies provide a population's current state at one particular moment, making them particularly useful for assessing the prevalence of conditions or identifying associations between variables at a specific moment. In a cross-sectional study, researchers collect data from a population to analyze the relationships between different variables, such as health behaviors, risk factors, and disease outcomes, all measured simultaneously. Cross-sectional studies are often used in public health to assess the burden of diseases within a community, understand health disparities, or identify potential risk factors for further investigation. For example, a cross-sectional study might analyze data on smoking habits and lung function in a population to assess the prevalence of respiratory conditions and explore the association between smoking and lung health. While cross-sectional studies are efficient and relatively easy to conduct, they are limited in their ability to establish causality because they do not follow participants over time. Instead, they provide valuable descriptive data that can guide further research and inform public health interventions (Puzzitiello et al. 2019).

1.3.3 Epidemiological Studies

The distribution of variables and factors that influence health and illness in populations are the main topics of epidemiological research. They are essential for identifying risk factors, assessing the impact of interventions, and guiding public health policy. These include descriptive epidemiology, which aims to describe the occurrence of a disease or health condition in terms of time, place, and person. It provides basic data on disease patterns, which is essential for public health planning. On the other hand, analytical epidemiology seeks to identify and quantify the relationship between exposure and disease, often using cohort, case-control, or cross-sectional study designs. Furthermore, in experimental epidemiology, researchers manipulate one or more variables to observe the effect on a health outcome. Clinical trials are a form of experimental epidemiology.

1.3.4 Translational Research

Translational research, often described as "bench to bedside" research, focuses on translating findings from basic science into practical applications that improve patient care. It involves taking discoveries made in the laboratory and developing them into treatments, diagnostics, or preventive measures that can be tested in clinical settings. Preclinical research is the early-stage study that involves laboratory and animal studies to explore the mechanisms of disease and the potential effects of new interventions before they are tested in humans. Once a new intervention has been shown to be safe and effective in clinical trials, translational research focuses on implementing it in the healthcare system, including developing guidelines, training healthcare providers, and ensuring accessibility for patients.

1.3.5 Patient-Centered Outcomes Research (PCOR)

PCOR places a strong emphasis on patient participation in the investigation process, concentrating on issues and results that are most important to patients and caregivers alike. It aims to compare the benefits and harms of different treatment options from the patient's perspective, helping them make informed healthcare decisions.

1.3.6 Genetic and Genomic Studies

These studies investigate the role of genetics and genomics in health and disease. By analyzing genetic variations and how they interact with environmental factors, researchers can identify genetic predispositions to certain conditions and develop personalized treatment strategies. Genome-Wide Association Studies (GWAS), which look across the whole genome to find genetic changes linked to certain diseases or characteristics, may be one of them. On the other hand, pharmacogenomics studies assess how genetic variations influence individual responses to medications, aiming to optimize drug efficacy and minimize adverse effects.

1.3.7 Behavioral and Social Science Research

This type of research focuses on understanding how behaviors, social structures, and cultural factors influence health outcomes. It encompasses studies on lifestyle interventions, mental health, health disparities, and the social determinants of health. These studies test strategies to promote healthy behaviors, such as smoking cessation, diet, and exercise. Also, these studies explore how factors like income, education, and community environments affect health and contribute to health disparities.

1.3.8 Health Services Research

The study of health services looks at how medical systems, policies, and organizational structures impact the quality, accessibility, and cost of healthcare. It intends to increase health facilities' efficiency and inform policy decisions. This includes cost-effectiveness analysis that evaluates the economic aspects of healthcare interventions, helping to determine whether the benefits justify the costs. Quality improvement studies are also studies that focus on strategies to enhance. The standard of treatment that patients get often involves the implementation of best practices and evidence-based guidelines (Figure 1.1).

1.4 SIGNIFICANCE OF CLINICAL RESEARCH

Clinical research plays a vital role in the healthcare system, advancing medical understanding, enhancing patient treatment, and influencing public health regulations. Its significance extends across multiple dimensions, including the development of new treatments, enhancement of patient care, contribution to public health, and support for regulatory processes.

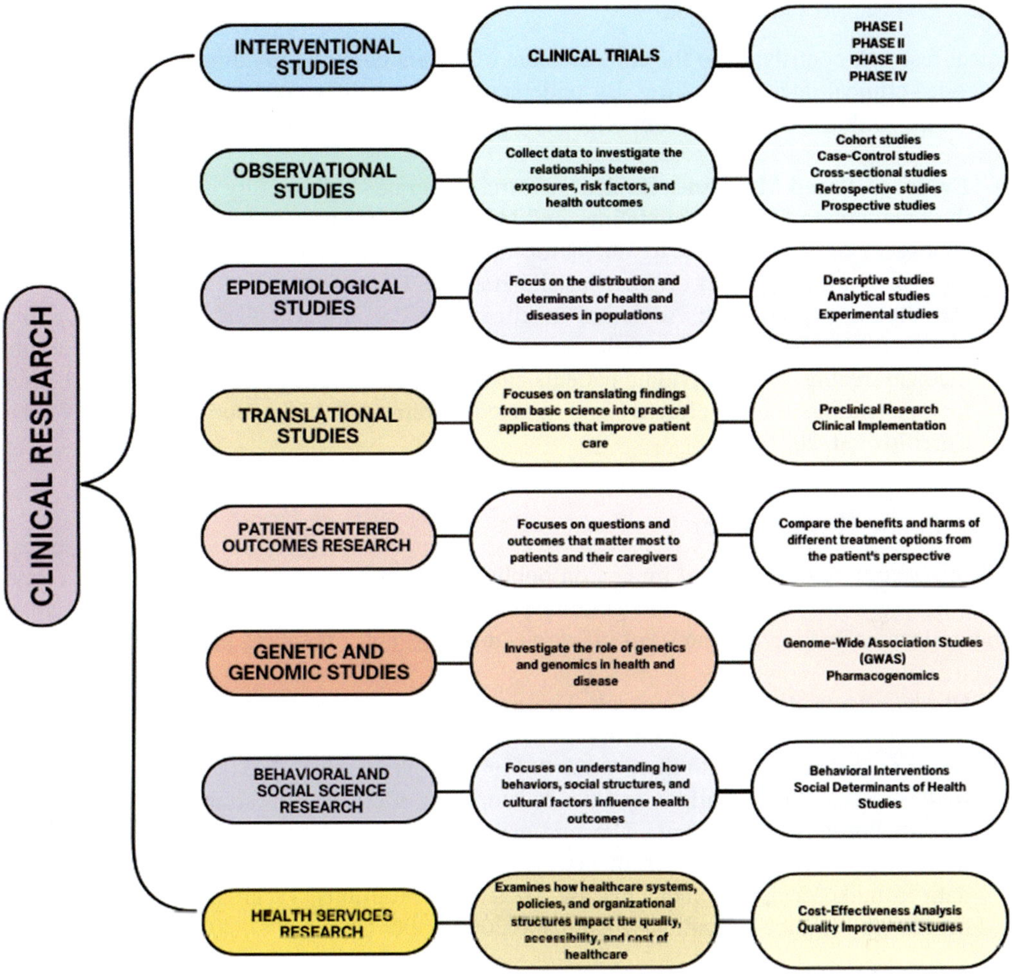

FIGURE 1.1 Clinical research and its associated methodologies and focuses.

1.4.1 Development of New Treatments

Clinical research is the base of developing new medical treatments, ranging from pharmaceutical drugs to medical devices and surgical procedures. Through systematic testing and rigorous evaluation in clinical trials, the best application of these novel therapies may be ascertained by research. This process is critical for bringing innovative treatments to the market that can address unmet medical needs, improve quality of life, and potentially cure diseases.

- **Pharmaceutical Development:** New drugs undergo multiple phases of clinical trials to guarantee their efficacy and safety for human usage. For example, the development of vaccines, such as those for COVID-19, relied heavily on clinical trials to establish their efficacy and safety before they could be widely distributed.
- **Medical Devices and Technologies:** Clinical research also facilitates the development of medical devices, such as pacemakers, prosthetics, and imaging technologies, which must be thoroughly tested to ensure they meet safety and performance standards (Floriani and Torri 2006; Kandi and Vadakedath 2023).

1.4.2 Enhancing Patient Care

Clinical research contributes to the enhancement of patient care by providing evidence-based data that guides clinical decision-making. By understanding how different treatments work in diverse populations, healthcare providers can offer more personalized and effective care.

- **Evidence-Based Medicine:** Clinical research generates high-quality evidence that forms the foundation of clinical guidelines and best practices. These guidelines help clinicians choose the most appropriate treatment for their patients, improving outcomes and reducing the risk of adverse effects (Whirl-Carrillo et al. 2021).
- **Personalized Medicine:** Advances in clinical research, particularly in genomics and pharmacogenomics, have paved the way for personalized medicine. This approach tailors medical treatments to individual patients based on their genetic profile, lifestyle, and other factors, leading to more effective and targeted therapies (J. A. Johnson et al. 2012; Whirl-Carrillo et al. 2021).

1.4.3 Public Health Impact

Clinical research has a profound impact on public health by identifying risk factors for diseases, evaluating preventive measures, and guiding public health policies. It is essential for managing chronic illnesses, halting the spread of infectious diseases, and enhancing public health in general.

- **Disease Prevention and Control:** Through epidemiological studies and clinical trials, researchers can identify risk factors for diseases and develop preventive measures, such as vaccines and public health interventions. For example, clinical research was instrumental in the eradication of smallpox and the development of effective treatments for HIV/AIDS.
- **Health Policy Development:** The findings from clinical research inform public health policies and strategies. Governments and health organizations rely on clinical research data to make decisions about disease prevention programs, vaccination schedules, and healthcare resource allocation (Health and 2006 2006; Leeuw et al. 2014).

1.4.4 Regulatory Approval and Safety

In order to satisfy the regulatory requirements imposed by organizations like the European Medicines Agency (EMA) in Europe or the Food and Drug Administration (FDA) in the United States, new medical goods must first pass stringent clinical research testing before being made accessible to the general public. This process ensures that only safe and effective treatments are approved for use.

- **Safety and Efficacy:** The purpose of clinical trials is to methodically assess the effectiveness and safety of novel therapies. This helps in identifying any potential side effects or risks associated with the treatment, ensuring that it is safe for widespread use.
- **Post-Market Surveillance:** Even after a product is approved, clinical research continues through Phase IV trials (post-marketing surveillance) to monitor long-term safety and effectiveness in a broader population. This ongoing research helps in detecting any rare or long-term adverse effects that may not have been apparent in earlier trials (Leeuw et al. 2014).

1.4.5 Advancement of Medical Knowledge

Clinical research advances medical knowledge by exploring new scientific questions, testing hypotheses, and uncovering novel insights into human health and disease. This continuous process of discovery is essential for the evolution of medicine and the development of innovative therapies.

- **Understanding Disease Mechanisms:** Finding novel treatment targets may result from clinical research's assistance in elucidating the underlying causes of illnesses. For example, tailored medicines that target cancer cells selectively while preserving healthy tissue have been developed as a result of studies understanding the molecular processes of cancer.
- **Innovative Treatment Approaches:** Clinical research fosters innovation by exploring new treatment modalities, such as gene therapy, immunotherapy, and regenerative medicine. These cutting-edge approaches have the potential to revolutionize the treatment of various diseases, offering hope to patients with conditions that were previously considered untreatable (Chen et al. 2012).

1.4.6 Economic Impact

Clinical research also has a significant economic impact. It drives the pharmaceutical and biotech industries, creates jobs, and contributes to the economy by bringing new products to market. Moreover, it reduces healthcare costs by improving the efficiency and effectiveness of treatments.

- **Job Creation and Industry Growth:** The clinical research industry is a major contributor to the economy, providing employment opportunities for researchers, healthcare professionals, and support staff. The creation and marketing of novel medications and equipment also contribute to the growth of the pharmaceutical and biotech sectors.
- **Cost-Effective Healthcare:** By identifying the most effective treatments, clinical research helps to optimize healthcare resources and reduce unnecessary expenditures. For example, studies that compare the cost-effectiveness of different therapies can guide healthcare providers in selecting treatments that offer the best value for money (Lokhandwala et al. 2018; Lee et al. 2024).

1.4.7 Ethical Standards and Patient Safety

Strict ethical standards are followed when conducting clinical research to safeguard participants' rights, well-being, and safety. Institutional Review Boards (IRBs) supervise research activities to make sure they follow ethical guidelines, such as informed consent, risk reduction, and confidentiality.

- **Informed Consent:** Clinical research participants must get complete information about the study's objectives, methods, any risks and rewards, and their freedom to discontinue participation at any moment. This guarantees that individuals are able to decide whether or not to join with knowledge.
- **Risk Minimization:** The goal of clinical research procedures is to maximize possible benefits while minimizing participant hazards. Studies are closely monitored, and any adverse events are promptly addressed to protect participants' safety (Emanuel et al. 2024).

1.4.8 Global Health and Collaboration

Clinical research fosters international collaboration and contributes to global health initiatives. Research conducted in one country can have far-reaching implications for public health worldwide, resulting in the creation of remedies and therapies that help individuals all over the world. Many clinical research studies involve collaboration between institutions and researchers from different countries, pooling resources and expertise to address complex health challenges. The reliability and generalization of study findings are improved by this worldwide method. In order to deal with global health concerns, including epidemics of infectious diseases, resistance to antibiotics, and non-transmissible disorders, medical research is essential. By developing new treatments and preventive measures, clinical research contributes to improving health outcomes on a global scale ("Global Patient Safety Action Plan 2021–2030" 2024; AlQassimi et al. 2020; Piot et al. 2001).

1.4.9 Patient Empowerment and Engagement

Through patient participation in the research process and access to novel treatments prior to their general release, clinical research empowers patients. The problems and issues that patients and their caregivers care about the most are the focus of patient-centered outcomes research in particular.

- **Access to New Treatments:** Clinical trial participants frequently get access to innovative therapies that are not yet generally available. This can be particularly beneficial for patients with rare or difficult-to-treat conditions.
- **Patient-Centered Research:** By focusing on outcomes that are important to patients, such as quality of life and functional status, clinical research ensures that the findings are relevant and meaningful to those who will ultimately benefit from the treatments (L. B. Johnson and Smalley 2019; Lauver et al. 2002).

1.5 REGULATORY AUTHORITIES

Clinical research involves a wide array of stakeholders; each is essential to making sure that research is carried out in a legitimate, successful, and productive manner. These stakeholders include regulatory authorities, sponsors, research institutions, investigators, patients, and more. Each group has specific responsibilities that contribute to the overall success of clinical research. Regulatory authorities are government agencies responsible for overseeing the conduct of clinical research to ensure the safety and well-being of participants, as well as the scientific validity and ethical standards of the studies.

- **Approval and Oversight:** Regulatory authorities review and approve clinical trial protocols before the studies can begin. They ensure that the research is scientifically sound and that the rights and safety of participants are protected. Examples include the Food and Drug Administration (FDA) in the United States, the European Medicines Agency (EMA) in Europe, and the Central Drugs Standard Control Organisation (CDSCO) in India.
- **Monitoring Compliance:** These agencies monitor ongoing trials for compliance with regulatory requirements, including Good Clinical Practice (GCP) guidelines. They may conduct inspections and audits of clinical trial sites to ensure adherence to approved protocols.
- **Review of Results:** Regulatory bodies examine the data from a clinical study to decide if the investigational product is safe and suitable for general use. The approval of novel medications, equipment, or therapies depends on this review procedure.

1.5.1 Stakeholders

1.5.1.1 Sponsors

Sponsors are organizations or individuals who initiate, manage, and finance clinical research. They can be pharmaceutical companies, biotechnology firms, academic institutions, government agencies, or nonprofit organizations.

- **Funding and Resource Allocation:** Sponsors provide the financial resources necessary to conduct clinical trials, including funding for the development of protocols, recruitment of participants, and analysis of data. They are responsible for budgeting and ensuring that adequate resources are available for the study's duration.

- **Study Design and Management:** Sponsors are involved in the design of the clinical trial, including the development of protocols and selection of research sites. They work closely with investigators to ensure that the study is conducted according to plan and that data is collected accurately.
- **Regulatory Submissions:** Sponsors are responsible for submitting clinical trial applications to regulatory authorities and ensuring that all regulatory requirements are met throughout the trial. This includes the submission of safety reports, amendments to protocols, and final study reports.
- **Data Analysis and Reporting:** After the trial is completed, sponsors analyze the data to determine the outcomes of the study. They are responsible for preparing and submitting the results to regulatory authorities and, often, for publishing the findings in scientific journals.

1.5.1.2 Institutional Review Boards (IRBs)/Ethics Committees (ECs)

IRBs (in the U.S.) or Ethics Committees (in other regions) are independent bodies that review and oversee clinical research to ensure the protection of human subjects involved in the study.

- **Ethical Review:** IRBs/ECs review clinical trial protocols to ensure that the research is ethically sound. They assess the risks and benefits of the study, the adequacy of the informed consent process, and the measures in place to protect participants' privacy and confidentiality.
- **Approval and Monitoring:** IRBs/ECs must approve a study before it can begin. Additionally, they keep updated on the study's development, examining any protocol modifications, shifts in the risk profile, or reports of unfavorable outcomes.
- **Informed Consent Process:** IRBs/ECs ensure that participants understand the purpose of the study, including any possible risks and benefits, and that the informed consent procedure is comprehensive. They check the permission papers to make sure they are adequate and clear.

1.5.1.3 Investigators and Research Teams

Investigators, often physicians or researchers, are responsible for conducting the clinical trial according to the study protocol. They lead the research team, which may include sub-investigators, nurses, and clinical research coordinators.

- **Conducting the Study:** The operational oversight of the clinical study is under the purview of the investigators. This includes recruiting and enrolling participants, administering the investigational product, and collecting and recording data.
- **Participant Safety and Care:** Throughout the study, researchers make sure that participants are safe and healthy. They keep an eye out for negative outcomes, offer medical attention as required, and make sure participants are updated on any new information that can influence their decision to stay in the research.
- **Compliance with Protocol:** Investigators are responsible for following the study protocol exactly as approved by the IRB/EC and regulatory authorities. Any deviations from the protocol must be documented and reported.
- **Data Collection and Reporting:** Investigators ensure that data is collected accurately and reported in a timely manner. They are responsible for maintaining detailed records of the study, including case report forms, informed consent documents, and correspondence with regulatory authorities.

1.5.1.4 Participants (Patients)

Participants are individuals who volunteer to take part in clinical research. They can be patients with a specific condition or healthy volunteers, depending on the study's objectives.

- **Informed Consent:** Prior to being included in research, participants must give their informed permission. This includes being aware of the goals of the study, the methods being used, the possible dangers and advantages, and their rights as participants, including the freedom to leave the study at any moment.
- **Adherence to Protocol:** Participants are expected to follow the study procedures as outlined in the protocol, which may include taking medication, attending follow-up visits, and undergoing tests or assessments.
- **Reporting Experiences:** Participants provide crucial data by reporting their experiences, including any side effects or changes in their health. Their feedback is essential for evaluating the safety and efficacy of the intervention being studied.

1.5.1.5 Contract Research Organizations (CROs)

CROs are organizations that provide outsourced research services to sponsors. Among the many services they provide are statistical evaluation, handling data, research design, and filings with regulators.

- **Study Management:** CROs often manage the operational aspects of clinical trials, including site selection, recruitment of participants, and coordination of study activities across multiple sites.
- **Data Collection and Analysis:** CROs are responsible for collecting, managing, and analyzing data from clinical trials. They guarantee that the data is precise, comprehensive, and in line with the study's procedure.
- **Regulatory Compliance:** CROs assist sponsors in preparing and submitting regulatory documents. They ensure that the trial complies with regulatory requirements and that all necessary documentation is in place for regulatory review.
- **Monitoring and Auditing:** CROs monitor clinical trial sites to ensure that the study is conducted according to GCP guidelines and the approved protocol. They may also conduct audits to verify the integrity of the data and adherence to regulatory standards.

1.5.1.6 Data Monitoring Committees (DMCs)

DMCs, also known as Data Safety Monitoring Boards (DSMBs), are independent groups that monitor the safety and efficacy data collected during a clinical trial. They have the authority to recommend modifications or early termination of a study based on their findings.

- **Safety Monitoring:** DMCs review data at regular intervals to monitor the safety of participants. They assess the frequency and severity of adverse events and determine whether the study should continue as planned.
- **Interim Analysis:** DMCs conduct interim analyses of efficacy data to determine whether the study is meeting its objectives. Based on their findings, they may recommend changes to the study design, such as adjusting the sample size or stopping the trial early if the results are overwhelmingly positive or negative.
- **Independent Decision-Making:** DMCs function independently of the sponsor and researchers, guaranteeing that their suggestions are objective and exclusively concerned with participant safety and the trial's scientific integrity.

1.5.1.7 Clinical Research Organizations and Academic Institutions

Academic institutions and clinical research organizations often serve as research sites for clinical trials. They provide the infrastructure, resources, and expertise needed to conduct high-quality clinical research.

- **Research Environment:** Academic institutions provide a research environment that fosters scientific inquiry and innovation. They offer access to specialized equipment, laboratories, and expertise in various fields of medicine and science.
- **Education and Training:** These institutions are involved in the education and training of future clinical researchers, ensuring that they have the skills and knowledge needed to conduct ethical and scientifically rigorous studies.
- **Collaboration and Networking:** Academic institutions often collaborate with industry sponsors, government agencies, and other research organizations. These collaborations can enhance the scope and impact of clinical research by bringing together diverse expertise and resources.

1.5.1.8 Patients' Advocacy Groups

When it comes to clinical research, patient advocacy organizations speak for patients as well as their close companions. They advocate for patient-centered research, greater transparency, and improved access to clinical trials.

- **Advocacy and Awareness:** Patient advocacy groups raise awareness about clinical trials and the importance of patient participation in research. They may advocate for more inclusive trial designs that reflect the diversity of the patient population.
- **Patient Education:** These groups provide educational resources to patients and their families, helping them understand the clinical trial process, the potential risks and benefits, and how to make informed decisions about participation.
- **Influencing Research Priorities:** Patient advocacy groups often work with sponsors, investigators, and regulatory authorities to ensure that research priorities align with the needs and concerns of patients. They may advocate for the inclusion of patient-reported outcomes in clinical trials and for studies that address unmet medical needs (August 2009; Step 2015; Rockhold 2002; technical 1994; Med and 2001 2024).

1.6 CONCLUSION

Clinical research is the bedrock of modern medicine, playing an essential function in expanding our knowledge of illnesses, creating novel therapies, and enhancing patient outcomes. Through rigorous scientific inquiry, ethical oversight, and collaboration among diverse stakeholders, clinical research ensures that medical interventions are both safe and effective before they are widely adopted.

The continuous evolution of clinical research methodologies, along with advancements in technology and data analytics, has greatly enhanced our ability to conduct more precise and personalized studies. Moreover, the increasing emphasis on ethical standards and patient-centered approaches has helped align research objectives with the needs and well-being of participants, thereby fostering greater trust and engagement. As we move forward, the challenges and opportunities in clinical research will continue to evolve, driven by emerging technologies, global health priorities, and the complex regulatory landscape. However, the core mission remains unchanged: to advance medical science in a way that improves the well-being and standard of living of people everywhere. Through ongoing innovation and collaboration, clinical research will continue to be a powerful force for progress in healthcare.

REFERENCES

AlQassimi, Sarah, Safiya AlBrashdi, Hassan Galadari, and Muhammad Jawad Hashim. 2020. "Global Burden of Psoriasis—Comparison of Regional and Global Epidemiology, 1990 to 2017." *International Journal of Dermatology* 59 (5). John Wiley & Sons, Ltd: 566–71. https://doi.org/10.1111/IJD.14864.

August, ICHHT Guideline—Q8 (2R). As revised in, and undefined. 2009. "Pharmaceutical Development." *Vnras.Com.* https://vnras.com/wp-content/uploads/2017/05/Q8R2_PHARMACEUTICAL-DEVELOPMENT.pdf.

Chalmers, I,. . . LV Hedges—Evaluation & the health, and undefined 2002. 2024. "A Brief History of Research Synthesis." *Journals.Sagepub.Com.* Accessed September 9. https://journals.sagepub.com/doi/abs/10.1177/0163278702025001003.

Chen, Rui, George I. Mias, Jennifer Li-Pook-Than, Lihua Jiang, Hugo Y.K. Lam, Rong Chen, Elana Miriami, et al. 2012. "Personal Omics Profiling Reveals Dynamic Molecular and Medical Phenotypes." *Cell* 148 (6). Elsevier B.V.: 1293–1307. https://doi.org/10.1016/J.CELL.2012.02.009.

education, G Norman—Medical, and undefined. 2005. "Research in Clinical Reasoning: Past History and Current Trends." *Wiley Online Library* 39 (4): 418–27. https://doi.org/10.1111/j.1365-2929.2005.02127.x.

Emanuel, E.J., D. Wendler, C. Grady—Jama, and undefined 2000. 2024. "What Makes Clinical Research Ethical?" *Jamanetwork.Com.* Accessed August 27. https://jamanetwork.com/journals/jama/article-abstract/192740.

Floriani, Irene, and Valter Torri. 2006. "Methodology of Clinical Research: An Overview." *Drug Development Research* 67 (3): 183–7. https://doi.org/10.1002/DDR.20075.

"Global Patient Safety Action Plan 2021-2030." 2024. Accessed March 21. https://www.who.int/teams/integrated-health-services/patient-safety/policy/global-patient-safety-action-plan.

Health, T.R. Oliver—Annu. Rev. Public, and undefined. 2006. "The Politics of Public Health Policy." *Annualreviews.Org* 27: 195–233. https://doi.org/10.1146/annurev.publhealth.25.101802.123126.

Johnson, J.A., B.M. Burkley, T.Y. Langaee, M.J. Clare-Salzler, T.E. Klein, and R.B. Altman. 2012. "Implementing Personalized Medicine: Development of a Cost-Effective Customized Pharmacogenetics Genotyping Array." *Clinical Pharmacology and Therapeutics* 92 (4): 437–9. https://doi.org/10.1038/CLPT.2012.125.

Johnson, Lorraine B., and Jaye Bea Smalley. 2019. "Engaging the Patient: Patient-Centered Research." *Strategies for Team Science Success: Handbook of Evidence-Based Principles for Cross-Disciplinary Science and Practical Lessons Learned from Health Researchers* (January). Springer International Publishing: 135–47. https://doi.org/10.1007/978-3-030-20992-6_10.

Kandi, Venkataramana, and Sabitha Vadakedath. 2023. "Clinical Trials and Clinical Research: A Comprehensive Review." *Cureus* 15 (2). Cureus Inc. https://doi.org/10.7759/CUREUS.35077.

Lauver, Diane R., Sandra E. Ward, Susan M. Heidrich, Mary L. Keller, Barbara J. Bowers, Patricia Flatley Brennan, Karin T. Kirchhoff, and Thelma J. Wells. 2002. "Patient-Centered Interventions." *Research in Nursing and Health* 25 (4): 246–55. https://doi.org/10.1002/NUR.10044.

Lee, B.Y., B.A. Norman, T.M. Assi, S.I. Chen, R.R. Bailey—Vaccine, and undefined 2010. 2024. "Single Versus Multi-Dose Vaccine Vials: An Economic Computational Model." *Elsevier.* Accessed August 24. https://www.sciencedirect.com/science/article/pii/S0264410X10007462.

Leeuw, E. De, C. Clavier, E. Breton—Health research policy and systems, and undefined. 2014. "Health Policy–Why Research It and How: Health Political Science." *Springer* 12 (1). BioMed Central Ltd.: 55. https://doi.org/10.1186/1478-4505-12-55.

Lokhandwala, T., N. Smith,. . . C. Sternhufvud—Journal of Medical, and undefined 2016. 2018. "A Retrospective Study of Persistence, Adherence, and Health Economic Outcomes of Fixed-Dose Combination vs Loose-Dose Combination of Oral Anti-Diabetes Drugs." *Taylor & Francis* 20 (4). Blackwell Publishing Inc.: 705–15. https://doi.org/10.1111/jch.13240.

Med, ICHHT Guideline—J Postgrad, and undefined 2001. 2024. "Guideline for Good Clinical Practice." *Math. Ku.Dk.* Accessed September 9. https://web.math.ku.dk/~richard/download/RW/GCP.pdf.

Obs, D. Berger—MLO Med Lab, and undefined 1999. 2024. "A Brief History of Medical Diagnosis and the Birth of the Clinical Laboratory: Part 1—Ancient Times through the 19th Century." *Ascls-Pa.Org.* Accessed September 9. http://ascls-pa.org/uploads/2/4/2/1/24211033/meddiagandlab.pdf.

Piot, P., M. Bartos, P.D. Ghys, N. Walker, and B. Schwartländer. 2001. "The Global Impact of HIV/AIDS." *Nature 2001 410:6831* 410 (6831). Nature Publishing Group: 968–73. https://doi.org/10.1038/35073639.

Puzzitiello, Richard N., Avinesh Agarwalla, Brian Forsythe, and Natalie L. Leong. 2019. "Principles of Clinical Research." *Orthopedic Practice Management: Strategies for Growth and Success* (December). Springer, Cham: 187–212. https://doi.org/10.1007/978-3-319-96938-1_15.

research, A Bhatt—Perspectives in clinical, and undefined 2010. 2024. "Evolution of Clinical Research: A History before and beyond James Lind." *Journals.Lww.Com*. Accessed September 9. https://journals.lww.com/picp/fulltext/2010/01010/evolution_of_clinical_research__a_history_before.2.aspx.

Rockhold, Frank W. 2002. "Industry Perspectives on ICH Guidelines." *Statistics in Medicine* 21 (19): 2949–57. https://doi.org/10.1002/SIM.1299.

Step, ICHH Guideline—Current, and undefined. 2015. "Integrated Addendum to ICH E6 (R1): Guideline for Good Clinical Practice E6 (R2)." *Fom.Kdu.Ac.Lk*. https://fom.kdu.ac.lk/wp-content/uploads/2024/04/pdf-3-GCP-draft-addendum-ICH-2015.pdf.

technical, ICHHT Guideline—International conference on harmonisation of, and undefined. 1994. "Clinical Safety Data Management: Definitions and Standards for Expedited Reporting E2A." *Fercsl.Lk*. http://fercsl.lk/wp/wp-content/uploads/2019/04/Clinical-Safety-Data-Management-Definitions-Standards-for-Expedited-Reporting-ICH-Harmonised-Tripartite-Guideline-1994.pdf.

Thiese, Matthew S. 2014. "Observational and Interventional Study Design Types; An Overview." *Biochemia Medica* 24 (2). Hrvatsko društvo za medicinsku biokemiju i laboratorijsku medicinu: 199–210. https://doi.org/10.11613/BM.2014.022.

Update, S. Junod—FDLI, and undefined 2008. 2024. "FDA and Clinical Drug Trials: A Short History." *HeinOnline*. Accessed September 9. https://heinonline.org/hol-cgi-bin/get_pdf.cgi?handle=hein.journals/fdliup2008&section=37.

Whirl-Carrillo, Michelle, Rachel Huddart, Li Gong, Katrin Sangkuhl, Caroline F. Thorn, Ryan Whaley, and Teri E. Klein. 2021. "An Evidence-based Framework for Evaluating Pharmacogenomics Knowledge for Personalized Medicine." *Clinical Pharmacology & Therapeutics* 110 (3). John Wiley & Sons, Ltd: 563–72. https://doi.org/10.1002/CPT.2350.

2 Historical Background

Haya Majid and Nidhi
Department of Translational and Clinical Research, School of Chemical and Life Sciences, Jamia Hamdard, New Delhi, India

2.1 INTRODUCTION

Clinical research represents a fundamental mechanism for generating evidence to guide medical interventions, improve patient outcomes, and inform public health policies. Its historical trajectory reflects a progressive refinement of methodologies, ethical considerations, and regulatory frameworks, shaped by cultural, scientific, and technological advancements across civilizations (Lloyd and White 2011).

The origins of clinical research can be traced back to ancient civilizations, where early medical practitioners in regions such as Egypt, India, China, and Mesopotamia relied on empirical observation, anecdotal evidence, and trial-and-error methods to understand diseases and develop treatments. Texts such as the *Ebers Papyrus* in Egypt, the *Charaka Samhita* in India, and the *Huangdi Neijing* in China document some of the earliest recorded medical experiments and therapeutic interventions (Figure 2.1). The medieval period saw the preservation and expansion of ancient medical knowledge, particularly through the contributions of scholars from the Islamic Golden Age and medieval Europe. Physicians like Avicenna and Al-Razi emphasized systematic observation, drug testing, and ethical responsibility in medical practice. During the Renaissance, a renewed focus on human anatomy, empirical observation, and controlled experimentation revolutionized medical understanding, with pioneers like Andreas Vesalius and William Harvey laying foundational principles in anatomy and physiology (Carpenter et al. 2006; "Companion Encyclopedia of the History of Medicine" 2013).

The 19th century marked the emergence of evidence-based medicine, characterized by the integration of statistical methods and the establishment of randomized controlled trials (RCTs) as the gold standard for evaluating medical interventions. This period also saw significant advancements in microbiology, pharmacology, and surgical techniques, driven by figures such as Louis Pasteur, Robert Koch, and Joseph Lister. In the 20th century, clinical research underwent formalization with the development of robust regulatory frameworks, ethical guidelines, and standardized methodologies. Landmark events, including the Nuremberg Code, the Declaration of Helsinki, and the Belmont Report, addressed ethical violations and established principles of informed consent, beneficence, and justice. In the 21st century, clinical research has been revolutionized by technological advancements, including artificial intelligence, big data analytics, genomics, and decentralized clinical trials. These innovations have enhanced data accuracy, trial efficiency, and patient-centric approaches, while regulatory and ethical standards continue to evolve to address emerging challenges (Castiglioni 2019; Magner and Kim 2017).

This chapter provides a comprehensive overview of the historical background of clinical research, analyzing its evolution through distinct historical epochs, identifying key contributors and milestones, and discussing the enduring principles that continue to shape contemporary clinical research practices.

DOI: 10.1201/9781003533085-2

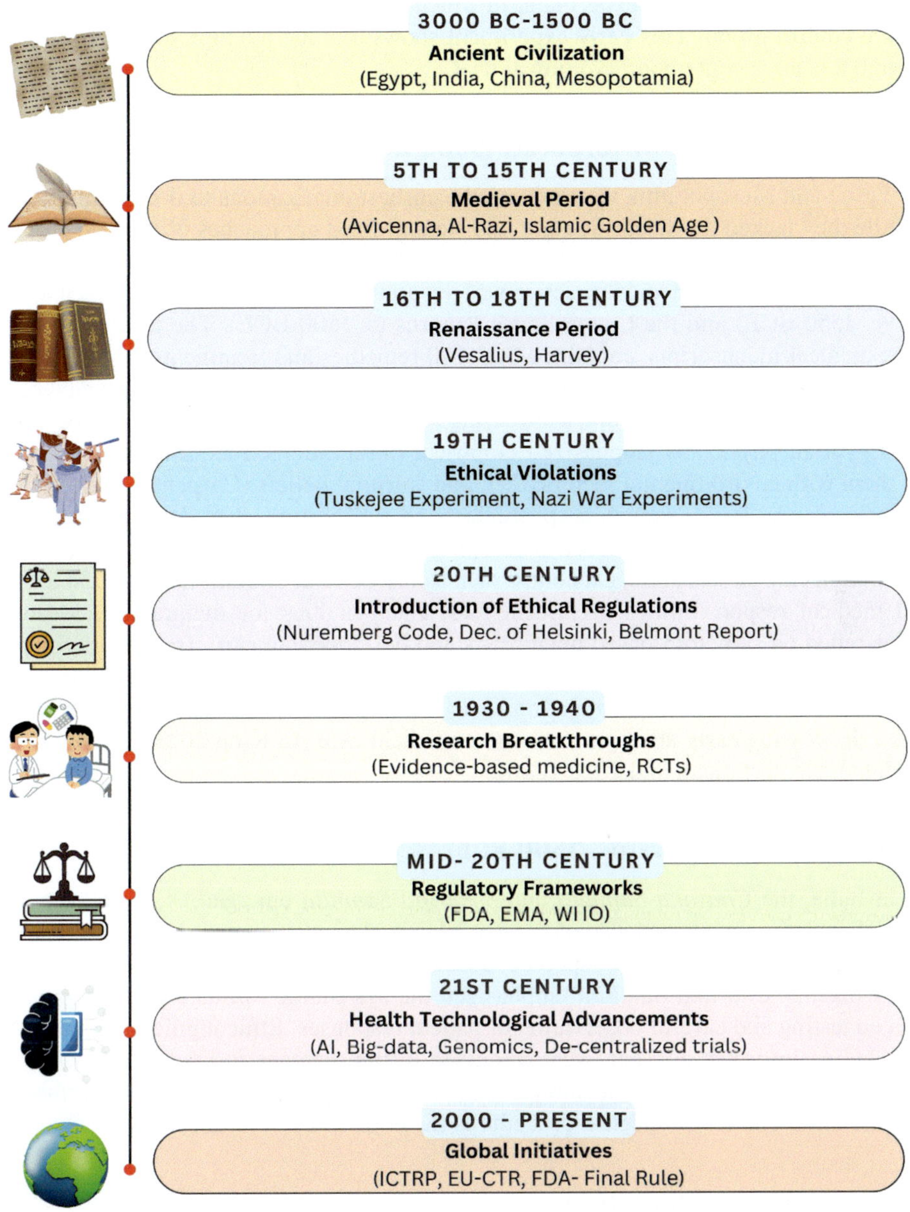

FIGURE 2.1 Historical evolution of clinical research.

2.2 ANCIENT FOUNDATIONS OF CLINICAL RESEARCH (BEFORE THE COMMON ERA)

2.2.1 Early Experimentation in Ancient Civilizations

Early clinical testing dates back to ancient civilisations, as evidenced by records indicating nutritional and health-related trials and observations. The Bible's "Book of Daniel" is a well-known example, detailing a nutritional experiment in which a vegetarian diet was contrasted with a royal diet, with a control group. This early experiment shows a crude attempt at outcome comparison, even though it is not a contemporary clinical trial.

2.2.2 Ancient Egypt and Mesopotamia (3000 BCE–1500 BCE)

Ancient Egypt and Mesopotamia were among the earliest civilizations to document medical practices. While they lacked the scientific rigor and standardized approaches of modern clinical trials, their contributions laid the foundation for empirical observation and documentation, essential elements of clinical research. Medical practice was documented extensively in texts such as the Ebers Papyrus (c. 1550 BCE) and the Edwin Smith Papyrus (c. 1600 BCE). The Ebers Papyrus, one of the oldest medical manuscripts, contained over 700 remedies and treatments for various ailments, addressing diseases, their symptoms, and potential interventions. The Edwin Smith Papyrus focused on surgical practices and trauma care, showcasing a systematic approach to classifying and treating injuries. Egyptian physicians emphasized empirical observations, recording symptoms and correlating them with environmental factors, diet, and spiritual beliefs (Carpenter et al. 2006). While these practices were deeply rooted in spirituality and superstition, they demonstrated attempts at structured medical interventions based on empirical observations. Clinical practices were documented through clay tablets and legal codes, such as the Code of Hammurabi (c. 1754 BCE), which outlined medical responsibilities, treatment fees, and penalties for malpractice. Mesopotamian physicians relied on symptom-based diagnostics and developed an early framework for prognosis. The role of healers and priests was central in both societies, often blending religious rituals with medicinal treatments. Surgical interventions, such as trepanation, were performed with rudimentary tools, showcasing early attempts at invasive medical care (L. King 2023; medycyny and 2004 2024; Adamo, Geotechnical, and 2020 2020).

2.2.3 Ancient India (Ayurveda, 1500 BCE)

In ancient India, the *Charaka Samhita* and *Sushruta Samhita* emerged as pivotal medical texts. Ayurveda, translating to "the science of life," emphasized a holistic approach to health and disease prevention. Treatments were patient-specific, considering an individual's physical and mental constitution (*Prakriti*). *Charaka Samhita* emphasized the systematic evaluation of drugs, advocating for repeated testing and careful observation of patient responses. Ethical guidelines for experimentation, including informed consent, were discussed in rudimentary forms. The *Sushruta Samhita* went further by detailing surgical techniques and antiseptic practices. The text described over 120 surgical instruments and 300 surgical procedures (Lr et al. 2024; Asaram Budhnar et al. 2022).

2.2.4 Ancient China (2000 BCE)

The *Huangdi Neijing* (*The Yellow Emperor's Classic of Internal Medicine*) is one of the earliest Chinese medical texts. It laid the foundation for traditional Chinese medicine (TCM), introducing concepts such as *yin* and *yang*, *qi* (energy flow), and the five-element theory. While not clinical trials in the modern sense, ancient Chinese healers meticulously recorded symptoms and treatment outcomes. Acupuncture and herbal medicine were developed during this period. Observation of patient responses played a critical role in refining treatments, marking an early form of empirical clinical research (Medicine and 2023 2024).

2.2.5 Early Controlled Experiments: The Babylonian Trial (600 BCE)

One of the earliest documented controlled experiments occurred in Babylon under King Nebuchadnezzar II. The king, concerned about his soldiers' health, conducted a dietary experiment.

Two groups of soldiers were given different diets: one group consumed only vegetables and water, while the other consumed meat and wine. After a defined period, the soldiers on the vegetarian diet appeared healthier and more physically fit. This trial is significant because it showcased a rudimentary understanding of experimental design: comparison groups, dietary intervention, and outcome observation. Though lacking statistical analysis, it demonstrated the importance of systematic comparison. This practice, while ethically questionable, marked an early attempt to determine which remedies were most effective based on direct observation and comparison. Physicians and healers were expected to keep records of their treatments and were held accountable for negative outcomes, including facing severe punishments for malpractice as described in the Code of Hammurabi (Gynecology and 1995 2024; "The Babylonian World" 2009; Abdul-Sahib 2024; Kiger 2022; praksa and 2022 2022).

2.3 CONTRIBUTIONS OF ANCIENT GREECE

Ancient Greece (c. 5th–4th centuries BCE) is regarded as the cradle of modern medical thought and practice. Greek physicians made significant contributions to the understanding of human health, disease, and treatment, shifting the focus from supernatural explanations to natural causes. Their legacy laid the groundwork for evidence-based medicine and clinical research methodologies still in use today. One of the most prominent figures in ancient Greek medicine was Hippocrates of Kos (c. 460–370 BCE), often referred to as the "Father of Medicine." He revolutionized medical practice by rejecting the widely accepted belief that diseases were caused by divine punishment or supernatural forces. Instead, Hippocrates emphasized the importance of empirical observation, logical reasoning, and clinical documentation. His most significant contribution was the Hippocratic Corpus, a collection of medical texts detailing disease symptoms, treatment approaches, and ethical guidelines. Among these, the Hippocratic Oath stands as a cornerstone of medical ethics, advocating for principles such as patient confidentiality, non-maleficence, and the duty to do no harm (Fox 2020).

Another major contribution of Ancient Greece was the development of the humoral theory, which proposed that the human body was governed by four bodily fluids: blood, phlegm, yellow bile, and black bile. Health was believed to result from the balance of these humors, while disease arose from their imbalance. While modern science has long since disproven this theory, it served as an essential framework for medical understanding for centuries and encouraged physicians to approach treatment holistically (H. King 2020; French 2024).

The Greeks also advanced clinical observation and case studies. Physicians like Galen of Pergamon (c. 129–216 CE), who built upon Hippocratic principles, meticulously recorded patient symptoms, disease progression, and the effects of treatments. Although Galen's work was often speculative and sometimes flawed, his emphasis on systematic observation and documentation had a lasting influence on both Eastern and Western medicine. Philosophy also deeply influenced Greek medical thought (Cellular and 2014 2014; Singer 2019). Thinkers like Aristotle (384–322 BCE) contributed to the study of anatomy, physiology, and biology. Aristotle's comparative studies of animal and human anatomy laid the foundation for future discoveries in medical science. Similarly, philosophers such as Plato explored the mind-body connection, highlighting the psychosomatic aspects of health—a concept increasingly recognized in modern medicine (Baker 2021; Schmitt and Webster 2024; Stackle 2021).

2.4 CLINICAL RESEARCH IN THE MEDIEVAL PERIOD (5TH–15TH CENTURY)

2.4.1 Monastic Medicine in Europe

During the early medieval period, monasteries became vital centers for preserving and transmitting medical knowledge. Monks meticulously copied ancient Greek and Roman medical manuscripts. The *Rule of Saint Benedict* emphasized care for the sick, and many monasteries established infirmaries where basic medical treatments were provided. Herbal gardens, maintained by monks, supplied medicinal plants used in treatments. Although much of monastic medicine relied on religious practices and spiritual healing, the emphasis on documentation and record-keeping contributed to the preservation of ancient medical wisdom (Fry 2016).

2.4.2 Translation Movement in the Islamic World

The Islamic Golden Age (8th to 13th centuries) was instrumental in preserving and expanding medical knowledge. In centers like Baghdad's *House of Wisdom*, scholars translated medical texts from Greek, Syriac, Persian, and Sanskrit into Arabic. Figures such as *Hunayn ibn Ishaq* and *Al-Kindi* played key roles in translating and annotating works by Hippocrates, Galen, and other ancient scholars. These translations were not mere reproductions but included extensive commentaries, corrections, and original insights, advancing the understanding of diseases and treatments. By the 12th century, the establishment of universities marked a significant advancement in formal medical education. Institutions like the *Schola Medica Salernitana* in Italy, the University of Montpellier in France, and the University of Bologna played pivotal roles in training physicians. The curriculum often included works from both ancient and Islamic scholars (Graeco-Roman, Ancient, and 2021 2024; Martiniana and 2024 2024; Belhandouz 2024).

2.4.2.1 Avicenna (Ibn Sina, 980–1037 CE)

Avicenna's *Canon of Medicine* became one of the most influential medical texts of the medieval period. It served as a comprehensive encyclopedia, covering medical theories, pharmacology, and treatment protocols. Avicenna emphasized the importance of observation, experimentation, and systematic documentation. His insights into dosage standardization, disease classification, and therapeutic approaches had a lasting impact on both Eastern and Western medicine (Ghaffari et al. 2024).

2.4.2.2 Al-Razi (Rhazes, 854–925 CE)

Al-Razi, another towering figure of medieval medicine, made significant contributions through works such as *Kitab al-Hawi* (The Comprehensive Book on Medicine) and *Kitab al-Mansuri*. He is credited with distinguishing smallpox from measles, marking one of the earliest examples of differential diagnosis. Al-Razi's emphasis on evidence-based treatments and his detailed case studies showcased a commitment to empirical observation (Science and 2019 2024; Tibi 2006).

2.4.2.3 Hildegard of Bingen (1098–1179 CE)

A prominent abbess, Hildegard of Bingen, combined spirituality, herbal medicine, and observation in her medical writings, including *Physica* and *Causae et Curae*. She documented numerous herbal remedies, dietary advice, and treatments for various ailments. Hildegard's holistic approach to medicine emphasized the connection between physical health, mental well-being, and spirituality (Mews 2020).

2.4.2.4 Paracelsus (1493–1541 CE)

Toward the end of the medieval period, Paracelsus challenged established medical authorities by advocating for hands-on experimentation and observation. He introduced the concept of dose-response relationships and emphasized the chemical composition of medicines. His famous maxim, "The dose makes the poison," remains foundational in pharmacology (Michaleas et al. 2021).

2.5 THE RENAISSANCE AND SCIENTIFIC REVOLUTION (16TH–18TH CENTURY)

2.5.1 The Decline of Galenic Medicine

For centuries, medical practice in Europe was dominated by the teachings of Galen, whose theories of humoral balance and disease causation were rarely questioned. Diseases were believed to result from imbalances in these humors, and treatments often involved bloodletting, purging, and herbal remedies. During the Renaissance, scholars began challenging these doctrines through direct observation, anatomical dissections, and controlled experiments.

Andreas Vesalius (1514–1564), in his monumental work, *De humani corporis fabrica* (On the Fabric of the Human Body), published in 1543, marked a turning point in anatomical studies. Vesalius conducted detailed dissections on human cadavers, directly observing and documenting the structures of the human body. His findings corrected numerous errors in Galenic anatomy, including misconceptions about the human liver, heart, and vascular system. Vesalius' emphasis on observation over-reliance on ancient texts laid the foundation for evidence-based anatomical research ("Andreas Vesalius: Anatomy and the World of Books—Sachiko Kusukawa—Google Books" 2024).

The scientific method emerged as a systematic framework for investigating natural phenomena. Pioneers such as Francis Bacon in his *Novum Organum* (1620), along with René Descartes, promoted inductive reasoning, where conclusions are drawn from carefully collected empirical evidence. This method became the foundation for scientific and medical inquiry, enabling structured experimentation and reproducible results. Physicians and researchers began applying these principles to clinical research, moving away from anecdotal evidence and unfounded traditions ("The Works of Francis Bacon: Vol. II—Francis Bacon—Google Books" 2024).

2.5.2 The Birth of Controlled Clinical Trials

James Lind and the Scurvy Trial (1747) experiment aboard the HMS Salisbury is widely regarded as the first controlled clinical trial. Lind aimed to find a cure for scurvy, a disease that plagued sailors on long voyages. He divided affected sailors into six groups and provided different treatments, including cider, vinegar, seawater, and citrus fruits. The group receiving citrus fruits showed rapid improvement, providing clear evidence of their efficacy. Lind's trial highlighted the importance of control groups and systematic observation in clinical research (Upadhyayula and Kasliwal 2020).

2.6 THE 19TH CENTURY: THE BIRTH OF EVIDENCE-BASED MEDICINE

2.6.1 The Role of Observation and Experimentation

The 19th-century physicians began to systematically document patient symptoms, disease progression, and treatment outcomes. Clinical records, previously sporadic and anecdotal, became structured tools for analyzing disease patterns and evaluating treatment efficacy. Case studies, longitudinal studies, and comparative methods were introduced, enabling better evaluation of interventions. Surgeons and physicians like John Snow and Pierre-Charles-Alexandre Louis demonstrated the power of methodical observation. For example, Louis used case studies and statistical methods to challenge bloodletting as a universal treatment, proving its limited effectiveness in many cases (PARK 2005).

2.6.2 Statistical Methods in Medicine

Pierre-Charles-Alexandre Louis is considered one of the earliest proponents of numerical medicine, systematically collecting data from large patient groups and analyzing outcomes to assess treatment efficacy. His studies on bloodletting were among the first examples of medical research relying on statistical data. Additionally, statistical tools were used to map and analyze disease outbreaks, track mortality rates, and identify risk factors. These advancements laid the foundation for modern epidemiology and clinical trial design (Best and Neuhauser 2005).

2.7 THE 20TH CENTURY: FORMALIZATION AND ETHICAL CHALLENGES

2.7.1 The Tuskegee Syphilis Study (1932–1972)

The Tuskegee Syphilis Study remains one of the darkest chapters in medical ethics. African American men with syphilis were deliberately left untreated, even after effective therapies became available. This unethical study highlighted systemic racism and the exploitation of vulnerable populations (Tobin 2022).

2.7.2 Nazi War Experiments: A Dark Chapter in Medical History

During World War II (1939–1945), under Adolf Hitler's leadership, Nazi physicians conducted some of the most horrific and unethical medical experiments in history. These experiments took place in concentration camps, particularly Auschwitz, Dachau, Ravensbrück, and Buchenwald, and were carried out on prisoners, including Jews, Romani people, disabled individuals, and political dissidents. The experiments were driven by a mix of pseudoscience, military objectives, and racial ideology, often under the guise of advancing scientific knowledge or improving military efficiency. Thousands of victims suffered unspeakable pain, mutilation, and death in the name of what the Nazis claimed was scientific research (Weindling 2022).

The objectives behind these experiments can be divided into three main categories. First, military and survival research aimed to improve the resilience of German soldiers in extreme combat conditions. Second, racial and genetic studies sought to reinforce Nazi ideology by "proving" the superiority of the Aryan race and exploring methods of eugenics. Third, infectious disease and pharmaceutical testing aimed to find vaccines, antibiotics, and treatments for soldiers and the general population. Despite their stated goals, these experiments were riddled with cruelty, lacked scientific merit, and had devastating human consequences (Hohonu and 2010, 2024; Novak 2020). One category of these experiments focused on survival and military research. At the Dachau concentration camp, prisoners were subjected to freezing experiments to simulate the effects of extreme cold on German pilots and soldiers. Victims were immersed in icy water or left exposed to sub-zero temperatures while scientists observed their reactions and attempted revival techniques, such as hot water baths or forced physical contact. Similarly, high-altitude experiments involved placing prisoners in low-pressure chambers to simulate conditions at high altitudes. Many died from oxygen deprivation or suffered permanent brain damage. Additionally, seawater experiments forced prisoners to drink only seawater, causing severe dehydration and hallucinations (De Leeuw 2020).

In another set of experiments, infectious diseases and pharmaceutical testing, prisoners were deliberately infected with diseases such as typhus, malaria, and tuberculosis. Scientists observed the progression of these diseases and tested experimental drugs, often with no regard for the immense suffering endured by their subjects. At Buchenwald, prisoners were exposed to toxic substances and chemical agents to study antidotes and treatments for chemical warfare injuries. Many victims died from the diseases themselves or from the toxic side effects of untested treatments (Mills 2020).

The genetic and racial experiments conducted by Dr. Josef Mengele, infamously known as the "Angel of Death," represent some of the most disturbing acts of the Nazi era. At Auschwitz, Mengele performed cruel experiments on twins, including blood transfusions between siblings, forced organ removals, and chemical injections into their eyes to change their iris color. When one twin died, the other was often killed for comparative autopsy purposes. These experiments were intended to support Nazi racial theories but had no scientific value (Halioua and Marmor 2020).

Equally disturbing were the sterilization and reproductive experiments. In the pursuit of eugenic ideals, Nazi doctors performed forced sterilizations on prisoners, particularly women, using methods such as radiation exposure, chemical injections, and invasive surgeries—often without anaesthesia. Many women were left infertile, while others died from complications. These inhumane procedures aimed to prevent reproduction among groups deemed "racially impure." The chemical and poison experiments added another layer of cruelty. Prisoners were exposed to toxic substances, including phenol, cyanide, and mustard gas, to study their effects and test antidotes. These experiments were often fatal, causing excruciating deaths. At Buchenwald, chemical injections were administered directly into prisoners' hearts, highlighting the sadistic nature of these so-called scientific studies (Weindling 2014; Mellanby and Reader 1947).

Dr. Sigmund Rascher was a Nazi physician infamous for conducting freezing and high-altitude experiments on prisoners at the Dachau concentration camp during World War II. His freezing experiments aimed to study hypothermia and methods of rewarming for German soldiers exposed to freezing conditions on the Eastern Front. Prisoners were submerged in ice-cold water tanks or left exposed to sub-zero temperatures outdoors, often naked, until they lost consciousness or died. Attempts at revival included immersion in hot water baths or forced physical contact with warm female prisoners. In his high-altitude experiments, Rascher used a low-pressure chamber to simulate conditions faced by Luftwaffe pilots at high altitudes. Prisoners were subjected to extreme drops in air pressure and oxygen levels, causing agonizing deaths from suffocation, embolisms, or brain damage. These brutal experiments resulted in the deaths of hundreds of prisoners and provided little scientific value. Rascher's work epitomizes the inhumanity of Nazi medical experiments and serves as a stark reminder of the catastrophic consequences of science devoid of ethics (Farron 2017).

Karl Brandt, Hitler's personal physician and a key figure in Nazi medical operations, played a central role in overseeing the "Aktion T4" euthanasia program during World War II. Initiated in 1939, Aktion T4 aimed to systematically exterminate individuals deemed "unworthy of life," including the mentally ill, disabled, and other vulnerable populations. Brandt, as the head of this program, authorized the use of gas chambers, lethal injections, and starvation to kill thousands of people in psychiatric institutions and care facilities. Under the guise of "mercy killing" and reducing the financial burden on society, the program became a model for the later mass exterminations carried out in concentration camps. Despite attempting to justify these actions as acts of compassion and scientific advancement, Brandt was ultimately held accountable for his crimes at the Nuremberg Doctors' Trial (1946–1947), where he was found guilty of crimes against humanity and sentenced to death. His involvement in Aktion T4 remains one of the most chilling examples of how medical authority can be distorted for genocidal purposes (Farron 2017). After the war, the world learned the full extent of these crimes during the Nuremberg Doctors' Trial. Out of 23 defendants, 16 were found guilty, and 7 were sentenced to death by hanging. This trial exposed the atrocities committed under the guise of science and established a legal precedent for holding medical professionals accountable for unethical conduct (Mills 2020; Novak 2020). As a direct outcome, the Nuremberg Code was established, outlining ten key principles for ethical human experimentation, including informed consent, the right to withdraw, and the obligation to minimize harm.

The Nazi medical experiments profoundly influenced modern medical ethics and research standards. The Declaration of Helsinki (1964) built upon the Nuremberg Code, creating internationally accepted guidelines for human research. Institutional Review Boards (IRBs) and ethics committees now oversee clinical trials to ensure compliance with ethical standards. Pharmacovigilance systems were also strengthened to monitor drug safety post-approval (Faden et al. 1996; Moreno et al. 2017).

2.7.2.1 The Nuremberg Code (1947)

The Nuremberg Code is a foundational document in medical ethics, established in response to the horrific Nazi medical experiments revealed during the Nuremberg Doctors' Trial. It outlines 10 key principles to ensure the ethical conduct of human experimentation. The code emphasizes voluntary informed consent as a fundamental requirement, ensuring participants fully understand the risks and can withdraw at any time. It mandates that experiments must have scientific merit, minimize harm, and avoid unnecessary suffering. Researchers must be qualified professionals, and the benefits of the research must outweigh the potential risks ("The Oxford Textbook of Clinical Research Ethics—Google Books" 2024).

2.7.3 The Streptomycin Trial (1946–1947)

The Streptomycin Trial conducted by the Medical Research Council (MRC) in the United Kingdom was the first-ever RCT and a landmark in clinical research history. It aimed to evaluate the effectiveness of streptomycin, the first antibiotic effective against tuberculosis (TB). Patients with pulmonary tuberculosis were randomly assigned to either a streptomycin treatment group or a control group receiving standard care without the drug. The trial introduced key methodological innovations, including randomization to reduce bias, blinding to minimize subjective influences, and careful statistical analysis of results. The findings demonstrated that streptomycin significantly reduced mortality and improved patient outcomes compared to standard care, although resistance to the drug emerged as a concern. This trial not only established streptomycin as a breakthrough TB treatment but also set the gold standard for clinical trial design, emphasizing the importance of randomization, control groups, and statistical rigor in evaluating medical interventions (Crofton 2006).

2.7.4 Pharmaceutical Industry and Drug Development

2.7.4.1 The Thalidomide Tragedy (Late 1950s–1960s)

The Thalidomide tragedy remains one of the most devastating pharmaceutical disasters in history. Marketed as a sedative and treatment for morning sickness in pregnant women, Thalidomide caused severe birth defects, including phocomelia (shortened or absent limbs), heart defects, and organ malformations, affecting over 10,000 infants worldwide. In response, governments implemented stricter regulations, including mandatory preclinical testing, comprehensive clinical trials, and post-market surveillance. The disaster exposed critical gaps in drug safety testing, particularly regarding reproductive toxicity, and highlighted the absence of stringent regulatory oversight in many countries. In the United States, Dr. Frances Kelsey of the Food and Drug Administration (FDA) prevented the approval of Thalidomide, saving countless lives and earning national recognition for her diligence (Kim and Scialli 2011).

2.7.4.2 Establishment of Regulatory Bodies

The Thalidomide disaster prompted the establishment of robust regulatory frameworks. The Kefauver-Harris Drug Amendments (1962) in the United States mandated that drug manufacturers demonstrate both safety and efficacy before marketing their products. The U.S. FDA and the European Medicines Agency (EMA) emerged as central figures in ensuring drug safety and efficacy (Greene and Podolsky 2012).

2.7.4.3 The Rise of Blockbuster Drugs

The latter half of the 20th century saw the development of revolutionary drugs, including penicillin, insulin, statins, and antiviral medications. These drugs transformed the treatment landscape for infectious diseases, chronic conditions, and previously untreatable illnesses. Blockbuster drugs not only saved millions of lives but also fueled economic growth in the pharmaceutical industry, solidifying its central role in healthcare (Berghauser Pont et al. 2021).

2.7.5 The Declaration of Helsinki (1964)

The Declaration of Helsinki, adopted in 1964 by the World Medical Association (WMA), is a cornerstone document in medical ethics that builds upon the principles of the Nuremberg Code. It provides ethical guidelines for physicians and researchers conducting medical research involving human subjects. The declaration emphasizes the importance of informed consent, ensuring participants fully understand the purpose, risks, and benefits of the study. It stresses the need for scientific validity, requiring research to be based on sound scientific principles and prior laboratory or animal studies where applicable. The document also highlights the duty to prioritize participant welfare over scientific or societal interests and mandates IRBs to oversee research protocols. Regularly updated to address evolving challenges in clinical research, the Declaration of Helsinki remains a globally recognized standard for ethical research involving humans. The Declaration has undergone multiple revisions, reflecting evolving ethical standards and addressing emerging challenges in global clinical research (Association 2024).

2.7.6 The Belmont Report (1979)

The Belmont Report, published in 1979 by the National Commission for the Protection of Human Subjects of Biomedical and Behavioral Research, is a cornerstone document in bioethics that outlines ethical principles and guidelines for research involving human subjects. It was developed in response to historical abuses in research, most notably the Tuskegee Syphilis Study, where African American men with syphilis were deliberately left untreated without their informed consent. The public outrage from this study led to the establishment of the National Research Act (1974), which tasked the commission with identifying fundamental ethical principles to guide research. The Belmont Report articulates three core principles: Respect for Persons, Beneficence, and Justice. Respect for Persons emphasizes the need for voluntary informed consent, treating individuals as autonomous agents while providing additional protection for vulnerable populations, such as children or prisoners. Beneficence obligates researchers to maximize potential benefits and minimize potential harm, ensuring that the risks to participants are justified by the study's scientific or social value. Justice requires the fair distribution of research benefits and burdens, preventing the exploitation of vulnerable groups and ensuring equity in participant selection (Nagai et al. 2022).

2.7.7 Council for International Organizations of Medical Sciences (CIOMS) (1982)

It was established in 1949 by the World Health Organization (WHO) and UNESCO and plays a vital role in promoting ethical medical research and pharmacovigilance globally. Initially focused on fostering international collaboration, CIOMS expanded its mandate to address ethical challenges in clinical research, particularly in resource-limited settings. Its most significant contribution is the "International Ethical Guidelines for Health-Related Research Involving Humans," first issued in 1982 and last updated in 2016. These guidelines emphasize informed consent, risk minimization, transparency, and equitable distribution of research benefits, with special attention to vulnerable populations such as children, pregnant women, and prisoners. CIOMS also contributes significantly to pharmacovigilance standards, offering globally recognized guidelines for adverse drug reaction (ADR) reporting and collaboration with the WHO and ICH. The organization promotes capacity building through workshops and training programs, ensuring stakeholders can address ethical dilemmas and adhere to global research standards. By advancing ethical principles, transparency, and participant protection, CIOMS remains a cornerstone of medical research integrity, ensuring that scientific advancements align with human rights, dignity, and safety (Macrae 2007).

2.7.8 International Council for Harmonisation of Technical Requirements for Pharmaceuticals for Human Use (ICH, 1990)

It standardizes and harmonizes regulatory guidelines for drug development and approval across Europe, Japan, and the United States. Its primary goal is to ensure the safety, efficacy, and quality of pharmaceutical products while minimizing duplication of testing during drug development. The ICH guidelines cover various aspects of clinical research, including Good Clinical Practice (GCP), ethical considerations, clinical trial design, pharmacovigilance, and data integrity. Key guidelines like ICH E6 (R2) focus on GCP standards, emphasizing ethical trial conduct, participant protection, and data reliability. The ICH also addresses quality control (Q-series), safety assessments (S-series), and efficacy requirements (E-series). These globally accepted guidelines ensure consistency in pharmaceutical regulations, enhance patient safety, and facilitate faster approval of innovative medicines across international markets (Bhavna et al. 2022).

2.7.9 The Common Rule (1991)

The Common Rule (1991) is a key set of regulations in the United States designed to protect human subjects involved in federally funded research. Rooted in the ethical principles of the Belmont Report, it establishes standards for informed consent, risk-benefit assessment, and the equitable selection of participants. The rule mandates the oversight of research by IRBs, which are responsible for reviewing and approving study protocols to ensure ethical compliance. It emphasizes voluntary participation, transparency about risks and benefits, and the protection of vulnerable populations such as children, pregnant women, and prisoners. The Revised Common Rule (2018) introduced updates, including simplified informed consent forms, greater transparency in clinical trial reporting, and provisions for low-risk research flexibility. Together, the Common Rule ensures that research involving human subjects adheres to ethical standards, prioritizes participant safety, and promotes public trust in scientific research.

2.7.10 The Health Insurance Portability and Accountability Act (HIPAA, 1996)

HIPAA is a landmark U.S. legislation designed to protect the privacy, security, and integrity of individuals' health information while ensuring the portability of health insurance coverage. HIPAA introduced the Privacy Rule and Security Rule, establishing strict standards for the use, storage, and sharing of Protected Health Information (PHI) by healthcare providers, insurance companies, and research entities. In clinical research, HIPAA mandates that researchers obtain authorization from participants before accessing or using their health data, ensuring transparency, confidentiality, and data protection. It also sets requirements for data de-identification when PHI is used for research purposes. By balancing patient privacy with the need for data access in medical research, HIPAA plays a crucial role in fostering trust, compliance, and ethical standards in healthcare and clinical studies (et al. 2017).

2.7.11 The U.S. Food and Drug Administration Modernization Act (FDAMA, 1997)

The FDAMA was enacted to modernize and streamline the drug approval process while maintaining high standards for safety and efficacy. It introduced faster review pathways for drugs targeting serious or life-threatening conditions, including the Fast Track designation to accelerate the availability of critical treatments. FDAMA also emphasized increased transparency by mandating the registration of clinical trials on platforms like ClinicalTrials.gov, ensuring public access to trial information. Additionally, it provided incentives for pediatric research, encouraging pharmaceutical companies to conduct studies specifically for pediatric populations. By balancing regulatory flexibility with rigorous oversight, FDAMA aimed to improve patient access to innovative therapies, enhance public confidence in drug development, and foster greater accountability and transparency in clinical research.

2.8 MODERN CLINICAL RESEARCH (21ST CENTURY)

2.8.1 WHO International Clinical Trials Registry Platform (ICTRP, 2005)

This was established to ensure transparency, accountability, and accessibility of information related to clinical trials worldwide. The platform serves as a global initiative to standardize trial registration and improve public access to trial data, regardless of the study's outcomes. It requires researchers to register clinical trials before participant recruitment in publicly accessible databases and provide key details, including study design, objectives, interventions, and primary outcomes. ICTRP aims to prevent publication bias, promote ethical research practices, and enable better collaboration and data sharing among scientists, policymakers, and healthcare professionals. By enhancing global transparency and public trust in clinical research, the ICTRP plays a vital role in ensuring that medical advancements are based on comprehensive, unbiased evidence (Fernández-González 2023).

2.8.2 Good Pharmacovigilance Practices (GVP, 2012)

These are a set of guidelines established by the EMA to ensure the safety and efficacy of medicinal products throughout their lifecycle. These practices outline standards for monitoring, assessing, and preventing ADRs, both during clinical trials and post-marketing surveillance. GVP emphasizes the importance of risk management plans (RMPs), clear protocols for adverse event reporting, and robust systems for signal detection and analysis. It also mandates transparency and timely communication of safety findings to regulatory authorities, healthcare providers, and the public. By promoting a proactive approach to drug safety, GVP aims to minimize risks associated with medications, enhance patient safety, and strengthen public confidence in pharmaceutical products (Sathya Narayanan et al. 2020).

2.8.3 European Union Clinical Trials Regulation (EU-CTR, 2014)

This was introduced to streamline and standardize the approval and conduct of clinical trials across EU member states. It replaced the earlier Clinical Trials Directive (2001/20/EC) to address inefficiencies and inconsistencies in trial approvals. The regulation established a centralized online portal and database for clinical trial applications and approvals, simplifying the submission and review process across multiple countries. It emphasized transparency and public access to clinical trial data, including results, regardless of outcomes. EU-CTR also reinforced participant protection, requiring robust informed consent processes and enhanced safety monitoring throughout the trial lifecycle. By creating a harmonized regulatory framework, the EU-CTR aims to promote innovation, increase efficiency, and ensure the highest standards of safety and ethical conduct in clinical research across Europe.

2.8.4 U.S. FDA Final Rule on Clinical Trials Reporting (2017)

The U.S. FDA Final Rule on Clinical Trials Reporting, implemented in 2017, represents a significant step in enhancing transparency, accountability, and public trust in clinical research. Issued under the Food and Drug Administration Amendments Act (FDAAA) of 2007, this rule clarified and expanded the requirements for registering and reporting results from clinical trials on the publicly accessible platform ClinicalTrials.gov. It aims to address long-standing issues of selective reporting, publication bias, and incomplete data dissemination, ensuring that clinical trial findings—both positive and negative—are available for public scrutiny, scientific advancement, and evidence-based decision-making (DeVito et al. 2019).

At the core of the Final Rule is the mandate that all Applicable Clinical Trials (ACTs)—including interventional studies of FDA-regulated drugs, biologics, and medical devices—must be registered on ClinicalTrials.gov within 21 days of enrolling the first participant. Researchers are also required to submit summary results within 12 months of trial completion, regardless of whether the results are positive, negative, or inconclusive. These requirements close the loopholes that previously allowed some sponsors to withhold unfavorable outcomes, leading to distorted perceptions of a drug's efficacy and safety (DeVito et al. 2020).

A critical component of the Final Rule is its focus on data transparency and completeness. The rule specifies that submitted data must include key trial details, such as study design, primary and secondary endpoints, participant demographics, and adverse event summaries. This level of detail ensures that other researchers, healthcare providers, and policymakers have access to comprehensive trial data for independent analysis, comparison, and meta-research. Furthermore, the FDA explicitly clarified penalties for non-compliance, including financial penalties of up to $10,000 per day for failing to register trials or report results on time. These enforcement measures were put in place to deter negligence and ensure compliance among all stakeholders (Wittes et al. 2015; DeVito et al. 2019).

Another significant aspect of the Final Rule is its requirement for increased public accessibility of clinical trial information. All trial data reported on ClinicalTrials.gov is made publicly available, with safeguards to protect participant privacy, such as de-identification of personal health information. This transparency not only fosters public trust in clinical research but also helps prevent unnecessary duplication of studies, reduces research waste, and promotes collaboration among scientists (DeVito et al. 2020).

The Final Rule also addressed challenges related to retrospective compliance and accountability. Trials that were previously non-compliant under the original FDAAA requirements were brought under the scope of this regulation, ensuring historical data gaps were addressed. Additionally, it emphasized the role of sponsors and principal investigators in maintaining compliance and ensuring the accuracy and completeness of submitted data (Wittes et al. 2015).

The impact of the FDA Final Rule on Clinical Trials Reporting extends beyond regulatory enforcement. It has fostered a culture of transparency and scientific integrity in clinical research. Researchers and sponsors are now more accountable for their findings, and healthcare providers and policymakers have better access to unbiased evidence when making treatment and policy decisions. It also aligns the U.S. regulatory framework more closely with global initiatives for trial transparency, such as the ICTRP and the EU-CTR (DeVito et al. 2019, 2020; Wittes et al. 2015).

2.9 CONCLUSION

The historical evolution of clinical research reflects humanity's persistent quest to understand, treat, and prevent diseases while balancing scientific discovery with ethical responsibility. From the earliest medical practices in Ancient Egypt and Mesopotamia to the controlled dietary experiments under King Nebuchadnezzar II, and the systematic approaches of Hippocrates and Galen in Ancient Greece, each era laid a foundational stone in the development of clinical research methodologies. The dark chapters of medical history, including the Nazi medical experiments, the Tuskegee Syphilis Study, and the Thalidomide tragedy, exposed the catastrophic consequences of unethical research practices and became powerful catalysts for change. Key milestones such as the Nuremberg Code, the Declaration of Helsinki, the Belmont Report, and the establishment of frameworks like the ICH Guidelines and the Common Rule have shaped the modern ethical and regulatory landscape of clinical research. These frameworks emphasize principles like informed consent, participant safety, transparency, and data integrity, ensuring that scientific advancement does not come at the cost of human dignity.

The introduction of RCTs, beginning with the Streptomycin Trial, revolutionized clinical research by providing robust methodologies for evaluating treatments. Subsequent advancements, including the establishment of clinical trial registries like ClinicalTrials.gov and global oversight bodies like the WHO ICTRP, have further solidified transparency and accountability in research.

REFERENCES

Abdul-Sahib, Mahdi. 2024. "Patient Rights and Physician Responsibilities in Ancient Civilizations Codex Hammurabi Is a Model." *Researchgate.Net*. Accessed December 30. https://www.researchgate.net/profile/Mahdi-Abdul-Sahib/publication/380603162_Patient_rights_and_physician_responsibilities_in_ancient_civilizations_Codex_Hammurabi_is_a_model/links/6645afd2479366623af049a2/Patient-rights-and-physician-responsibilities-in-ancient-civilizations-Codex-Hammurabi-is-a-model.pdf.

Adamo, N, N Al-Ansari—Journal of Earth Sciences and Geotechnical, and undefined 2020. 2020. "In Old Babylonia: Irrigation and Agriculture Flourished under the Code of Hammurabi (2000–1600 BC)." *Diva-Portal.Org* 10 (3). online Scientific Press International Limited: 1792–9660. https://www.diva-portal.org/smash/record.jsf?pid=diva2:1412803.

"Andreas Vesalius: Anatomy and the World of Books—Sachiko Kusukawa—Google Books." 2024. Accessed December 30. https://books.google.co.in/books?hl=en&lr=&id=k2f7EAAAQBAJ&oi=fnd&pg=PT10&dq=Andreas+Vesalius+&ots=5ZdyzZKPZJ&sig=e928U9oANHU7SsamYlNAi4iWJOI&redir_esc=y#v=onepage&q=Andreas%20Vesalius&f=false.

Asaram Budhnar, Pravin, Aparna Raut, Ramesh Ahire, Ashish Hastak, and Shubhangi Wankhedkar. 2022. "Basic Shalya Ideologies of Sushruta Samhita-An Overview." *Certified Journal │ Pravin et al. World Journal of Pharmaceutical Research* 11: 1532. https://doi.org/10.20959/wjpr20227-24681.

Association, World Medical. 2024. "World Medical Association Declaration of Helsinki: Ethical Principles for Medical Research Involving Human Participants." *JAMA*, October. https://doi.org/10.1001/JAMA.2024.21972.

"The Babylonian World." 2009. *The Babylonian World*, June. Routledge. https://doi.org/10.4324/9780203946237.

Baker, Samuel H. 2021. "Aristotle on the Nature and Politics of Medicine." *Apeiron* 54 (4). De Gruyter Open Ltd: 411–49. https://doi.org/10.1515/APEIRON-2019-0052/HTML.

Belhandouz, Amina. 2024. "The Scientific Arabic Terminology in the Golden Age Period and the Modern Period." *Asjp.Cerist.Dz*, 244–56. Accessed December 30. https://www.asjp.cerist.dz/en/downArticle/160/17/3/187531.

Berghauser Pont, Lotte, Jiri Keirsse, Rachel Moss, Pawel Poda, Lucas Robke, and Stephan Wurzer. 2021. "Developing Blockbuster Drugs: Both Nature and Nurture." *Nature Reviews: Drug Discovery* 20 (6). NLM (Medline): 421–2. https://doi.org/10.1038/D41573-020-00061-9.

Best, M., and D. Neuhauser. 2005. "Pierre Charles Alexandre Louis: Master of the Spirit of Mathematical Clinical Science." *BMJ Quality & Safety* 14 (6). BMJ Publishing Group Ltd: 462–4. https://doi.org/10.1136/QSHC.2005.016816.

Bhavna, Samir Bhargava, and Abhijeet Ojha. 2022. "International Council for Harmonisation (ICH) Guidelines." *Regulatory Affairs in the Pharmaceutical Industry*, January. Academic Press, 47–74. https://doi.org/10.1016/B978-0-12-822211-9.00008-3.

Carpenter, Stephen, Michel Rigaud, Mary Barile, Tracy J. Priest, Luis Perez, and John B. Ferguson. 2006. "The Ebers Papyrus." *Dirzon.Com*. https://www.dirzon.com/file/telegram/Ancient_Egyptian_Language/An_Interlinear_Transliteration_and_English_Translation_of_Portions.pdf.

Castiglioni, Arturo. 2019. "A History of Medicine." *A History of Medicine*, January. Taylor and Francis, 1–1253. https://doi.org/10.4324/9780429019883/HISTORY-MEDICINE ARTURO-CASTIGLIONI.

Cellular, J.B. West—American Journal of Physiology-Lung, and undefined 2014. 2014. "Galen and the Beginnings of Western Physiology." *Journals.Physiology.Org* 307 (2). American Physiological Society. https://doi.org/10.1152/ajplung.00123.2014.

"Companion Encyclopedia of the History of Medicine." 2013. *Companion Encyclopedia of the History of Medicine*, June. Routledge. https://doi.org/10.4324/9781315002514/COMPANION-ENCYCLOPEDIA-HISTORY-MEDICINE-BYNUM-ROY-PORTER.

Crofton, J. 2006. "The MRC Randomized Trial of Streptomycin and Its Legacy: A View from the Clinical Front Line." *Https://Doi.Org/10.1177/014107680609901017* 99 (10). SAGE PublicationsSage UK: London, England: 531–4. https://doi.org/10.1177/014107680609901017.

DeVito, Nicholas J., Seb Bacon, and Ben Goldacre. 2019. "FDAAA TrialsTracker: A Live Informatics Tool to Monitor Compliance with FDA Requirements to Report Clinical Trial Results." *BioRxiv*, October. Cold Spring Harbor Laboratory, 266452. https://doi.org/10.1101/266452.

DeVito, Nicholas J., Seb Bacon, and Ben Goldacre. 2020. "Compliance with Legal Requirement to Report Clinical Trial Results on ClinicalTrials.Gov: A Cohort Study." *The Lancet* 395 (10221). Lancet Publishing Group: 361–9. https://doi.org/10.1016/S0140-6736(19)33220-9.

Faden, Ruth R., Susan E. Lederer, and Jonathan D. Moreno. 1996. "US Medical Researchers, the Nuremberg Doctors Trial, and the Nuremberg Code: A Review of Findings of the Advisory Committee on Human Radiation Experiments." *JAMA* 276 (20). American Medical Association: 1667–71. https://doi.org/10.1001/JAMA.1996.03540200053031.

Farron, Nichola. 2017. "Rascher and the 'Russians': Human Experimentation on Soviet Prisoners in Dachau—A New Perspective." *From Clinic to Concentration Camp*, April. Routledge, 257–71. https://doi.org/10.4324/9781315583310-12.

Fernández-González, Loreto. 2023. "Registering Transparency: The Making of the International Clinical Trial Registry Platform by the World Health Organization (2004–2006)." *Globalization and Health* 19 (1). BioMed Central Ltd: 1–12. https://doi.org/10.1186/S12992-023-00970-5/METRICS.

Fox, R.L. 2020. *The Invention of Medicine: From Homer to Hippocrates*. https://books.google.com/books?hl=en&lr=&id=HafIDwAAQBAJ&oi=fnd&pg=PP11&dq=Hippocrates&ots=o8sUATAfXb&sig=U6zewWs5bqzVp6a6GfVdv_7sKMI.

French, R. 2024. *Ancients and Moderns in the Medical Sciences: From Hippocrates to Harvey*. https://books.google.com/books?hl=en&lr=&id=1GI0EQAAQBAJ&oi=fnd&pg=PP9&dq=Hippocrates&ots=T8WY4vOU3x&sig=I7gM4loj851VES-AgYP6iZKuP5Y.

Fry, T. 2016. *The Rule of St. Benedict in English*. https://books.google.com/books?hl=en&lr=&id=KpkkDwAAQBAJ&oi=fnd&pg=PA9&dq=Rule+of+Saint+Benedict+&ots=lROc-X6gkR&sig=YVRaBSeJdo9iHNH3Lfpl1LIct9U.

Ghaffari, F., M. Taheri, A. Meyari,. . . Y. Karimi—Journal of Medicine, and undefined 2022. 2024. "Avicenna and Clinical Experiences in Canon of Medicine." *Ncbi.Nlm.Nih.Gov*. Accessed December 30. https://www.ncbi.nlm.nih.gov/pmc/articles/PMC8999087/.

Graeco-Roman, V. Cotesta—The Heavens and the Earth:, undefined Ancient, and undefined 2021. 2024. "Al-Kindi: Muhammad and Aristotle." *Brill.Com*. Accessed December 30. https://brill.com/downloadpdf/book/9789004464728/BP000035.pdf.

Greene, Jeremy A., and Scott H. Podolsky. 2012. "Reform, Regulation, and Pharmaceuticals—The Kefauver–Harris Amendments at 50." *New England Journal of Medicine* 367 (16). New England Journal of Medicine (NEJM/MMS): 1481–3. https://doi.org/10.1056/NEJMP1210007.

Gynecology, D.A. Grimes—Obstetrics &, and undefined 1995. 2024. "Clinical Research in Ancient Babylon: Methodologic Insights from the Book of Daniel." *Journals.Lww.Com*. Accessed December 30. https://journals.lww.com/greenjournal/abstract/1995/12000/clinical_research_in_ancient_babylon__methodologic.34.aspx.

Halioua, Bruno, and Michael F. Marmor. 2020. "The Eyes of the Angel of Death: Ophthalmic Experiments of Josef Mengele." *Survey of Ophthalmology* 65 (6). Elsevier: 744–8. https://doi.org/10.1016/J.SURVOPHTHAL.2020.04.007.

Hohonu, T. Gomes -, and undefined 2010. 2024. "Nazi Experiments." *Hilo.Hawaii.Edu*. Accessed December 30. https://www.hilo.hawaii.edu/campuscenter/hohonu/volumes/documents/Vol08x03NaziExperiments.pdf.

Kiger, J.P. 2022. *How the Code of Hammurabi Influenced Modern Legal Systems*. http://9ae2r36v53.remont-ehlektrostal.ru/6mn7uhcz0.pdf.

Kim, James H., and Anthony R. Scialli. 2011. "Thalidomide: The Tragedy of Birth Defects and the Effective Treatment of Disease." *Toxicological Sciences* 122 (1). Oxford Academic: 1–6. https://doi.org/10.1093/TOXSCI/KFR088.

King, H. 2020. *Hippocrates Now: The 'Father of Medicine'in the Internet Age*. https://library.oapen.org/handle/20.500.12657/23773.

King, L.W. 2023. *Codex Hammurabi*. https://books.google.com/books?hl=en&lr=&id=sm_iEAAAQBAJ&oi=fnd&pg=PT14&dq=Code+of+Hammurabi+&ots=cl3a_BpI_j&sig=axO4Yaj6fADU7fVZ8Pqn8FpDoqY.

Leeuw, Daan De. 2020. "'In the Name of Humanity': Nazi Doctors and Human Experiments in German Concentration Camps." *Holocaust and Genocide Studies* 34 (2). Oxford Academic: 225–52. https://doi.org/10.1093/HGS/DCAA025.

Lloyd, Keith, and Jo White. 2011. "Democratizing Clinical Research." *Nature* 474 (7351): 277–8. https://doi.org/10.1038/474277A.

Lr, Usharani, B.H. Katti, Venkatesh Goudar, and M.R. Sajjanshetty. 2024. "A Comprehensive Review on Basic Principles of Samkhya Darshana and Their Implications in Charaka Samhita." *Jaims.In* 6: 4. Accessed December 30. https://jaims.in/jaims/article/view/2698.

Macrae, Duncan J. 2007. "The Council for International Organizations and Medical Sciences (CIOMS) Guidelines on Ethics of Clinical Trials." *Proceedings of the American Thoracic Society* 4 (2): 176–8. https://doi.org/10.1513/PATS.200701-011GC.

Magner, Lois N., and Oliver J. Kim. 2017. "A History of Medicine, Third Edition." *A History of Medicine, Third Edition*, January. CRC Press, 1–446. https://doi.org/10.1201/9781315113814/HISTORY-MEDICINE-LOIS-MAGNER-OLIVER-KIM.

Martiniana, M.W. Worthing—Acta Medica, and undefined 2024. 2024. "Nestorian Christian Contributions to Medicine in the Golden Age of Islam Under the Abassid Caliphs of Baghdad 786–1258 CE." *Sciendo.Com* 24 (3): 116–26. https://doi.org/10.2478/acm-2024-0015.

Medicine, S.X. Ke—Journal of Ayurveda and Integrative, and undefined 2023. 2024. "The Principles of Health, Illness and Treatment-The Key Concepts from 'The Yellow Emperor's Classic of Internal Medicine.'" *Elsevier*. Accessed December 30. https://www.sciencedirect.com/science/article/pii/S0975947622000961.

medycyny, A Hallmann-Mikołajczak—Archiwum historii i filozofii, and undefined 2004. 2024. "Ebers Papyrus: The Book of Medical Knowledge of the 16th Century BC Egyptians." *Europepmc.Org*. Accessed December 30. https://europepmc.org/article/med/15586450.
Mellanby, Kenneth, and Sc D. Reader. 1947. "Medical Experiments on Human Beings in Concentration Camps in Nazi Germany." *British Medical Journal* 1 (4490): 148. https://doi.org/10.1136/BMJ.1.4490.148.
Menikoff, Jerry, Julie Kaneshiro, and Ivor Pritchard. 2017. "The Common Rule, Updated." *New England Journal of Medicine* 376 (7). New England Journal of Medicine (NEJM/MMS): 613–15. https://doi.org/10.1056/NEJMP1700736/SUPPL_FILE/NEJMP1700736_DISCLOSURES.PDF.
Mews, Constant J. 2020. "Hildegard of Bingen." *Encyclopedia of Medieval Philosophy*. Dordrecht: Springer, Dordrecht, 725–7. https://doi.org/10.1007/978-94-024-1665-7_214.
Michaleas, Spyros N., Konstantinos Laios, Gregory Tsoucalas, and Georges Androutsos. 2021. "Theophrastus Bombastus Von Hohenheim (Paracelsus) (1493–1541): The Eminent Physician and Pioneer of Toxicology." *Toxicology Reports* 8 (January). Elsevier: 411–14. https://doi.org/10.1016/J.TOXREP.2021.02.012.
Mills, James. 2020. "Pandora's Box Closed: The Royal Air Force Institute of Aviation Medicine and Nazi Medical Experiments on Human Beings during World War II." *Studies in History and Philosophy of Science Part C: Studies in History and Philosophy of Biological and Biomedical Sciences* 79 (February). Pergamon: 101190. https://doi.org/10.1016/J.SHPSC.2019.101190.
Moreno, Jonathan D., Ulf Schmidt, and Steve Joffe. 2017. "The Nuremberg Code 70 Years Later." *JAMA* 318 (9). American Medical Association: 795–6. https://doi.org/10.1001/JAMA.2017.10265.
Nagai, Hiroyuki, Eisuke Nakazawa, and Akira Akabayashi. 2022. "The Creation of the Belmont Report and Its Effect on Ethical Principles: A Historical Study." *Monash Bioethics Review* 40 (2). Springer: 157–70. https://doi.org/10.1007/S40592-022-00165-5/TABLES/1.
Novak, D. 2020. "Is the Use of Data from Nazi Medical Experiments Justifiable or Not?" *Ethics, Medicine and Public Health* 12 (January). Elsevier Masson: 100431. https://doi.org/10.1016/J.JEMEP.2019.100431.
PARK, K. 2005. "Park's Textbook of Preventive and Social Medicine." *Preventive Medicine in Obstet, Paediatrics and Geriatrics*. Ms Banarsidas Bhanot. https://cir.nii.ac.jp/crid/1574231875325750784.
praksa, D. Kovačević—Pravo teorija i, and undefined 2022. 2022. "A Historical–Legal Review of Hammurabi's Code." *Ceeol.Com*. https://doi.org/10.5937/ptp2201071K.
"The Oxford Textbook of Clinical Research Ethics—Google Books." 2024. Accessed December 30. https://books.google.co.in/books?hl=en&lr=&id=vKFYAtcLAxgC&oi=fnd&pg=PA136&dq=nuremberg+code+ethics&ots=In2a1ZdZg0&sig=lQlev3K4fABB7rvf9SDHYApF9Q0&redir_esc=y#v=onepage&q=nuremberg%20code%20ethics&f=false.
Sathya Narayanan, A.S., K.S. Lakshmi, and Raju Kamaraj. 2020. "An Overview on Good Pharmacovigilance Practices and New Operational Plan Milestones of Eudravigilance in European Union." *Research Journal of Pharmacy and Technology* 13 (4). Research Journal of Pharmacy and Technology: 1793–8. https://doi.org/10.5958/0974-360X.2020.00323.6.
Schmitt, Charles B., and Charles Webster. 2024. "Aristotle among the Physicians." *Reappraisals in Renaissance Thought*, August. Routledge, VII-1-VII–279. https://doi.org/10.4324/9781003554592-7/ARISTOTLE-AMONG-PHYSICIANS-CHARLES-SCHMITT CHARLES-WEBSTER
Science, H.N. Wasti—Muslim Contribution to, and undefined 2019. 2024. "Muslim Contribution to Medicine." *Books.Google.Com*. Accessed December 30. https://books.google.com/books?hl=en&lr=&id=xenuPgbyXRcC&oi=fnd&pg=PA191&dq=Kitab+al-Hawi+Medicine+&ots=W6Mmqb56h4&sig=hr_YSFUng4hvTGiubvjM3oCYq38.
Singer, P.N. 2019. *Galen and the Culture of Pergamon: A View of Greek Medical-Intellectual Life in Roman Asia*. https://www.academia.edu/download/64991845/Singer.Galen_and_Culture_of_Pergamon.pdf.
Stackle, Erin C. 2021. "Aristotle the Virtue Doctor." *Heythrop Journal—Quarterly Review of Philosophy and Theology* 62 (3). Blackwell Publishing Ltd: 431–43. https://doi.org/10.1111/HEYJ.12347.
Tibi, Selma. 2006. "Al-Razi and Islamic Medicine in the 9th Century." *Journal of the Royal Society of Medicine* 99 (4). SAGE Publications: 206–7. https://doi.org/10.1177/014107680609900425.
Tobin, Martin J. 2022. "Fiftieth Anniversary of Uncovering the Tuskegee Syphilis Study the Story and Timeless Lessons." *American Journal of Respiratory and Critical Care Medicine* 205 (10). American Thoracic Society: 1145–58. https://doi.org/10.1164/RCCM.202201-0136SO/SUPPL_FILE/DISCLOSURES.PDF.
Upadhyayula, Satyanarayana, and RaviR Kasliwal. 2020. "Commemorating James Lind: The Man Who Gave Us the Concept of Controlled Clinical Trials." *Journal of Clinical and Preventive Cardiology* 9 (3). Medknow: 92. https://doi.org/10.4103/JCPC.JCPC_40_20.

Weindling, Paul. 2014. "Victims and Survivors of Nazi Human Experiments." *Victims and Survivors of Nazi Human Experiments: Science and Suffering in the Holocaust*, January. Bloomsbury Publishing, 1–256. https://doi.org/10.1093/gerhis/ghv070.

Weindling, Paul. 2022. "Painful and Sometimes Deadly Experiments Which Nazi Doctors Carried out on Children." *Acta Paediatrica* 111 (9). John Wiley & Sons, Ltd: 1664–9. https://doi.org/10.1111/APA.16310.

Wittes, Janet, Brenda Crowe, Christy Chuang-Stein, Achim Guettner, David Hall, Qi Jiang, Daniel Odenheimer, et al. 2015. "The FDA's Final Rule on Expedited Safety Reporting: Statistical Considerations." *Statistics in Biopharmaceutical Research* 7 (3). Taylor & Francis: 174–90. https://doi.org/10.1080/19466315.2015.1043395.

"The Works of Francis Bacon: Vol. II—Francis Bacon—Google Books." 2024. Accessed December 30. https://books.google.co.in/books?hl=en&lr=&id=YuHbEAAAQBAJ&oi=fnd&pg=PR1&dq=Francis+Bacon+&ots=nGZYpNWXe8&sig=1r0fa09-8gvKHahwmbU21Xx9jIo&redir_esc=y#v=onepage&q=Francis%20Bacon&f=false.

3 Protocol in Clinical Research

Atiya Sahar[1] *and Kamlesh Garg*[2]
[1]Department of Translational and Clinical Research, School of Chemical and Life Sciences, Jamia Hamdard, New Delhi, India
[2]Department of Pharmacology, Vardhman Mahavir Medical College & Safdarjung Hospital, Ansari Nagar West, New Delhi, India

3.1 INTRODUCTION

For conducting a clinical research study, every researcher requires proper and meticulous planning to ensure its success. A well-structured protocol acts as a roadmap providing a foundation for designing, implementing, and conducting a clinical trial in a systematic and ethical manner. It helps to outline the study's objective, methodology, participant criteria, safety measures, and statistical plan. It also ensures transparency, compliance, and effective communication among sponsors, investigators, ethics committees, and regulatory authorities by providing clear guidelines, minimizing risk, and enhancing integrity, which is necessary for generating meaningful and reliable results.

Clinical research study requires a protocol explaining the purpose of the study. Transparent, thorough, and well-written protocols are crucial for conducting clinical trials as they allow for study evaluation. High-quality protocol promotes proper conduct of a clinical trial. It is a key tool for all aspects of clinical trials, being necessary for all reasons as it presents study schedule, manages the conduct of the trial that should be strictly followed by all the study administrators, and informs study administrators who are Contact Research Organizations (CRO). It is required to get ethical approval from the Institutional Ethics Committee (IEC) or Institutional Review Board (IRB). Protocol also contains the information of previously conducted phases, schedules of tests and procedures, and duration of study (Nikam et al. 2022;D'errico et al. 2023).

Every protocol needs a research question, providing knowledge gaps along with the planned research. The development of research question is extremely important. When developing a research question, patient/problem, intervention/exposure, comparison, and outcome (PICO) may be helpful for drafting testable questions, and generating a hypothesis is of utmost importance in order to pre-specify what results are expected (Rosenthal et al. 2014).

3.2 DEFINITIONS

According to the New Drugs and Clinical Trials Rules, 2019, clinical trial protocol is defined as "a document containing the background, objective, rationale, design, methodology including matters containing performance, management, conduct, analysis, adverse event, withdrawal, statistical considerations and record keeping pertaining to clinical trial" (*New Drugs and Clinical Trials Rules, 2019*, 2019).

ICH GOOD CLINICAL PRACTICE (ICH GCP) E6 (R3) guidelines define protocol as "a document that describes the objective(s), design, methodology, statistical considerations and organization of trial" ("INTERNATIONAL COUNCIL FOR HARMONISATION OF TECHNICAL REQUIREMENTS FOR PHARMACEUTICALS FOR HUMAN USE ICH HARMONISED GUIDELINE GOOD CLINICAL PRACTICE (GCP) E6(R3)," n.d.).

Central Drug Standard Control Organization's (CDSCO) GCP guidelines describe protocol as "a document that states the background, objectives, rationale, design, methodology (including the methods for dealing with Adverse Effects (AEs), withdrawals etc.) and statistical considerations

DOI: 10.1201/9781003533085-3

of the study. It also states the conditions under which the study shall be performed and managed" ("Clinicalgcpguide," n.d.).

To be ethically accepted, a clinical study protocol must be reviewed and approved by the IEC/IRB. The IEC/IRB frequently asked whether the planned study by the investigator is scientifically valid, and whether the rights and safety of research participants will be protected. The potential risks to which the participants are likely to be exposed, as well as the planned measures to reduce those risks, are given careful consideration (Orimadegun AE 2020).

Developing a clinical trial protocol following guidelines ensures that a clinical trial is well-planned, scientifically and ethically sound, and protects patient safety, while also producing reliable results.

3.3 FORMAT OF PROTOCOL

ICH GCP E6 (R3) recommends that a protocol follow a specific format, including the following contents, which may vary depending upon the study.

3.3.1 General Information

General information provides essential details of a clinical trial, including its title, unique identification number, sponsor information, and key personnel responsible for protocol amendments. These details enhance communication between stakeholders such as regulatory bodies, ethics committees, and researchers, ensuring clarity, transparency, and traceability throughout the study.

3.3.1.1 Protocol Title, Unique Identification Number, Date

Protocol title should be clear, concise, short, and accurate, highlighting the purpose of the research. The title should clearly state the main objective, significance of the research, and target population without any abbreviations. The title of the protocol should be written in such a way that it provides a short overview of the techniques being used (Saluja and Modi 2021).

A unique identification number is given to each protocol, which helps in distinguishing it from similar studies. Publication references, internal documentation, and regulatory submissions all use this number. It guarantees that various versions of the protocol may be systematically tracked.

The date of protocol version is crucial for compliance and record keeping. Any protocol modifications should contain a new version number and date so that stakeholders can distinguish between the original and revised versions.

3.3.1.2 Name and Address of the Sponsor

It is the sponsor's responsibility to initiate, manage, and finance the clinical trial. It is essential that the protocol include the sponsor's name and complete address for establishing accountability and contact details for regulatory bodies and ethics committees, ensuring proper adherence to Good Clinical Practice (GCP) guidelines, and facilitating communication in case of safety concerns, trial updates, or regulatory inquiries.

3.3.1.3 Name and Title of the Person Authorized to Sign the Protocol and Amendments for the Sponsor

The name and title of the authorized person must be included in the protocol to maintain legal and regulatory compliance. The authorized individual has the authority to approve and sign the protocol and any future versions on behalf of the sponsor.

3.4 BACKGROUND

This section provides scientific and clinical justification for conducting a clinical trial. It includes an overview of the investigational product (IP), relevant preclinical and clinical findings of previously conducted studies, potential risks and benefits that were observed in previous phases of the study, description and justification of the dosage, route of administration, and treatment period.

The protocol must begin with a detailed description of the disease, its pathophysiology, existing therapies, and description of IP, including name composition, pharmacological properties, mechanism of action, intended therapeutic use, and population to be studied.

3.4.1 Review of Literature

Review of literature provides an overview of the current state of knowledge by describing the previous research to assess the research area and to justify the aim, research question, and hypotheses of the study. Conducting a review of literature helps to identify the actual research gap instead of conducting the same research repeatedly and improves the quality of the research. It begins by summarizing the previous studies and existing studies to develop a scientific background and relevance of the study. This can be done thoroughly by using databases such as PubMed, Medline, Cochrane, and Embase, which highlight the key research gaps and areas requiring further research from published and ongoing research. Protocol review of literature determines what is already known and what remains unexplored, ensuring that the study addressed an unanswered scientific and clinical questions. The review of literature could conclude by clearly defining the rationale for performing the study while ensuring that the study is scientifically justified (Snyder 2019).

3.4.2 Trial Objective and Purpose

According to ICH GCP E6(R3), a well-defined scientific objective is crucial in a clinical trial protocol as it establishes the primary purpose and focus of the study. Research questions and hypotheses give rise to the study's objective and purpose. They should answer the research question and hypotheses that are being measured and analysed. Aim or objective and purpose should be reasonable, coherent, feasible, concise, realistic, and meet the purpose of the study and be related to the intended research. The aim of the study should be rational and feasible with respect to time and budget. It is not recommended to include too many aims/objectives (preferably 2–5 are most appropriate). The objectives should be Specific, Measurable, Achievable, Relevant, and Time based (SMART). Aims and objectives should start with action verbs like to determine, to compare, to calculate, and to measure. In case of estimands, quantities should be precisely defined that describe the treatment effect in a target population (Al Jundi and Sakka 2016).

3.5 TRIAL DESIGN

This is a description of the research's strategies and is most likely the easiest section to prepare. It is preferable to use the active voice instead of passive so that it is easier to read and understand. According to ICH GCP E6(R3) guidelines, a well-defined trial design is crucial for producing valid, reproducible, and meaningful clinical evidence while ensuring participants' safety and regulatory compliance (O'brien and Wright, n.d.).

3.5.1 Primary and Secondary Endpoint, if Any, during the Trial

One of the core elements of trial design is to define the study endpoints. The protocol must divide endpoints into major types such as clinical endpoints, surrogate endpoints, patient-reported outcomes, and biomarkers. Primary endpoints are generally efficacy measures that should address the research questions. The selection of the primary endpoint should align with the clinical relevance, disease characteristics, and regulatory guidance, ensuring that they provide reliable results. Secondary endpoints may support the efficacy by providing additional effects or by supporting a causal mechanism, but they are typically insufficient to influence the decision-making alone. These may include exploratory measures, biomarker analysis, safety evaluations, or patient-reported outcomes (PROs). Secondary endpoints help in understanding the broader impact of the treatment. For trial results to be significant and relevant to the target population, the protocol must justify endpoints based on previous research, disease pathophysiology, and statistical considerations (D'errico et al. 2023; McLeod et al. 2019).

3.5.2 Description of Trial Design

Trial design should be clearly outlined in the protocol, whether it follows a randomized, double-blind, placebo-controlled, parallel group, adaptive, or decentralized model. The selection of trial design should depend upon the trial objective, intervention type, disease characteristics, and ethical considerations. To provide a clear understanding, the protocol should include a schematic diagram illustrating the study design, procedures, trial stages, and participant flow.

3.5.3 Description of Measures to Minimize/Avoid Bias in Randomization and Blinding

It is essential that the protocol include all the measures that will be taken to minimize or avoid bias during randomization and blinding by providing the randomization method and type of blinding so as to ensure and enhance the comparability of the study groups.

3.5.4 Description of Trial Treatment

To standardize administration, patient safety, protocol should clearly outline, with detailed description of IP, its dosage regimen, route of administration (oral, intravenous, subcutaneous, etc.), frequency, duration of treatment, formulation, dosage form (tablet, capsule, syrups, etc.), packaging, labelling, storage conditions, batch numbers, expiration date, and handling instructions to maintain accuracy in treatment delivery.

3.5.5 Description of Sequence and Duration of Trial

The protocol must provide a clear timeline outlining the expected duration of the participant's involvement in the trial. This should describe the sequence and duration of all trial periods, including screening, baseline visit, treatment, washout (if applicable), and follow-up phases or visits to monitor the outcome of the IP.

3.5.6 Description of Discontinuation Criteria, Dose Adjustment, Stopping Rules, Dose Interruptions

It is important in the protocol to include discontinuation criteria and stopping rules, and to ensure that individual participants may be withdrawn from the trial study due to any serious adverse events (SAEs), safety concerns, disease progression, lack of treatment efficacy, protocol violation, or voluntary withdrawal. Protocol should include that the entire trial study should be modified—by making dose reduction, escalation, based on participants' response, safety, or pharmacokinetics findings, paused, or terminated—to optimize the therapeutic benefits.

3.5.7 Accountability Procedures

Protocol should include information about the accountability of IP, placebo/comparator, by providing the details of procedures of receipt, storage, dispensing, return, and disposal of all the study drugs.

3.5.8 Maintenance of Breaking Randomization Codes and Procedures

Protocol must include details of how the randomization codes are generated, assigned, stored, and protected throughout the trial process. It should also include the procedures for breaking the randomization of codes in cases where unblinding is necessary, such as in emergencies like death, where information on treatment is necessary for participant's safety, and also who is responsible for breaking these randomization codes.

3.6 SELECTION OF PARTICIPANTS

Details of inclusion and exclusion criteria are important parts that should be explained in the protocol. For inclusion criteria, specify the predefined characteristics that participants must meet to be eligible for the trial. These include factors such as age, gender, disease condition or status, details of laboratory values, and prior treatments. For exclusion criteria, specify the conditions or factors of participants that must be excluded from enrolling in the trial, such as comorbid conditions, concurrent treatment, pregnancy, alcohol, and history of adverse drug reactions.

This section in the protocol should also explain how the potential participants will be identified, screened, assessed, enrolled, and followed throughout the trial process.

3.7 WITHDRAWAL AND DISCONTINUATION OF PARTICIPANTS

Protocol should provide detailed information on the withdrawal of consent or discontinuation of participation, as well as clear procedures for handling such procedures, including documentation requirements and any follow-up assessment. The protocol should also specify whether previously collected data can be used in the data analysis or not, and how the missing data will be managed.

3.8 TREATMENT AND INTERVENTION FOR PARTICIPANTS

Treatment and intervention strategy should outline treatment(s) to be administered, dosing regimens, permitted and prohibited medications, and adherence monitoring strategies.

3.8.1 Details of Treatment

In this section, details of all interventions and any placebo/comparator must be included with names of all the investigational products, along with their doses, dosing schedules, criteria for dose adjustment, route and mode of administration, treatment period for each trial arm or group, the duration of administration, and any applicable follow-up period. It is essential that the investigator develop a clear and structured plan for treatment administration.

3.8.2 Treatment Permitted and Not Permitted before or during the Trial

It is important to describe in the protocol which treatment/medication is permitted and which is not permitted before and during the trial so as to prevent possible drug interactions. This includes concomitant medications, rescue medications which are used to alleviate the adverse effects, timeframe before and during the trial in which these medications should be avoided.

3.8.3 Treatment Adherence

Ensuring participants' adherence to the treatment regimen is important. It is necessary to describe the strategies to monitor adherence, such as blood sampling, biomarker analysis, or drug level measurements to confirm whether the investigational product has been taken as prescribed, participant diaries, pill counts, electronic medication monitoring systems, and adherence questionnaires, which help track compliance trends over time. Scheduled follow-up visits and counselling sessions, allow investigators to reinforce adherence and identify barriers to compliance.

3.9 ASSESSMENT OF EFFICACY

This section describes the methods which will be used to determine the effectiveness of the intervention.

3.9.1 Efficacy Parameters

Describing efficacy parameters is essential for assessing the intervention's impact. The protocol should explain how the efficacy will be measured and specify timepoints for parameter assessment.

3.9.2 Methods for Assessing Efficacy Parameters

It is important for investigators to include a detailed plan for assessing efficacy parameters in the protocol, along with specific techniques and tools that will be used, frequency and time points at which the efficacy data will be collected, the process of documenting efficacy findings, and statistical methods applied for data analysis.

3.10 ASSESSMENT OF SAFETY

A structured safety assessment ensures early detection of AE and supports risk mitigation.

3.10.1 Safety Parameters

Protocol should provide specific clinical, laboratory, and imaging assessments used to monitor participant safety, including vital signs, biochemical markers, and adverse event reporting. It should also outline a schedule for regular safety evaluations and describe the documentation process for AE and serious adverse events (SAEs), including causality assessment and timelines.

3.10.2 Methods for Assessing Safety Parameters

For capturing safety-related data, protocol must specify the methods, extent, and timing that will be used to assess safety parameters.

It is the responsibility of the investigator to specify in the protocol who is responsible for collecting, verifying, and entering safety data.

3.11 STATISTICAL CONSIDERATIONS

Statistical methodologies are used to analyse both efficacy and safety data, ensuring that the results are scientifically justified.

3.11.1 Description of Statistical Methods

Statistical methods used to analyse the collection of data, handling of missing data, assessing treatment effects, and adjustments of potential bias should be explained in this section. Statistical techniques that will be used for primary and secondary endpoint analyses should be explained, such as mean, median, standard deviation, confidence interval, t-test, ANOVA, and chi-square test.

Details of the interim analysis, timing for conducting the interim analysis before the trial is completed, and the role of the Independent Data Monitoring Committee (DMC) in evaluating the interim analysis should be explained in the protocol.

3.11.2 Sample Size

This section provides a planned number of participants to be enrolled in the trial. Description of the total number of participants to be enrolled, as well as the allocation ratio, is extremely important in protocol. However, the sample size should depend on the primary endpoint and the expected treatment effect.

It is important to describe the justification that the sample size of participants includes the target population, considering the disease prevalence, expected dropout rates, and feasibility of recruitment.

It is essential to include the specific sample size formula to get the desired number of participants in this section.

General formula for calculating population mean:

$$n = Z^2\sigma^2/d2$$

where, n = sample size

Z = critical value of the normal distribution at the required confidence level

σ = estimated standard deviation of the population

d = precision/margin of error

3.11.3 Criteria for Termination

Termination or stopping of the trial must be predefined in the protocol, describing who has the authority to stop the trial, communicating the decision to stakeholders, and participants' follow-up after termination.

3.11.3.1 Access to Source Record

The protocol must ensure that the investigator, sponsor, or CRO is required to permit direct access to source records for authorized personnel, including monitors, auditors, and regulatory authorities. By documenting these requirements, the protocol ensures that all essential documents, medical records, case reports, and other trial-related material are available for review.

3.11.3.2 Quality Control and Quality Assurance

This section is dedicated to addressing quality control measures, risk identification, monitoring approach, and handling non-compliance. This should describe key quality factors and potential risks related to the study. It should also describe whether the trial will use on-site monitoring, centralized monitoring, or a risk-based monitoring approach, as well as procedures for identifying, documenting, and addressing protocol deviations or GCP non-compliance. This includes defining corrective and preventive actions (CAPA), reporting mechanisms, and potential consequences.

3.11.3.3 Ethics

In order to ensure that the study complies with ethical and regulatory requirements and safeguards human rights, the protocol must specify that the trial will only be conducted after obtaining IRB/IEC approval, and it should also describe the ongoing ethical oversight throughout the study duration.

3.11.3.4 Data Handling and Record Keeping

This section must include all data points, including demographic details, clinical outcomes, adverse events, laboratory results, and treatment response that should be included in the data collection tools, such as case report forms (CRF), either paper or electronic, and their procedures. It also includes data specifications that must be documented in trial-related document, such as the Data Management Plan (DMP). It also states which record will be directly entered into the data collection tool. These entries are considered source data and must be properly managed.

It should include a clear statement regarding the retention of trial-related records, the duration for which records will be maintained, and ensuring that they are available for audits, inspections, and future reference.

3.11.3.5 Financing and Insurance

Finance and insurance considerations ensure that the study is adequately funded and include a section detailing funding sources and insurance coverage. It should explain how financial resources will be allocated to cover study-related costs, including investigational products, site operations, investigator fees, participant reimbursements, and data management, and also describe the insurance provisions covering the trial. The protocol should also mention whether compensation will be provided for trial-related harms.

3.11.3.6 Publication Policy

Publication policy is essential to ensure that the findings of clinical trial are accurately reported, ethically distributed, and accessible to the scientific community. If not covered in a separate agreement, the protocol must include a section outlining the terms, responsibilities, and guidelines for publishing trial results.

It must define the criteria for authorship based on internationally accepted guidelines. It should clarify the roles and responsibilities of investigators, sponsors, and collaborators in drafting, reviewing, and submitting manuscripts for publication; expected timeline for publication and whether the study results will be made publicly available through peer-reviewed journals, clinical trial registries (e.g., ClinicalTrials.gov, EudraCT), or conference presentations; and whether the sponsor has any role in reviewing and approving publications before submission.

3.12 CONCLUSION

The clinical trial protocol is an important document for planning and conducting clinical research. It should be developed in a multidisciplinary setting, approved, and rigorously followed by all the study personnel involved in the conduct of the clinical trial. Any modifications need to be amended and approved by an IEC and the regulatory authorities. The ultimate goal of the protocol is to facilitate the conduct of scientifically and ethically sound research, providing high-quality evidence relevant to health care decision-making.

REFERENCES

Al Jundi, Azzam Al, and Salah Sakka. 2016. "Protocol Writing in Clinical Research." *Journal of Clinical and Diagnostic Research: JCDR* 10 (11). Journal of Clinical and Diagnostic Research: ZE10. https://doi.org/10.7860/JCDR/2016/21426.8865.

"Clinicalgcpguide." n.d.

D'errico, Stefano, Matteo Bolcato, Jonathan Cimino, and Claude Braun. 2023. "Design a Clinical Research Protocol: Influence of Real-World Setting." *Healthcare 2023, Vol. 11, Page 2254* 11 (16). Multidisciplinary Digital Publishing Institute: 2254. https://doi.org/10.3390/HEALTHCARE11162254.

"International Council for Harmonisation of Technical Requirements for Pharmaceuticals for Human Use ICH Harmonised Guideline Good Clinical Practice (GCP) E6(R3)." n.d.

McLeod, Charlie, Richard Norman, Edward Litton, Benjamin R. Saville, Steve Webb, and Thomas L. Snelling. 2019. "Choosing Primary Endpoints for Clinical Trials of Health Care Interventions." *Contemporary Clinical Trials Communications* 16 (December). Elsevier: 100486. https://doi.org/10.1016/J.CONCTC.2019.100486.

"New Drugs and Clinical Trials Rules, 2019." 2019.

Nikam, Supriya, Akash Inde, Anjali Jambhulkar, and Abhilasha Ghule. 2022. "Development and Writing of Clinical Trial Protocol." *International Journal of Pharmaceutical Sciences Review and Research* 72 (1). Global Research Online. https://doi.org/10.47583/ijpsrr.2022.v72i01.011.

O'brien, Kevin, and Jean Wright. n.d. "How to Write a Protocol."

Orimadegun A.E. 2020. "Protocol and Researcher's Relationship with Institutional Review Board." *African Journal of Biomedical Research* 23. www.ajbrui.org.

Rosenthal, Rachel, Juliane Schäfer, Matthias Briel, Heiner C. Bucher, Daniel Oertli, and Salome Dell-Kuster. 2014. "How to Write a Surgical Clinical Research Protocol: Literature Review and Practical Guide." *American Journal of Surgery*. https://doi.org/10.1016/j.amjsurg.2013.07.039.

Saluja, Satish, and Manoj Modi. 2021. "Guidelines for Writing Research Protocol." *Current Medicine Research and Practice* 11 (1). Medknow: 53–61. https://doi.org/10.4103/CMRP.CMRP_4_21.

Snyder, Hannah. 2019. "Literature Review as a Research Methodology: An Overview and Guidelines." *Journal of Business Research* 104 (November). Elsevier: 333–9. https://doi.org/10.1016/J.JBUSRES.2019.07.039.

4 Diversity in Clinical Trials

Dipika Bansal[1], *Akanksha Singh*[1], *Mamidi Niveditha*[1], *and Debashish Hota*[2]
[1]National Institute of Pharmaceutical Education and Research (NIPER), SAS Nagar, Punjab, India
[2]Department of Pharmacology, All India Institute of Medical Sciences, Bhubaneswar Orissa, India

4.1 INTRODUCTION

Clinical trials are the cornerstone of evidence-based medicine, with the data from trial outcomes providing critical insights that inform optimal clinical decision-making across the continuum of patient care (1).

Randomized controlled trials (RCTs) have long been regarded as the gold standard in evidence-based medicine for assessing the safety and efficacy of new medical therapies. Historically, their results were presumed to apply universally across populations. However, recent evidence challenges this assumption, revealing that excluded and underrepresented groups may exhibit unique disease presentations and varied responses to investigational treatments.

Participants in clinical trials have predominantly been younger, healthier white males. This skewed representation raises concerns about the generalizability of trial results, particularly regarding the safety and efficacy of new therapies for minority populations (2).

Marginalized ethnic and racial communities, as well as other disenfranchised groups, continue to be significantly underrepresented in clinical trials (3). For instance, in U.S. drug trials, just 8% of 32,000 participants were Black, 6% were Asian, 11% were Hispanic, and 30% were over the age of 65, underscoring the lack of diversity (4).

In 1977, the United States Food and Drug Administration (USFDA) issued a policy advising the exclusion of women of childbearing age from Phase I and Phase II drug trials. However, the National Institute of Health Sciences (NIH) revitalized the Act of 1993 and introduced amendments and key provisions, advocating the inclusion of women and minority groups in clinical research (5), realizing that men and women differ genetically and physiologically, leading to sex-based variations in drug pharmacokinetics and dynamics. Factors such as renal clearance, body weight, and fat percentage contribute to different outcomes in men and women (6). Women generally have a lower body weight than men, so taking the same dose of a drug results in Higher Plasma concentrations and greater drug exposure (7). Furthermore, lipophilic agents may have a greater distribution in females due to high fat content in females (8).

Inadequate representation of minority groups limits our understanding of the safety and efficacy of novel therapy, hindering the ability to generalize findings and perpetuating health disparities (9). To ensure the generalizability of clinical trial results, including a diverse participant pool that reflects the patients who will ultimately use the treatment is essential (10).

Various barriers impede participation in clinical trials, especially among underrepresented groups, as highlighted by researchers and government reports. Major challenges include the financial strain on participants; insufficient training for trial personnel in engaging diverse populations, biases, stereotypes held by staff; and a lack of institutional policies supporting diversity in trial recruitment. Additionally, medical mistrust among potential participants, inflexible and restrictive eligibility criteria, and ineffective community outreach efforts further complicate participation.

DOI: 10.1201/9781003533085-4

These obstacles often lead to limited patient awareness and understanding of clinical trials and reduce their likelihood of enrolling in available studies. Efforts to address these disparities have been initiated at various levels. At the site level, strategies include building relationships with healthcare providers who serve underrepresented populations, offering language support services and conducting targeted risk assessments (11–16). Few initiatives focus on organizational-level changes aimed at reshaping how clinical trials are envisioned and implemented. Some recent examples include increasing workforce training and development as well as promoting racial and ethnic diversity in clinical trial leadership to better reflect the broader patient population (17). Recognizing these persistent gaps, the USFDA issued new guidance in November 2020, entitled "Enhancing the Diversity of Trial Populations—Eligibility Criteria, Enrollment Practices, and Trial Designs Guidance for Industry" aimed to address the barriers to create more inclusive and representative trial populations (18). Furthermore, regulatory reforms in the United States have led to the emergence of "recruitmentology": a field dedicated to empirically studying recruitment techniques to include minority populations. However, only a few studies allow for subgroup analysis, which is crucial to compare treatment outcomes across diverse groups. Despite ongoing efforts to improve diversity in clinical trials, there is still a paucity of evidence on the effectiveness of therapy across diverse population, resulting in a lack of comprehensive guidelines for professionals (19).

Addressing diversity in clinical trials is a shared challenge among pharmaceutical companies, academic institutions, and clinical research organizations. It is essential to increase diversity in a sustainable and scalable way to improve insights into the variability of drug responses and ensure equitable health outcomes. In reflection on these considerations, this chapter sheds light on the relevance of diversity in clinical trials, identifies important barriers to participation, and addresses developing strategies for doing more inclusive, representative, and meaningful research. The goal is to create a research environment that represents the full spectrum of the population, ensuring that findings apply to all demographic groups, and improving health outcomes through more equitable and inclusive clinical practices.

4.2 WHY DIVERSITY IN CLINICAL TRIALS IS IMPORTANT

Lack of representation threatens the overarching goal of clinical research, which is to improve the health and well-being of the population. Diversity in clinical trials is essential for several reasons:

4.2.1 Generalizability of Findings

Diverse populations help ensure that research findings apply to a broader range of individuals. This is crucial for understanding how different groups respond to treatment, as biological and environmental factors can influence efficacy and safety (20). As findings may vary from population to population, the lived experience of interpersonal racism, along with factors like lower socioeconomic status and reduced educational opportunities, has been linked to increased blood pressure and higher cardiovascular risk (21–24). Including participants from all races and groups in research is essential for exploring the factors that may vary the response or outcome, ensuring that findings are generalizable to broader populations (25).

4.2.2 Building Trust

Historically, marginalized groups have faced mistrust in medical research due to past abuses and ongoing inequities. Research on vaccine hesitancy among Black populations revealed that greater awareness and confidence in the vaccine development and testing process were linked to higher rates of vaccine acceptance (26). Increasing diversity in trials can help rebuild trust in medical institutions, making these communities more likely to participate in research and seek medical care (27).

4.2.3 Promoting Fairness

Ensuring that all demographic groups have equitable access to participate in clinical trials promotes fairness. This can help address health disparities and ensure that the benefits of medical advancements are distributed more equitably across different populations (20).

4.2.4 Advancing Biomedical Knowledge

Diverse populations can lead to new biological insights and targeted therapeutic strategies. It allows researchers to identify and understand heterogeneous treatment effects, which can improve the development of effective interventions for all groups (20).

4.2.5 Addressing Health Disparities

Healthy people describe health disparities as differences that are strongly tied to social, economic, or environmental disadvantages. These disparities disproportionately affect groups that have historically faced greater challenges in achieving good health due to factors such as race or ethnicity, religion, socioeconomic status, gender, age, mental health, cognitive, sensory, or physical disabilities, sexual orientation, or gender identity, geographic location, or other characteristics linked to discrimination or exclusion. Health disparities are widespread and hinder the achievement of health equity, which is achieved by ensuring the highest possible level of health for all individuals. By focusing on diseases disproportionately affecting underrepresented groups, researchers can generate knowledge that can directly benefit these populations, ultimately leading to better health outcomes (20, 28).

4.3 POPULATION DIVERSITY

The true effectiveness of a drug in terms of safety and efficacy is more accurately ensured in clinical trials that include a diverse population. Furthermore, patients' trust in the safety and effectiveness of medications is strengthened when their characteristics are reflected in the trial, fostering a sense of reliability in the treatment (29). Participant/population diversity includes demographic characteristics like race, ethnicity, sex, age, and genetics. It also includes health status, cultural and behavioral differences, and socioeconomic and educational diversity.

4.3.1 Race

Race is a social construct mostly generated from physical or phenotypic traits that individuals tend to rely on to differentiate and identify themselves, as well as the way these individuals make themselves known within the hierarchies of a society. There are five racial categories defined by the U.S. Office of Management and Budget—White, Black or African American, American Indian or Alaska Native, Asian, and Native Hawaiian or Other Pacific Islander (30). Participants underreporting their race restricts the evaluation of how treatments perform across different racial groups. For instance, in a review of 281 articles, 138 (49%) gave no information about the race of the research participants. In the studies conducted in 2000–2001, 32% reported on participants' race, and White participants were disproportionately represented in the trials conducted from 2000 to 2001 and 2020 to 2021 (31). This pattern holds in further studies that investigate diversity in clinical trials. A review of 1,005 GSK-sponsored intervention trials, with a total of 460,707 participants, found that the overall percentage of African American and non-Hispanic White participants slightly exceeded their U.S. Census representation, but the representation of Asian and Hispanic or Latino individuals was below national levels (32). A similar review of diversity at AstraZeneca-sponsored clinical trials, implementing 246 trials with 95,372 U.S.-based participants, revealed that American Indian or

Alaska Native and Native Hawaiian or Other Pacific Islander participants were underrepresented, aligning with their small proportions in the U.S. Census (33). The disparities show that there is still a long way to go toward a more inclusive clinical trial set in a diverse population, which should provide for more inclusive and more effective healthcare solutions.

4.3.2 Ethnicity

Ethnicity can be understood as a fundamental concept in understanding human diversity, not allied with race but based on social and cultural reflections rather than physical traits. Ethnicity is a social construct identified with a common culture and language. Overall, ethnicity is a sense of belonging that connects individuals to a larger group through shared historical and cultural experiences. The U.S. Office of Management and Budget categorized ethnicity as Hispanic or Latino, not Hispanic or Latino. As a result, two ethnic constructs serve as the foundation for the FDA's data standards for clinical trial participant diversity (30).

A comprehensive review of the 281 articles highlighted the global pattern of ethnic representation of clinical trial participants and found that 79.2% of clinical trial participants were non-Hispanic, while North America, having the highest percentage of Hispanic participants, showed a lack of Hispanic representation in trials (31). AstraZeneca-sponsored clinical trials further illustrated how Hispanic patients are not accurately represented in differing therapeutic areas. Hispanic representation of 19.1% is greater than the national U.S. Census proportion in cardiovascular and renal as well as in metabolic trials. But even in respiratory and immunology trials, Hispanic representation was only 13.4% (33).

4.3.3 Gender

Participants of both sexes should be well represented in research, particularly when testing treatments that may have different effects on patients based on their gender (34). Gender, encompassing social, environmental, cultural, and behavioral factors, has been linked to individual medication responses. Men and women differ from one another in terms of body weight, body fat percentage, and renal clearance due to sex's influence on how the body processes medications (35, 36). For example, autosomal chromosomes contain genes encoding CYP enzymes, causing sex-related differences in expression and activity, with women having 20–50% higher CYP3A4 activity, facilitating faster drug clearance (37, 38).

Likewise, a Bøttern et al., 2023 found a persistent gender diversity, with 34% of trials in 2000–2001 including only men and 39 explicitly listing female sex as an exclusion criterion. Despite slight improvements in 2020–2021, 20% of trials involved only male participants, with 20 excluding women (31). The proportion of female participants in trials without explicit exclusion criteria remained unchanged over time. Additionally, a demographic diversity study conducted in Singapore revealed that 56.3% of trials underrepresented women, compared to the 2020 Singapore Census (39). This highlights the global challenge of ensuring balanced gender representation in clinical trials for optimal treatment outcomes.

4.3.4 Age

Including participants of various age groups increases the generalizability of trial results across larger populations. Age-related diversity in clinical trials is important to making sure investigational therapies are safe and effective across life stages. It is especially crucial for diseases with disproportionately high frequencies in specific age groups, including pediatric and geriatric populations (40, 41). Aging in geriatric populations often leads to polypharmacy, where patients require more prescribed medications due to their complex comorbid conditions (42). A review of 33 clinical trials found age diversity is a concern, with 14 trials excluding older participants, ranging from 45 to

85 years old. This exclusion limits understanding of how treatments interact with age-related factors like comorbidities and polypharmacy, which are common in older adults (39). Moreover, a study by a renowned company found that U.S. clinical trial participants are underrepresented in age groups 5–17 and 18–64, while those under 5 and 65 and older are overrepresented (32). This highlights the need for age diversity in trials to better understand therapies' interactions with different age groups and develop more effective treatments.

4.3.5 Genetic

In clinical trials, genetic diversity refers to the recruitment of participants with diverse genetic backgrounds. By employing this approach, we get more generalizable outcomes, discover which genetic factors influence drug effectiveness, and improve personalized medicine by tailoring treatments to individual profiles (30). Often, it happens that individuals with distinct ancestries have undergone significant genetic mixing, thereby producing differences within and between populations (30). For example, the effectiveness of clopidogrel was diminished by CYP2C19 loss-of-function variants that are more prevalent in Asian populations, underscoring the need for enhanced metabolite conversion in these groups (43). Furthermore, the metabolism of drugs varies between men and women, regardless of gender, due to variations in how enzymes metabolize drugs. For example, the CYP3A4 drug-metabolizing enzyme is more active in females, thus clearing the drug away faster (44). Because of this difference in drug clearance rates, dosing strategies and safety and therapeutic outcomes may be different in genders.

4.3.6 Geography

Geographic diversity in clinical trials is critical for ensuring that study findings apply to diverse populations from various regions. Including participants from diverse geographic areas helps account for variations in genetic backgrounds, environmental factors, healthcare access, and cultural practices that can affect treatment responses (45). Researchers can improve trial outcomes' external validity and generalizability by recruiting participants from different locations. This ensures that therapies are effective and safe for global populations (46). This is particularly crucial when addressing diseases that vary in prevalence or impact across different regions. Geographic diversity also helps identify potential differences in drug metabolism and effectiveness that may arise due to environmental factors such as climate, diet, or regional healthcare standards (47). In doing so, it contributes to the development of more equitable and comprehensive healthcare solutions (46).

4.3.7 Pregnant and Lactating Individuals

Very few drugs are approved for use during pregnancy, and there is a shortage of data on safety and efficacy during this key window of time (48). This is because pregnant and lactating individuals are being excluded from clinical trials, as the risks to their health are unknown, and the infamous case of thalidomide has complicated the understanding of the medications in pregnant and breastfeeding women (49).

At the same time, the design of clinical trials for the COVID-19 vaccine in pregnant and breastfeeding women has been hampered due to safety concerns and potential risks to the mother and fetus and excluded early from trials due to complications (50). For pregnant and lactating individuals, uncertainty arises about whether they could receive COVID-19 vaccines and worries about birth defects or harmful transmission into breast milk (51). This lack of data-driven guidance made it difficult for healthcare providers in decision-making.

Yet, the federal efforts to include pregnant and lactating individuals in clinical trials are significantly underrepresented. Only 0.32% of registered trials actively focus on pregnant participants, highlighting the continued neglect of this group in clinical research (52). Another study of 338 Phase III and Phase IV NIH-funded trials found that 68% excluded pregnant women and 47.3% excluded lactating women, underscoring the greater need for better evidence about medications and treatments in critical life stages (53). To date, gaps in understanding the results from trials are complicated due to a lack of representation in medical decision-making for healthcare providers and patients.

4.4 BARRIERS TO ENROLLMENT OF PARTICIPANTS IN CLINICAL TRIALS

Historically, clinical trials have been largely composed of specific demographic groups, mainly white, male, and middle-aged individuals. This limited diversity arises from numerous barriers, including socioeconomic disparities, cultural influences, and systemic issues. As per the existing literature, these barriers to participation in clinical trials are broadly categorized into three main themes: patient-related, physician-related, and system-related.

4.4.1 Patient-Related Barriers

First is mistrust, which leads to skepticism toward the research process. This includes fear of randomization into control groups, not receiving the required medical intervention (54), and concern about potential risks and adverse events; for example, in some cases, prospective participants expressed concerns about potential negative health repercussions from participation in the study (55). Deeply held beliefs about illness, treatment, and the healthcare system as, in a study, most of the respondents believed that women of childbearing age should not participate in clinical research (56), which presents challenges in recruiting diverse populations. Second, time and resource constraints make it difficult for the underrepresented population to participate in clinical trials, with time and travel commitments often outweighing the perceived benefits of the trial. For example, in a study, assessing the willingness of post-menopausal breast cancer patients to participate in acupuncture trials for pain relief, investigators found women who declined to participate were most likely to report transportation concerns as their reason for not participating (57).

Third, lack of accessible information about clinical trials, often due to literacy and language barriers, limits participation. A study of American female cancer patients indicated that 62% had no understanding of clinical trials and had negative sentiments toward them (58).

Fourth, potential participants may feel uncomfortable with the process, and a preference for herbal or alternative medicine among some ethnic minorities further reduces their willingness to participate in clinical trials. Lastly, a lack of awareness about the significance of clinical trials further deters participation (10).

4.4.2 Physician-Related Barriers

Lack of communication is the major barrier to the recruitment of minority groups into clinical trials, as illustrated in Figure 4.1. Communication issues stem from the interpretation and presentation of clinical trials by physicians/healthcare providers, along with their consideration of patients' ability to understand the complexities of the proposed trial. Inadequate communication can occur due to cultural, educational, and health literacy differences among patients (59).

The attitude of healthcare providers contributes to low enrolment, which is related to the perception of patients' circumstances or preferences, patients' suitability for the study, and their ability to comply with the protocols and the anticipated quality of the outcome (60).

One of the healthcare provider/physician-related barriers is a lack of information or awareness about the ongoing trials, which prevents them from discussing trial participation with patients. As a result, patients miss out on opportunities to participate in trials, especially in certain populations like minorities who are already underrepresented (58).

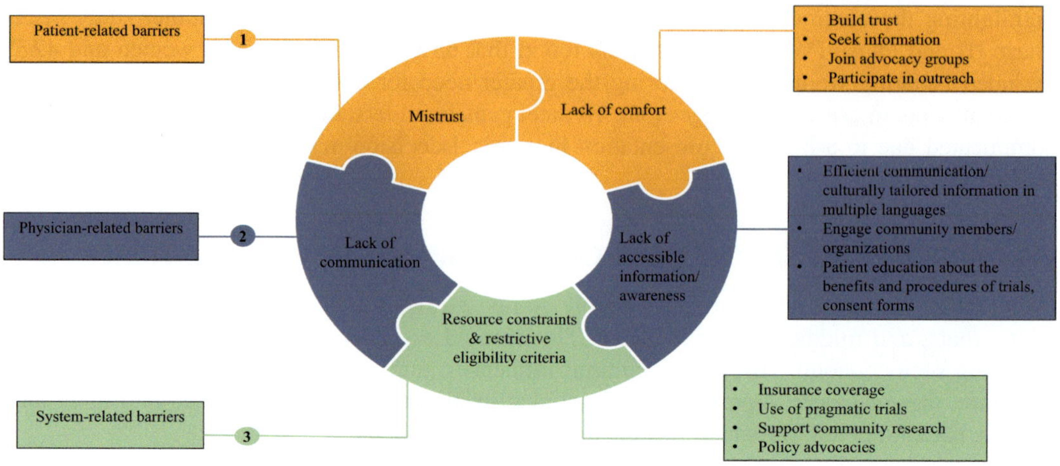

FIGURE 4.1 Major barriers to diversity and inclusion in clinical trials and strategies for addressing them. The diagram illustrates three primary categories of barriers (left), with key barriers represented in a central puzzle circle. Corresponding strategies for overcoming these barriers are outlined in the boxes on the right.

4.4.3 System-Related Barriers

System-related barriers include restrictive eligibility criteria for clinical trials, which exclude most of the population (61, 62). Lack of resources, infrastructure, and funds also restricts the inclusion of diverse populations in trials. A concern over insurance denial is a significant factor contributing to patients opting out of clinical trial participation, and it seems to be an increasing worry among those considering enrolment. Data indicates that individuals with private insurance are statistically less likely to participate in clinical trials than those with government insurance. Patients with private coverage often fear that their third-party insurers may not provide sufficient coverage if they join a trial (63, 64).

4.5 ACTIONABLE STEPS TO OVERCOME BARRIERS

4.5.1 Fostering Trust

The foundation for achieving equity in clinical research is to build trust among minority populations (65). Building trust over time requires consistent engagement in the community beyond the confines of the study itself, developing meaningful relationships with study participants, and contribute to the well-being of the community. Participants in an HIV study valued research professionals who were respectful, experienced, adaptable, and empathic, as well as possessing strong community skills. Several studies found that the researchers' capacity to build favorable interactions with study participants was beneficial (66). Ensuring patient safety is crucial for building trust. Introducing participants to the role of data safety and monitoring committees (DSMCs), which oversee safety and integrity, can help foster confidence in the research process. DSMCs ensure that studies are conducted safely and produce reliable outcomes. They also reassure participants that using investigational medicines either poses no harm or is so beneficial that continuing with conventional treatment would be questioned (67).

4.5.2 Patient and Community Engagement

Community-based programming and networking successfully enhance ethnic minorities' participation in research and clinical trials by increasing awareness. Building relationships with key community leaders, spokespersons, and networks (e.g., political leaders, religious organizations, respected elders, and civic members) can provide insight into recruitment barriers and improve effectiveness in overcoming them. Patient- and community-engaged research has been discovered to be feasible in many contexts with careful planning, suitable training, and appropriate funding for collaboration. Community-based participatory research, a type of community-engaged scholarship that emphasizes rigorous collaborative methods and focuses on community concerns, has been associated with significantly higher recruitment and retention of minority participants in research (68). A feasibility study of a breast cancer screening strategy for rural Hawaiian women revealed that recruitment through rural churches exceeded expectations, and retention rates were equivalent to other clinical trials (69).

4.5.3 Recruiting Staff from Diverse Backgrounds

Nurses coordinate cancer clinical studies, recruit patients, and ensure all team members adhere to trial protocols and practice guidelines. Including ethnic minority nurses and clinical trial coordinators in research teams can reduce language barriers, mistrust of healthcare providers, lack of comfort, and minority patients' concerns about clinical trials. It can also improve communication between cancer patients and health professionals and promote understanding of clinical trial availability and accessibility among ethnic minority patients and their families (70). One study found that hiring culturally appropriate data collectors, such as Arab Muslim mothers, and having a member of the study population serve as an investigator effectively establishes culturally appropriate connections with participants (71).

4.5.4 Flexible Research Visits and Accommodation

To address patients' travel, time, and resource concerns, as well as other study-related challenges. Research visits can be more versatile. Telephonic communication can be preferred over clinical visits, and accommodations can be provided whenever possible. Subject retention for a physical activity intervention with African-American women was high, probably due to flexible scheduling, regular contact, and a supportive setting (72).

4.5.5 Providing Resources and Support

To achieve a representative sample, various resources are essential. 80% of participants identified time and financial support as the most critical material resources for successfully conducting this work. Low-income population, primarily women, often struggle to cover study-related expenses, including transportation. As a result, funding for recruitment efforts became a key priority in specific announcements targeting underrepresented populations. To retain female volunteers in longitudinal research, financial incentives such as cash, gift cards, and presents were found to be effective (73). Expanded budgets for teams working on recruiting and retaining these populations, along with flexibility in budgeting to foster deeper collaboration with community partners, were also emphasized (25).

4.5.6 Communication and Patient Education

Clear communication can enhance participant knowledge and alleviate mistrust and anxiety. The communication initiative promotes clear language and culturally appropriate information for target

TABLE 4.1
Studies Highlighting Approaches to Improve Diversity in Clinical Trial Enrollment

Study ID	Objective	Suggestions to Enhance Diversity
Filbey et al. 2023 (76)	Strategies that may increase representativeness in Cardiovascular Diseases clinical trial populations	• Recruiting from underrepresented population • Providing salary/funding • Avoid restrictive criteria based on sex, age, and comorbidities. • Supportive follow-up • Include diverse trial leadership teams
Haider et al. 2023 (77)	Importance of diversity, identifying gaps, and addressing them using real-world data	• Collaboration with underrepresented communities • Raising awareness and education • Implementing guidelines and enforcement mechanisms • Hiring racially & ethnically diverse staff
Masters et al. 2022 (78)	Clinical pharmacology-driven actions for enabling diversity with regard to race and ethnicity in patient trials	• Continuous monitoring of trial participation • Increasing awareness and understanding among the population • Implement model-informed drug development plans • Use patient-centric sampling technologies
Palumbo et al. 2022 (79)	Enhancing diversity in clinical trial participation by identifying barriers and proposing strategies	• Hiring diverse clinical trial coordinators • Build trust among minority communities • Provide targeted funding and support • Use flexible trial designs • Maintain transparent communication with participants
Garrick et al. 2022 (80)	Addressing the clinical research barriers and recommendations	• Development programs to increase diversity • Covering out-of-pocket patient costs • Educating benefits of trial participation • Design patient-centric trials
Oyer et al. 2022 (81)	Recommendations to improve racial and ethnic diversity in cancer clinical trials	• Provide recurring education and training for trial conductors • Forming long-standing partnerships with patients • Establishing trial sites in communities • Consistent screening for eligibility • Develop programs & policies to increase diversity
Brathwaite et al. 2023 (82)	Enhance diversity in clinical trial participants to improve treatment efficacy and safety	• Diversification of trial workforce • Adoption of a diversity site assessment tool • Incorporation of decentralized trial design
Marrie et al. 2023 (83)	Recommendations for enhancing diversity and inclusion in clinical trials in multiple sclerosis	• Developing a diversity plan • Engaging with community groups • Train principal investigators and study staff to understand norms • Target appropriate population

audiences. Effective communication among investigators, providers, and participants improved recruitment results (74). Participants valued the clinician's ability to clearly express the trial's worth, advantages, and address patient concerns and side effects. Women who accepted randomization were more likely to follow their doctors' advice, highlighting the need to discuss the benefits of clinical trials and randomization with patients to make educated decisions about study participation (75). Practices to improve diversity in clinical trial settings are supported by evidence and are outlined in Table 4.1.

4.6 GOVERNMENT POLICIES TO ADDRESS DIVERSITY IN CLINICAL TRIALS

4.6.1 FDA Initiative to Assure Racial and Ethnic Diversity in Clinical Trials

The FDA released guidance on April 13, 2022, aimed at increasing the representation of ethnic and racial minority groups in clinical trials, acknowledging the long-standing underrepresentation of these populations in biomedical research (84). The initiative focuses on developing strategies to enhance the recruitment and retention of diverse participants in collaboration with industry stakeholders, advocacy groups, and other relevant entities to create effective diversity plans. By identifying and mitigating barriers to participation, such as health literacy, transportation issues, and cultural differences, the FDA seeks to ensure that clinical trial outcomes better reflect the broader population, leading to improved health outcomes, through more inclusive research practices (85).

4.6.2 Contribution of the National Institute of Health (NIH)

NIH is the largest federal sponsor of clinical trials in the United States, allocates approximately $3 billion every year to fund trials, and plays a vital role in shaping clinical trial policies that influence rigor and inclusivity (86). The journey of NIH toward clinical trial policies began in response to the 1985 U.S. Public Health Service Task Force on Women's Health, leading to mandating the inclusion of women and minorities in 1986; however, the initial implementation was slow. The Women's Health Equity Act and NIH Office of Research on Women's Health (ORWH) to promote female inclusion were created after the 1990 GAO report of inconsistent application of the 1986 (87). NIH Revitalization Act of 1993 expanded the inclusion policy, ensuring minorities and women are represented in clinical research, by emphasizing sufficient participation in Phase III trials for minority groups. In 1998, NIH implemented policies to include children in clinical research, to improve access for children while protecting vulnerable populations (88). Minority Health and Health Disparities Research and Education Act of 2000 and subsequent legislation expanded NIH efforts to address health disparities. In 2015, the NIH Sexual and Gender Minority Research Office was created to support participation in LGBTQ+ health. The NIH has established working groups and programs to address the hurdles that underrepresented demographics and individuals with disabilities confront in the biomedical research workforce; yet, inequities in career development and representation persist (89).

4.6.3 Role of Centers for Disease Control and Prevention (CDC)

The agency plays a role in regulating the recruitment of diverse populations, although the contribution to funding clinical trials is small from the CDC's research budget. Federal legislation has been a key driver behind CDC policies that promote diversity in research. CDC did not have a direct role in the 1993 NIH Revitalization Act, but it encouraged CDC to develop its guidelines aimed at increasing the inclusion of women and underrepresented racial and ethnic groups in research (90).

In 1995 CDC implemented the "Policy on the Inclusion of Women and Racial and Ethnic Minorities in Externally Awarded Research." Later in the same year, the CDC introduced that policy for intramural research as well. These policies mandated adequate representation of women and minority groups in all human-subject research conducted by the CDC unless a strong justification for exclusion existed. Furthermore, they emphasized that women of childbearing age should not be excluded from research without valid reasons. It also provided guidance for researchers on achieving diverse representation. For instance, if it is not feasible to include every single population in the same study, conducting multiple studies could be an alternative (91).

4.6.4 Centers for Medicare and Medicaid Services (CMS)

In addition to the CDC, CMS funds and regulates clinical trials (92). Historically, there were no government mandates for clinical trial participation, making it excessively costly for many Medicaid patients to join (93). In 2000, the financing administration responded to the president's memorandum on covering costs related to clinical trials and medical complications by stating that Medicaid would pay for "routine" expenses that follow clinical trial participation, such as diagnostic tests, hospitalization charges, and physician fees, but would exclude coverage for "items and amenities provided exclusively for data collection," affecting underrepresented groups (94). CMS updated its policies, requiring clinical trial protocols that allow it to provide coverage of service only for clinical study (95). Furthermore, in 2020, omnibus package coverage expanded to Medicaid recipients, making trials more accessible to low-income participants. Ancillary costs like missed work and transportation still limit participation, and little research exists on the impact of reimbursement policies. CMS also runs demonstration projects to test the effectiveness of strategies and reimbursement incentives for improving the quality of outcomes with diverse enrollment (96).

4.6.5 Indian Council of Medical Research (ICMR)

The ICMR and the Department of Health Research (DHR) have invited expressions of interest from government and private hospitals to establish a pan-India network of clinical research institutes known as the Indian Clinical Trial & Education Network (INTENT). "INTENT" aims to deliver evidence-based, cost-effective, scientifically robust, and culturally relevant solutions to address disease and health challenges of national or regional significance. It will serve as a unified platform for conducting a variety of RCTs, facilitating the standardization of trial methodologies, pooling of results, and ensuring timely project completion, while ensuring inclusive representation of India's diverse communities (97).

4.7 CURRENT STATUS AND FUTURE TRENDS OF DIVERSITY IN CLINICAL TRIALS

The current state of clinical trial participation shows significant disparities, particularly for underrepresented racial and ethnic minorities (URiM). Recent studies show that Black, Asian/Pacific Islander, and Hispanic/Latinx populations continue to be underrepresented in U.S. clinical trials. While 79% of participants are white, only 11% are African American/Black, and a mere 4% are Hispanic/Latinx. Older adults were generally well represented in trials, with a trial participation rate of 71%; however, younger adults had much lower representation at 27% (98). Notably, larger trials showed a significantly lower representation of Black participants, though Hispanic/Latinx have increased over time (99). This emphasizes the need for targeted interventions, such as patient navigation programs and culturally tailored education programs, to improve URiM participation. While progress has been made, more research is needed to develop effective strategies for reducing these disparities and ensuring that clinical trial results apply to diverse populations. An emerging trend in clinical trials is using digital solutions. Incorporating Artificial Intelligence (AI) in site selection and patient recruitment and retention can revolutionize efforts to overcome patient diversity challenges. AI-driven tools such as natural language processing (NLP) can streamline site selection by analyzing metadata, medical claims, and patient demographics, reducing biases and ensuring access to diverse populations. Currently, 86% of trials fail to meet their enrollment timelines, with nearly one-third of Phase III trials stalling due to slow recruitment. Additionally, 40% of patients become non-adherent within 150 days of a trial. Once a site is selected, NLP also significantly eases core clinical trial design challenges, ranging from patient recruitment to follow-up and retention (100). Another option is decentralized clinical trials (DCTs), which benefit both participants and researchers. DCTs enable remote monitoring of participants and reduce transportation barriers, which promotes better self-management of health conditions and leads to improved clinical outcomes for participants (101). Additionally, AI paired with devices such as wearables, sensors, and video-monitoring solutions may help reduce the burden on participants by automating tasks such as disease diaries and self-monitoring, gathering more accurate data. Generative AI tools will likely become integral to the clinical trial process, automating patient identification and eligibility assessments, personalizing recruitment efforts, and tracking patient care, ensuring diversity is maintained throughout (100).

REFERENCES

1. Mahmud A, Zalay O, Springer A, Arts K, Eisenhauer E. Barriers to participation in clinical trials: A physician survey. *Curr Oncol.* 2018;25(2):119–25.
2. Varma T, Jones CP, Oladele C, Miller J. Diversity in clinical research: Public health and social justice imperatives. *J Med Ethics.* 2023;49(3):200–3.
3. Schwartz AL, Alsan M, Morris AA, Halpern SD. Why Diverse Clinical Trial Participation Matters. *N Engl J Med.* 2023;388(14):1252–4.
4. U.S. Food and Drug Administration. 2020 Drug Trials Snapshots Summary Report. [Available from: https://www.fda.gov/media/145718/download]
5. Institute of Medicine Committee on the E, Legal Issues Relating to the Inclusion of Women in Clinical S. The National Academies Collection: Reports funded by National Institutes of Health. In: Mastroianni AC, Faden R, Federman D, editors. Women and Health Research: Ethical and Legal Issues of Including Women in Clinical Studies: Volume 2: Workshop and Commissioned Papers. Washington (DC): *National Academies Press (US)* 1999.
6. Institute of Medicine Committee on E, Legal Issues Relating to the Inclusion of Women in Clinical S. In: Mastroianni AC, Faden R, Federman D, editors. Women and Health Research: Ethical and Legal Issues of Including Women in Clinical Studies: Volume I. Washington (DC): *National Academies Press (US)* 1994.
7. Parekh A, Fadiran EO, Uhl K, Throckmorton DC. Adverse Effects in Women: Implications for Drug Development and Regulatory Policies. *Expert Rev Clin Pharmacol.* 2011;4(4):453–66.
8. Institute of Medicine Committee on Women's Health R. Women's Health Research: Progress, Pitfalls, and Promise. Washington (DC): *National Academies Press* (US) 2010.
9. Corneli A, Hanlen-Rosado E, McKenna K, Araojo R, Corbett D, Vasisht K, et al. Enhancing Diversity and Inclusion in Clinical Trials. *Clin Pharmacol Ther.* 2023;113(3):489–99.
10. Clark LT, Watkins L, Pina IL, Elmer M, Akinboboye O, Gorham M, et al. Increasing Diversity in Clinical Trials: Overcoming Critical Barriers. *Curr Probl Cardiol.* 2019;44(5):148–72.
11. Amorrortu RP, Arevalo M, Vernon SW, Mainous AG, 3rd, Diaz V, McKee MD, et al. Recruitment of Racial and Ethnic Minorities to Clinical Trials Conducted within Specialty Clinics: An Intervention Mapping Approach. *Trials.* 2018;19(1):115.
12. Gabler BS, Barrios A, Kakishita S, Cufino D, Frost CJ. Increasing Diversity in Research through Dedicated Language Access Services. *Contemp Clin Trials.* 2021;106:106439.
13. Tilley BC, Mainous AG, 3rd, Smith DW, McKee MD, Amorrortu RP, Alvidrez J, et al. Design of a Cluster-Randomized Minority Recruitment Trial: Recruit. *Clin Trials.* 2017;14(3):286–98.
14. Vaswani PA, Tropea TF, Dahodwala N. Overcoming Barriers to Parkinson Disease Trial Participation: Increasing Diversity and Novel Designs for Recruitment and Retention. *Neurotherapeutics.* 2020;17(4): 1724–35.
15. Bylund CL, Weiss ES, Michaels M, Patel S, D'Agostino TA, Peterson EB, et al. Primary Care Physicians' Attitudes and Beliefs about Cancer Clinical Trials. *Clin Trials.* 2017;14(5):518–25.
16. McCaskill Stevens W, Wilson JW, Cook ED, Edwards CL, Gibson RV, McElwain DL, et al. National Surgical Adjuvant Breast and Bowel Project Study of Tamoxifen and Raloxifene Trial: Advancing the Science of Recruitment and Breast Cancer Risk Assessment in Minority Communities. *Clin Trials.* 2013;10(2):280–91.
17. Bierer BE, White SA, Meloney LG, Ahmed HR, Strauss DH, Clark LT. Achieving Diversity, Inclusion, and Equity in Clinical Research Guidance Document Version 1.1 (Multi-Regional Clinical Trials Center of Brigham and Women's Hospital and Harvard (MRCT Center). Accessed October 11, 2024).
18. Gross AS, Harry AC, Clifton CS, Della Pasqua O. Clinical Trial Diversity: An Opportunity for Improved Insight into the Determinants of Variability in Drug Response. *Br J Clin Pharmacol.* 2022;88(6):2700–17.
19. Stronks K, Wieringa NF, Hardon A. Confronting Diversity in the Production of Clinical Evidence Goes Beyond Merely Including under-Represented Groups in Clinical Trials. *Trials.* 2013;14:177.
20. Alsan M, Wanamaker M. Tuskegee and the health of Black Men. *Q J Econ.* 2018;133(1):407–55.
21. Hamad R, Nguyen TT, Bhattacharya J, Glymour MM, Rehkopf DH. Educational Attainment and Cardiovascular Disease in the United States: A Quasi-Experimental Instrumental Variables Analysis. *PLoS Med.* 2019;16(6):e1002834.
22. Hamad R, Penko J, Kazi DS, Coxson P, Guzman D, Wei PC, et al. Association of Low Socioeconomic Status with Premature Coronary Heart Disease in US Adults. *JAMA Cardiol.* 2020;5(8):899–908.

23. King JB, Pinheiro LC, Bryan Ringel J, Bress AP, Shimbo D, Muntner P, et al. Multiple Social Vulnerabilities to Health Disparities and Hypertension and Death in the REGARDS Study. *Hypertension*. 2022;79(1):196–206.
24. Krieger N, Sidney S. Racial Discrimination and Blood Pressure: The CARDIA Study of Young Black and White Adults. *Am J Public Health*. 1996;86(10):1370–8.
25. National Academies of Sciences, Engineering, and Medicine; Policy and Global Affairs; Committee on Women in Science, Engineering, and Medicine; Committee on Improving the Representation of Women and Underrepresented Minorities in Clinical Trials and Research; Bibbins-Domingo K, Helman A, editors. Improving Representation in Clinical Trials and Research: Building Research Equity for Women and Underrepresented Groups. Washington (DC): *National Academies Press (US)* 2022 May 17. 2, Why Diverse Representation in Clinical Research Matters and the Current State of Representation within the Clinical Research Ecosystem.
26. Quinn SC, Jamison A, An J, Freimuth VS, Hancock GR, Musa D. Breaking Down the Monolith: Understanding Flu Vaccine Uptake among African Americans. *SSM Popul Health*. 2018;4:25–36.
27. National Academies of Sciences E, Medicine, Policy, Global A, Committee on Women in Science E, Medicine, et al. The National Academies Collection: Reports Funded by National Institutes of Health. In: Bibbins-Domingo K, Helman A, editors. Improving Representation in Clinical Trials and Research: Building Research Equity for Women and Underrepresented Groups. Washington (DC): *National Academies Press (US)* 2022
28. Alsan M, Durvasula M, Gupta H, Schwartzstein J, Williams H. Representation and Extrapolation: Evidence from Clinical Trial. Q J Econ. 2024;139(1):575–635.
29. Borno HT, Zhang S, Gomez S. COVID-19 Disparities: An Urgent Call for Race Reporting and Representation in Clinical Research. *Contemp Clin Trials Commun*. 2020;19:100630.
30. Rodney RA. The Attainment of Patient Diversity in Clinical Trials: Race, Ethnicity, *Genetics. Am J Med*. 2021;134(12):1440–1.
31. Bottern J, Stage TB, Dunvald AD. Sex, Racial, and Ethnic Diversity in Clinical Trials. *Clin Transl Sci*. 2023;16(6):937–45.
32. Reid MM, Davis SP, Henry ON, Mathew AA, McCallister S, Nero TT, et al. Demographic Diversity of US-based Participants in GSK-Sponsored Interventional Clinical Trials. *Clin Trials*. 2023;20(2):133–44.
33. Cabrera C, Fernandez-Llaneza D, Ghazoui Z, D'Abrantes S, Esparza-Franco MA, Sopp C, et al. Diversity of US Participants in AstraZeneca-Sponsored Clinical Trials. *Contemp Clin Trials*. 2024;140:107496.
34. National Institutes of Health. NIH Policy and Guidelines on The Inclusion of Women and Minorities as Subjects in Clinical Research. [updated 6/12/2017. Available from: https://grants.nih.gov/policy/inclusion/women-and-minorities/guidelines.htm]
35. Soldin OP, Mattison DR. Sex Differences in Pharmacokinetics and Pharmacodynamics. *Clin Pharmacokinet*. 2009;48(3):143–57.
36. Spoletini I, Vitale C, Malorni W, Rosano GM. Sex Differences in Drug Effects: Interaction with Sex Hormones in Adult Life. *Handb Exp Pharmacol*. 2012(214):91–105.
37. Anderson GD. Sex and Racial Differences in Pharmacological Response: Where Is the Evidence? Pharmacogenetics, Pharmacokinetics, and Pharmacodynamics. *J Womens Health (Larchmt)*. 2005;14(1): 19–29.
38. Franconi F, Brunelleschi S, Steardo L, Cuomo V. Gender Differences in Drug Responses. *Pharmacol Res*. 2007;55(2):81–95.
39. Bin WJJ, Chow A, Smith HE, Lee ES. Demographic Diversity of Participants in Clinical Trials Conducted in Singapore. *Ann Acad Med Singap*. 2024;53(7):446–53.
40. Moore KL, Patel K, Boscardin WJ, Steinman MA, Ritchie C, Schwartz JB. Medication Burden Attributable to Chronic Co-Morbid Conditions in the Very Old and Vulnerable. *PLoS One*. 2018;13(4):e0196109.
41. Vitale C, Fini M, Spoletini I, Lainscak M, Seferovic P, Rosano GM. Under-Representation of Elderly and Women in Clinical Trials. *Int J Cardiol*. 2017;232:216–21.
42. Mangoni AA. Cardiovascular Drug Therapy in Elderly Patients: Specific Age-Related Pharmacokinetic, Pharmacodynamic and Therapeutic Considerations. *Drugs Aging*. 2005;22(11):913–41.
43. Writing Committee M, Holmes DR, Dehmer GJ, Kaul S, Leifer D, O'Gara PT, et al. ACCF/AHA Clopidogrel Clinical Alert: Approaches to the FDA "Boxed Warning". Circulation. 2010;122(5):537–57.
44. Sex as a Biological Variable. [updated 12/29/2023. Available from: https://www.fda.gov/consumers/about-owh/sex-biological-variable]
45. Su SC, Kanarek N, Fox MG, Guseynova A, Crow S, Piantadosi S. Spatial Analyses Identify the Geographic Source of Patients at a National Cancer Institute Comprehensive Cancer Center. *Clin Cancer Res*. 2010;16(3):1065–72.

46. Clougherty JE, Kinnee EJ, Cardet JC, Mauger D, Bacharier L, Beigelman A, et al. Geography, Generalisability, and Susceptibility in Clinical Trials. *Lancet Respir Med.* 2021;9(4):330–2.
47. Richardson DB, Volkow ND, Kwan MP, Kaplan RM, Goodchild MF, Croyle RT. Medicine: Spatial Turn in Health Research. Science. 2013;339(6126):1390–2.
48. Blehar MC, Spong C, Grady C, Goldkind SF, Sahin L, Clayton JA. Enrolling Pregnant Women: Issues in Clinical Research. Womens Health Issues. 2013;23(1):e39–45.
49. Becker J Harvard Law "Bill of Health" (blog) 2021 [April 16, 2021] Excluding Pregnant People from Clinical Trials Reduces Patient Safety and Autonomy. [Available from: https://blogpetrieflomlawharvardedu/2021/04/16/pregnant-clinical-trials-safety-autonomy/[Internet]]
50. Szabo L. Kaiser Health News. 2022. Why Pregnant People Were Left behind While Vaccines Moved at 'Warp Speed' to Help the Masses. [Available from: https://khn.org/news/article/why-pregnant-people-were-left-behind-while-vaccines-moved-at-warp-speed-to-help-the-masses/]
51. Michos ED, Van Spall HGC. Increasing Representation and Diversity in Cardiovascular Clinical Trial Populations. *Nat Rev Cardiol.* 2021;18(8):537–8.
52. Spong CY, Bianchi DW. Improving Public Health Requires Inclusion of Underrepresented Populations in Research. *Jama.* 2018;319(4):337–8.
53. Scaffidi J, Mol BW, Keelan JA. The Pregnant Women as a Drug Orphan: A Global Survey of Registered Clinical Trials of Pharmacological Interventions in Pregnancy. *Bjog.* 2017;124(1):132–40.
54. Avis NE, Smith KW, Link CL, Hortobagyi GN, Rivera E. Factors Associated with Participation in Breast Cancer Treatment Clinical Trials. *J Clin Oncol.* 2006;24(12):1860–7.
55. Schonfeld TL, Amoura NJ, Stoner JA, Gordon BG. Women and Contraception in Research: A Pilot Study. *J Womens Health (Larchmt).* 2009;18(4):507–12.
56. Russell SL, Katz RV, Kressin NR, Green BL, Wang MQ, Claudio C, et al. Beliefs of Women's Risk as Research Subjects: A Four-City Study Examining Differences by Sex and by Race/Ethnicity. *J Womens Health (Larchmt).* 2009;18(2):235–43.
57. Mao JJ, Tan T, Li SQ, Meghani SH, Glanz K, Bruner D. Attitudes and Barriers towards Participation in an Acupuncture Trial among Breast Cancer Patients: A Survey Study. *BMC Complement Altern Med.* 2014;14:7.
58. Tu SP, Chen H, Chen A, Lim J, May S, Drescher C. Clinical Trials: Understanding and Perceptions of Female Chinese-American Cancer Patients. *Cancer.* 2005;104(12 Suppl):2999–3005.
59. Howerton MW, Gibbons MC, Baffi CR, Gary TL, Lai GY, Bolen S, et al. Provider Roles in the Recruitment of Underrepresented Populations to Cancer Clinical Trials. *Cancer.* 2007;109(3):465–76.
60. Grunfeld E, Zitzelsberger L, Coristine M, Aspelund F. Barriers and Facilitators to Enrollment in Cancer Clinical Trials: Qualitative Study of the Perspectives of Clinical Research Associates. *Cancer.* 2002;95(7):1577–83.
61. Adams-Campbell LL, Ahaghotu C, Gaskins M, Dawkins FW, Smoot D, Polk OD, et al. Enrollment of African Americans onto Clinical Treatment Trials: Study Design Barriers. *J Clin Oncol.* 2004;22(4):730–4.
62. Lara PN, Jr., Higdon R, Lim N, Kwan K, Tanaka M, Lau DH, et al. Prospective Evaluation of Cancer Clinical Trial Accrual Patterns: Identifying Potential Barriers to Enrollment. *J Clin Oncol.* 2001;19(6):1728–33.
63. Klamerus JF, Bruinooge SS, Ye X, Klamerus ML, Damron D, Lansey D, et al. The Impact of Insurance on Access to Cancer Clinical Trials at a Comprehensive Cancer Center. *Clin Cancer Res.* 2010;16(24):5997–6003.
64. Ulrich CM, Zhou Q, Ratcliffe SJ, Ye L, Grady C, Watkins-Bruner D. Nurse Practitioners' Attitudes about Cancer Clinical Trials and Willingness to Recommend Research Participation. *Contemp Clin Trials.* 2012;33(1):76–84.
65. Barnes LL, Bennett DA. Alzheimer's Disease in African Americans: Risk Factors and Challenges for the Future. *Health Aff (Millwood).* 2014;33(4):580–6.
66. Loutfy MR, V LK, Mohammed S, Wu W, Muchenje M, Masinde K, et al. Recruitment of HIV-Positive Women in Research: Discussing Barriers, Facilitators, and Research Personnel's Knowledge. *Open AIDS J.* 2014;8:58–65.
67. Ensuring Patient Safety and Scientific Credibility in Clinical Trials. *J Oncol Pract.* 2008;4(2):83–4.
68. De las Nueces D, Hacker K, DiGirolamo A, Hicks LS. A Systematic Review of Community-based Participatory Research to Enhance Clinical Trials in Racial and Ethnic Minority Groups. *Health Serv Res.* 2012;47(3 Pt 2):1363–86.
69. Ka'opua LS, Park SH, Ward ME, Braun KL. Testing the Feasibility of a Culturally Tailored Breast Cancer Screening Intervention with Native Hawaiian Women in Rural Churches. *Health Soc Work.* 2011;36(1):55–65.

70. Hussain-Gambles M, Atkin K, Leese B. Why Ethnic Minority Groups Are Under-Represented in Clinical Trials: A Review of the Literature. *Health Soc Care Community.* 2004;12(5):382–8.
71. Aroian KJ, Katz A, Kulwicki A. Recruiting and Retaining Arab Muslim Mothers and Children for Research. *J Nurs Scholarsh.* 2006;38(3):255–61.
72. Staffileno BA, Coke LA. Recruiting and Retaining Young, Sedentary, Hypertension-Prone African American Women in a Physical Activity Intervention Study. *J Cardiovasc Nurs.* 2006;21(3):208–16.
73. McFarlane J. Strategies for Successful Recruitment and Retention of Abused Women for Longitudinal Studies. *Issues Ment Health Nurs.* 2007;28(8):883–97.
74. Dickson S, Logan J, Hagen S, Stark D, Glazener C, McDonald AM, et al. Reflecting on the Methodological Challenges of Recruiting to a United Kingdom-Wide, Multi-Centre, Randomised Controlled Trial in Gynaecology Outpatient Settings. Trials. 2013;14:389.
75. Mancini J, Genève J, Dalenc F, Genre D, Monnier A, Kerbrat P, et al. Decision-Making and Breast Cancer Clinical Trials: How Experience Challenges Attitudes. *Contemp Clin Trials.* 2007;28(6):684–94.
76. Filbey L, Zhu JW, D'Angelo F, Thabane L, Khan MS, Lewis E, et al. Improving Representativeness in Trials: A Call to Action from the Global Cardiovascular Clinical Trialists Forum. *Eur Heart J.* 2023;44(11):921–30.
77. Haider N. Improving Diversity in Clinical Trials: Identifying Gaps and the Role of Real-World Data. *J Artif Intell Mach Learn & Data Sci* 2023.1(3):393–5.
78. Masters JC, Cook JA, Anderson G, Nucci G, Colzi A, Hellio MP, et al. Ensuring Diversity in Clinical Trials: The Role of Clinical Pharmacology. *Contemp Clin Trials.* 2022;118:106807.
79. Poopat PPPHMMSOBC, Sanchez CTMAH. Diversity in Clinical Trials Participation: A Life Sciences Perspective. *WhitePaper.* 2022.
80. Garrick O, Mesa R, Ferris A, Kim ES, Mitchell E, Brawley OW, et al. Advancing Inclusive Research: Establishing Collaborative Strategies to Improve Diversity in Clinical Trials. *Ethn Dis.* 2022;32(1):61–8.
81. Oyer RA, Hurley P, Boehmer L, Bruinooge SS, Levit K, Barrett N, et al. Increasing Racial and Ethnic Diversity in Cancer Clinical Trials: An American Society of Clinical Oncology and Association of Community Cancer Centers Joint Research Statement. *J Clin Oncol.* 2022;40(19):2163–71.
82. Brathwaite J, Wolgast M, Bickhart S. Viable Strategies to Increase Clinical Trial Patient Diversity. *Al-Kindy College Med J.* 2023;19(2):133–6.
83. Marrie RA, Chataway J, Bierer BE, Finlayson M, Martinez-Lapiscina EH, Panagoulias J, et al. Enhancing Diversity of Clinical Trial Populations in Multiple Sclerosis. *Mult Scler J.* 2023;29(9):1174–85.
84. FDA Takes Important Steps to Increase Racial and Ethnic Diversity in Clinical Trials. [updated 13/04/2022. Available from: https://www.fda.gov/news-events/press-announcements/fda-takes-important-stepsincrease-racial-and-ethnic-diversity-clinical-trials]
85. Adashi EY, Cohen IG. The FDA Initiative to Assure Racial and Ethnic Diversity in Clinical Trials. *J Am Board Fam Med.* 2023;36(2):366–8.
86. NIH. Information about NIH Clinical Trial Stewardship. [updated 10/09/2024. Available from: https://grants.nih.gov/policy-and-compliance/policy-topics/clinical-trials/why-changes]
87. Nadel MV. Associate Director, National and Public Health Issues, Human Resources Division, before the Subcommittee on Housing and Consumer Interest, Select Committee on Aging, U.S. House of Representatives. Washington, DC: U.S. General Accounting Office; 1990. [July 24, 1990]. "National Institutes of Health: Problems in Implementing Policy on Women in Study Populations" Statement of Mark V. Nadel.
88. Mastroianni AC FR, Federman D, editors. B, NIH Institute of Medicine (US) Committee on Ethical and Legal Issues Relating to the Inclusion of Women in Clinical Studies. Women and Health Research: Ethical and Legal Issues of Including Women in Clinical Studies: Volume I Washington (DC*): National Academies Press* (US) 1994.
89. Institute of Medicine (US) Committee on Lesbian, Gay, Bisexual, and Transgender Health Issues and Research Gaps and Opportunities The Health of Lesbian, Gay, Bisexual, and Transgender People: Building a Foundation for Better Understanding Washington (DC*): National Academies Press (US)* 2011. [Available from: https://wwwncbinlmnihgov/books/NBK64806/https://doi.org/1017226/13128]
90. Geller SE, Koch A, Pellettieri B, Carnes M. Inclusion, Analysis, and Reporting of Sex and Race/Ethnicity in Clinical Trials: Have We Made Progress? *J Womens Health (Larchmt).* 2011;20(3):315–20.
91. Centers for Disease Control and Prevention (CDC) & Agency for Toxic Substances and Disease Registry (ATSDR). (1995). Policy on the Inclusion of Women and Racial and Ethnic Minorities in Externally Awarded Research; notice. *Fed Regist.* 1995;60(179):47947–51.
92. Department of Homeland Security, Department of Agriculture, Department of Energy, National Aeronautics and Space Administration, Department of Commerce, Social Security Administration,

Agency for International Development, Department of Housing and Urban Development, Department of Labor, Department of Defense, Department of Education, Department of Veterans Affairs, Environmental Protection Agency, Department of Health and Human Services, National Science Foundation, & Department of Transportation. Federal Policy for the Protection of Human Subjects: Final rule. *Fed Regist.* 2017;82(12):7149–274.
93. Winkfield KM, Phillips JK, Joffe S, Halpern MT, Wollins DS, Moy B. Addressing Financial Barriers to Patient Participation in Clinical Trials: ASCO Policy Statement. *J Clin Oncol.* 2018:Jco1801132.
94. CMS. Routine Costs in Clinical Trials. 2000. National Coverage Determination (NCD) [Available from: https://www.cms.gov/medicare-coverage-database/view/ncd.aspx?ncdid=1&ncdver=1&fromdb=true]
95. CMS. Decision Memo for Transcatheter Aortic Valve Replacement (TAVR) (CAG-00430N). [Available from: http://www.cms.gov/medicare-coverage-database/details/nca-decision-memo.aspx?NCAId=257&NcaName=Transcatheter+Aortic+Valve+Replacement+(TAVR)&bc=AiAAAAAACAAAAA%3d%3d&]
96. Takvorian SU, Guerra CE, Schpero WL. A Hidden Opportunity—Medicaid's Role in Supporting Equitable Access to Clinical Trials. *N Engl J Med.* 2021;384(21):1975–8.
97. Kumar A. To Conduct Large-Scale Clinical Trials, ICMR Calls for Entries in Indian *Clinical Trial & Education Network.* [Internet] [cited 2024 Oct 11] 2021.
98. Balakrishnan AS, Palmer NR, Fergus KB, Gaither TW, Baradaran N, Ndoye M, et al. Minority Recruitment Trends in Phase III Prostate Cancer Clinical Trials (2003 to 2014): Progress and Critical Areas for Improvement. *J Urol.* 2019;201(2):259–67.
99. Alcorn SR, Chino F. Current Trends for Diversity, Equity, and Inclusion Among Medical Faculty and Clinical Trial Participation. *Int J Radiat Oncol*Biol*Phys.* 2023;116(2):207–11.
100. CLINICAL TRIALS—The Power of AI in Overcoming Patient Diversity Challenges [Available from: https://drug-dev.com/clinical-trials-the-power-of-ai-in-overcoming-patient-diversity-challenges/]
101. Copland RR, Hanke S, Rogers A, Mpaltadoros L, Lazarou I, Zeltsi A, et al. The Digital Platform and Its Emerging Role in Decentralized Clinical Trials. *J Med Internet Res.* 2024;26:e47882.

5 Clinical Trial Protocol
The Backbone of a Clinical Trial

Shalini Dwivedi
Krystelis India Scientific Service

5.1 INTRODUCTION

The National Institutes of Health (NIH), a division of the US Department of Health and Human Services (DHHS), includes the National Institute of Allergy and Infectious Diseases (NIAID). From single-investigator, single-site natural history studies to multi-center, worldwide clinical trials spanning Phase 0 through Phase IV, NIAID grants research conducted by both intramural and extramural investigators in a range of contexts. A team headed by a principal investigator must create a protocol document that is not only scientifically sound but also complies with a number of regulatory, human subject safety, and data quality requirements that are subject to interpretation and are subject to frequent revisions in order to conduct clinical research, regardless of the setting.

5.2 PRELIMINARY STEPS OF PROTOCOL DEVELOPMENT

Writing a clinical trial protocol is not an easy task, specifically because the development and planning phase of the clinical trial involves several stakeholders. However, with careful planning, it is possible to develop a comprehensive, coherent, clear, and compelling protocol that will increase the likelihood of approval. First, it is important to identify a research question that is feasible, relevant, and worthy of investigation. Before drafting the protocol, it is crucial to define the research question and objectives clearly (Al-Jundi, 2016). A thorough review of existing literature and consultation with subject matter experts, including statisticians, clinicians, and drug regulatory professionals, ensures that the clinical trial is well-grounded in evidence and feasible in its design.

After identifying the research question, the next step is to consider a robust study design, which should be carefully selected to ensure that the question can be precisely answered. The study design should be appropriate for the research setting and the type of data that will be collected or created. It is important to consider the feasibility of the proposed design, including resource availability, the potential challenges and limitations, and the anticipated outcomes.

Based on the study design and statistical considerations, it is also important to evaluate the number of sites and participants required for the clinical trial. This involves an evaluation of patient flows in different hospitals (clinical trial sites), availability of investigators (particularly if they would like to consider research activities), and facilities at the prospective clinical trial sites. Feasibility evaluation is an important step that helps in the operational aspects of the clinical trials.

ICH E6 encourages an interdisciplinary approach in protocol development. These days, patients are increasingly being considered as an important stakeholder in clinical trial planning. Therefore, collaboration with patient representatives can provide insights into practical considerations, such as the acceptability of procedures and endpoints. Ethical concerns, such as risk minimization and equitable participant selection, should also be considered early on.

 DOI: 10.1201/9781003533085-5

5.3 STRUCTURE AND COMPONENTS OF A CLINICAL TRIAL PROTOCOL

A protocol's structure must adhere to ICH E6 guidelines while being adaptable to the specific needs of the study. Table 5.1 defines the sections outlined by ICH E6 as the critical components of a clinical trial protocol:

TABLE 5.1
Structure and Components of a Clinical Trial Protocol (According to ICH-GCP)

Sections according to ICH E6	Details
1. General information	• *Title page*: protocol title, version number, and date, along with details about the sponsor, investigators, and trial registration identifiers (e.g., ClinicalTrials.gov, EU Clinical Trial number). • *Administrative sections*: funding sources and potential conflicts of interest to maintain transparency and trust.
2. Background Information	• Includes the scientific and clinical context for the trial. • Should provide a comprehensive literature review, with gaps in current knowledge and how the trial aims to address these gaps. The rationale should justify the intervention, population, and endpoints selected for the study. • ICH E6 stresses the importance of this section in ensuring that the trial's design is both scientifically valid and ethically sound. • This section supports ethical decision-making by stakeholders.
3. Trial objective and purpose	Each objective should correspond to a specific hypothesis. • Primary objectives focus on the main research question, while secondary objectives explore additional aspects of the intervention's effects. • The hypotheses should be evaluable, based on existing evidence, and aligned with the trial's overall goals: the primary hypothesis might evaluate its efficacy compared to a standard treatment, while the secondary hypotheses could examine safety and tolerability.
4. Trial design	• The study design dictates the trial's structure and methodology. This section must specify whether the trial is randomized, controlled, double-blind, or observational. • The design should minimize bias and maximize the validity of the results. • A detailed description of the intervention, comparator, and control conditions should be provided, along with justifications for their selection. • A flowchart illustrating the study timeline can enhance clarity.
5. Selection and withdrawal of subjects	• The inclusion and exclusion criteria are crucial for defining the study population. ICH E6 mandates that these criteria should be provided to ensure the safety of participants while maintaining the generalizability of the results. • Recruitment strategies should aim to enroll a diverse and representative population, addressing barriers to participation where possible. • Ethical considerations, such as ensuring voluntary participation and protecting vulnerable groups, should be explicitly addressed.
6. Treatment of Subjects	• Describes the investigational product, including its formulation, dosage, administration, and storage requirements. • Procedures for managing side effects, adverse events, and deviations from the protocol must also be included. • ICH E6 emphasizes the need for standard operating procedures (SOPs) to ensure consistency in administering interventions and recording outcomes. • Detailed instructions help mitigate variability across sites and investigators.
7. Assessment of Efficacy	• Clear specification of the efficacy parameters and description of the methods and timing for assessing, recording, and analyzing efficacy parameters.

(Continued)

TABLE 5.1 (Continued)
Structure and Components of a Clinical Trial Protocol (According to ICH-GCP)

Sections according to ICH E6	Details
8. Assessment of Safety	• Specification of safety parameters, along with the methods and timing for assessing, recording, and analyzing safety parameters; procedures for eliciting reports of and for recording and reporting adverse events and intercurrent illnesses should be provided. • The protocol should also provide details of the type and duration of the follow-up of subjects after adverse events.
9. Statistics	• Sample size calculations must ensure the trial is adequately powered to detect meaningful differences between groups. • The protocol should describe the statistical methods for analyzing primary and secondary outcomes, handling missing data, and conducting interim analyses. • Endpoints should be measurable, clinically meaningful, and aligned with the study objectives. • Exploratory outcomes can also be included to generate hypotheses for future research. • ICH E6 recommends including validated measurement tools and clearly defining how outcomes will be assessed.
10. Direct access to source data/documents	• Specification of the written agreement that the investigator(s)/institution(s) will permit trial-related monitoring, audits, IRB/IEC review, and regulatory inspection(s), providing direct access to source data/documents.
11. Quality control and quality assurance	• A robust data management plan to ensure the integrity and confidentiality of trial data should be provided. • The protocol should specify how data will be collected, stored, and analyzed in compliance with regulatory standards. • ICH E6 emphasizes the need for quality assurance systems, including regular audits and risk-based monitoring strategies. These measures help identify and address issues promptly, ensuring the trial's integrity.
12. Ethics	• The protocol must describe how informed consent will be obtained, how participant confidentiality will be maintained, and how risks will be minimized. • ICH E6 requires the inclusion of measures to ensure participant safety, such as regular monitoring by an independent data monitoring committee. • Provisions for addressing adverse events, discontinuation criteria, and compensation for trial-related injuries should also be detailed.
13. Data Handling and Record Keeping	• The protocol should clearly describe how data will be recorded, whether electronically using validated systems or manually on case report forms (CRFs), and outline measures to safeguard data from unauthorized access or loss, such as encryption, password protection, and secure backups. • Details on how the data will be stored during and after the trial and the duration of retention, typically in compliance with regulatory requirements. • The protocol should also describe the procedures for monitoring and verifying data accuracy, such as source data verification (SDV) and audits. The protocol should state how discrepancies will be identified and resolved.
14. Financing and insurance	• Providing a clear and detailed description of the financial and insurance arrangements that will support the study is important. • This section ensures transparency about funding sources, allocates financial responsibilities, and addresses how participants will be compensated in the event of harm during the trial.

TABLE 5.1 (Continued)
Structure and Components of a Clinical Trial Protocol (According to ICH-GCP)

Sections according to ICH E6	Details
15. Publication policy	• Transparency in reporting trial results is essential for advancing medical knowledge and maintaining public trust. • The protocol should outline plans for registering the trial, sharing findings through publications, and making data available for secondary analyses. • ICH E6 encourages adherence to reporting standards to ensure that results are presented comprehensively and objectively. • Dissemination plans should prioritize accessibility to all stakeholders, including participants and the wider medical community.
16. Supplements	• Informed consent forms, questionnaires, and any other documents that support the trial conduct and that will be used in the clinical trial should be provided as an appendix.

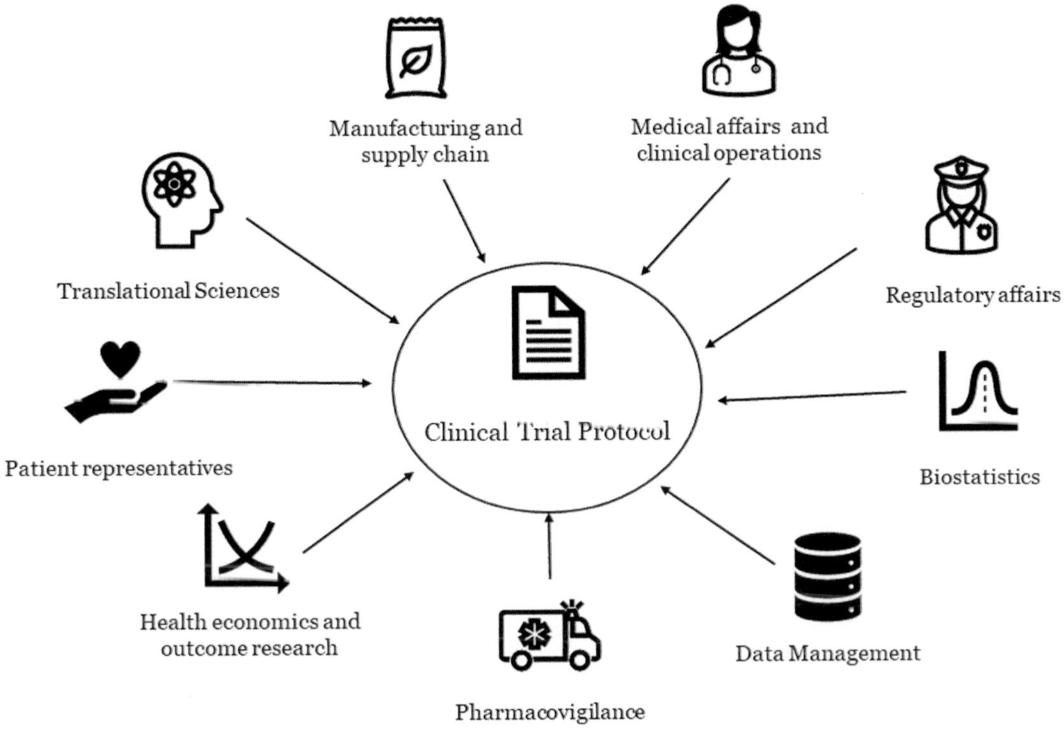

FIGURE 5.1 Functions involved in protocol development.

5.4 PROTOCOL DEVELOPMENT INVOLVES COORDINATION AMONG VARIOUS TEAMS

As you have observed in Table 5.1, a clinical trial protocol contains various inter-disciplinary elements and therefore requires inputs from multiple teams, such as, clinical operations, data management, biostatistics, medical affairs, regulatory affairs, pharmacovigilance, quality assurance, health economics and outcome research, translational sciences, and manufacturing and supply chain (Figure 5.1).

TABLE 5.2
Roles and Responsibilities of Different Stakeholders in Protocol Development

Function	Responsibilities
Clinical Operations and Medical Affairs	• Define the study objectives, endpoints, and overall trial design. • Ensure that the protocol aligns with the drug development strategy and regulatory requirements. • Determine patient population, inclusion/exclusion criteria, and study duration. • Select the trial phase (Phase I-IV) and study design (e.g., randomized controlled trial, open-label, crossover). • Provide insights on trial feasibility, site selection, patient recruitment, and operational challenges. • Ensure study logistics are feasible and cost-effective. • Provide insights on the clinical relevance of endpoints and study design from a medical and patient-centered perspective. • Help align the protocol with real-world clinical practice.
Biostatistics	• Design the statistical analysis plan (SAP), determine sample size calculations, and ensure appropriate endpoint selection. • Help in defining randomization strategies and stratification methods. • Define interim analyses and stopping rules (if applicable).
Pharmacovigilance	• Ensure safety monitoring and reporting requirements are included in the protocol. • Define adverse event reporting processes and risk mitigation strategies.
Data management	• Define data collection requirements, case report forms (CRFs), and electronic data capture (EDC) systems. • Ensure compliance with data integrity standards. • Develop data monitoring and cleaning strategies.
Health Economics and Outcome Research	• Ensure inclusion of health-economic and patient-reported outcome (PRO) measures where relevant. • Support protocol alignment with market access strategies. • Recommend inclusion of cost-effectiveness and quality-of-life measures. • Align trial design with payer expectations and reimbursement requirements. • Support real-world evidence (RWE) integration.
Quality Assurance	• Ensure that the protocol adheres to GCP guidelines and internal quality standards. • Review for potential compliance risks. • Conduct protocol compliance audits. • Identify and mitigate compliance risks.
Translational Sciences	• Provide input on biomarkers, genetic testing, and translational research elements. • Help design exploratory endpoints for personalized medicine approaches. • Support companion diagnostics development. • Optimize pharmacokinetics and pharmacodynamics assessments.
Manufacturing and Supply Chain	• Ensures the investigational product is available in required formulations and quantities. • Support packaging, labeling, and distribution planning. • Ensure compliance with Good Manufacturing Practices (GMP). • Plan and execute supply chain logistics for multiple trial sites.

Representatives from each of these teams should be involved since the concept stage of the protocol to ensure the protocol is scientifically sound, ethically appropriate, and operationally feasible. Effective collaboration between these teams helps streamline protocol development, enhances patient safety, and ensures regulatory compliance. Table 5.2 details functional requirements of these teams.

5.5 ROLE OF MEDICAL WRITERS IN PROTOCOL DEVELOPMENT

Medical writers function as a liaison among all these teams, taking feedback from all departments and putting together a draft protocol. They play a critical role in protocol development by ensuring that the document is scientifically accurate, regulatory-compliant, and clearly written for multiple stakeholders, including investigators, ethics committees, and regulatory agencies. Medical writers collaborate with clinical development, regulatory affairs, biostatistics, and clinical operations teams to translate complex scientific and statistical concepts into a structured, reader-friendly document.

The responsibilities of a medical writer include drafting the protocol based on input from subject matter experts, ensuring consistency with supporting documents such as the investigator's brochure and statistical analysis plan, and aligning the content with ICH-GCP and regulatory requirements. Medical writers also facilitate version control, incorporate feedback from internal and external reviewers, and ensure clarity to minimize ambiguity that could lead to protocol deviations. By maintaining scientific rigor and regulatory compliance while enhancing readability, they contribute to the development of a high-quality protocol that effectively guides study execution.

5.6 BEST PRACTICES FOR WRITING A PROTOCOL

A precise and consistent language is very important while preparing any regulatory document, as is the case for a clinical trial protocol. The information should be clear and free from ambiguity. Some experience-based best practices have been detailed next. Adhering to these best practices enhances the clarity and utility of the protocol.

5.6.1 Protocol Language and Contents

In the introduction section, providing a broader context and eventually focusing on the specific objectives is a good practice. A critical appraisal of the literature (just as in a review article) is important; however, overall, this section should be very concise. This helps the readers and reviewers to understand the significance of the trial. The introduction section should also provide the rationale of the trial.

The objectives should follow Specific, Measurable, Attainable, Relevant, and Time-bound (SMART) criteria and provide intended outcomes, their indicator, target level, and time frame. The criteria of qualification of these four parameters are provided in Figure 5.2.

A clear description of the proposed study design, including the population and methodology, and an explanation of why the specific study design was chosen and how this selection will effectively deliver the potential answers to the objectives, should be provided in the protocol. Stating the selection and qualifying factors should also be provided using references to previous clinical trials.

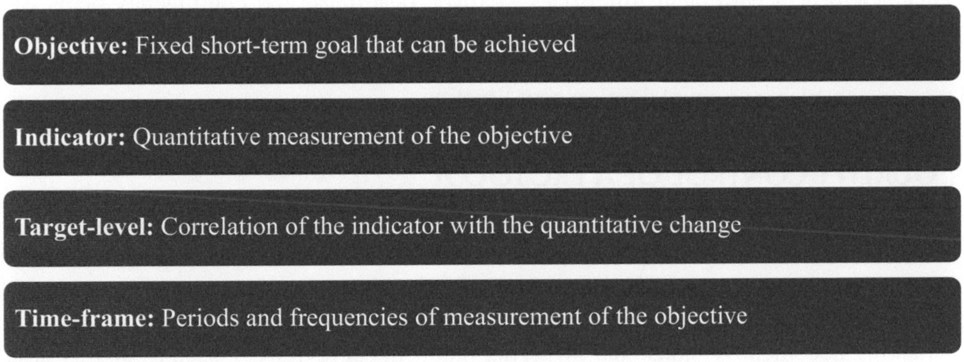

FIGURE 5.2 Criteria for defining SMART objectives.

5.6.2 Presenting the Information and Managing Reviews

Visual aids, such as diagrams and tables, can simplify complex information and improve understanding. A visit-wise schedule is very important to provide information on the study schedule, timelines, and parameters evaluated at each visit. A schedule of assessment table is a must in every clinical trial protocol. Similarly, a complex study design can be presented more lucidly by preparing a diagram rather than presenting information as text.

Iterative reviews with stakeholders to refine the protocol are helpful. Feedback from different stakeholders, such as clinicians, pharmacokinetic scientists (if pharmacokinetic endpoints are being measured), pharmacovigilance specialists (for safety sections), clinical operations leads (for trial procedures and conduct), biostatisticians, and patient representatives, ensures that the document is comprehensive and aligns with all requirements. Once reviews from internal stakeholders have been incorporated, the protocol undergoes reviews by ethics committees and regulatory authorities. Their feedback further strengthens the protocol and the study design.

5.6.3 Keeping Readers in Mind

Many stakeholders will use the protocol throughout the clinical trial procedure. The clinical investigators will be in charge of carrying out the protocol precisely as planned. The protocol will be used by the institutional review boards (IRBs) to ensure the safety and well-being of trial participants. Among the other participants in the study are statisticians, data managers, and the clinical study manager. A clearly written protocol helps in comprehending the defined procedures easily and accurately.

The clinical study protocol will ultimately also be used as a framework for developing the clinical study report, manuscripts, posters, and presentations to communicate the results to patients and other stakeholders. Therefore, developing a clear protocol with the end in mind is essential.

5.7 REALISTIC TIMELINES

Being realistic with protocol development timelines requires a strategic balance between scientific rigor, regulatory compliance, and operational feasibility. It is essential to factor in the complexity of the study design, the therapeutic area, and the number of stakeholders involved. Discussing timelines with the cross-functional teams early, such as clinical development, regulatory affairs, biostatistics, medical writing, and clinical operations, can help anticipate potential delays and streamline decision-making. Regulatory requirements, ethics committee approvals, and patient recruitment feasibility should also be assessed upfront to avoid unforeseen roadblocks.

Incorporating buffer time for reviews, revisions, and approvals ensures flexibility in handling unexpected challenges, such as protocol amendments or regulatory feedback. A well-defined project management plan with clear milestones, realistic deadlines, and contingency plans can help prevent overly aggressive timelines that compromise quality or lead to costly protocol amendments. Open communication among stakeholders and proactive risk management further contribute to a realistic and achievable protocol development timeline.

5.8 QUALITY CONTROL OF A PROTOCOL

A structured quality control checklist can help identify errors, inconsistencies, or missing information, while cross-referencing with other study documents, such as the investigator's brochure and statistical analysis plan, ensures coherence. Attention should also be given to clarity and readability, reducing ambiguity that could lead to protocol deviations at study sites. Utilizing electronic review tools, tracking document versions, and involving independent reviewers, such as quality assurance or external consultants, further enhances the reliability of the protocol.

Lastly, ensuring compliance with ICH-GCP guidelines and addressing regulatory or ethics committee feedback before finalization helps mitigate risks of protocol amendments, thereby maintaining efficiency and study integrity.

5.9 VERSION CONTROL

Maintaining a clear version control system helps track revisions and ensures consistency across documents. It is critical for managing updates and ensuring all stakeholders are working from the most recent version of the protocol. Therefore, each version of the protocol should be uniquely identified with a version number, date, and a brief description of the changes made. Any amendments made to the protocol should be well-documented, approved, and communicated to all stakeholders, including investigators, sponsors, ethics committees, and regulatory authorities. Including log summarizing changes across versions and detailing the rationale for amendments and their implications for the trial are helpful to maintain a history of changes. The outdated versions should be archived appropriately.

5.10 CONCLUSION

Writing a clinical trial protocol is a meticulous process that integrates scientific, ethical, and regulatory considerations. By adhering to ICH E6 guidelines and best practices, researchers can ensure that their protocols are robust, transparent, and capable of generating reliable and impactful data. Life-science students, as future contributors to clinical research, must appreciate the protocol's pivotal role in advancing patient care and medical knowledge.

REFERENCES

4 Best Practices for Clinical Protocol Writing, available from: https://blog.amwa.org/4-best-practices-for-clinical-protocol-writing, accessed on 24 Jan 2025.

Al-Jundi A, Sakka S. Protocol Writing in Clinical Research. J Clin Diagn Res. 2016 Nov;10(11):ZE10-ZE13. https://doi.org/10.7860/JCDR/2016/21426.8865. Epub 2016 Nov 1. Erratum in: J Clin Diagn Res. 2016 Dec;10(12):ZZ03. https://doi.org/10.7860/JCDR/2016/21426.9316. PMID: 28050522; PMCID: PMC5198475.

ICH Harmonised Guideline Guideline for Good Clinical Practice E6(R3), available from: ICH_E6(R3)_Step4_FinalGuideline_2025_0106.pdf, accessed on 08 Feb 2025.

The Ultimate Guide to Clinical Trial Protocol Writing, available from: The Ultimate Guide to Clinical Trial Protocol Writing, accessed on 29 Jan 2025.

6 Informed Consent in Health Research

Pooja Gupta[1], *Nikita Gupta*[2], *and Juhi Mittal*[1]
[1]Department of Pharmacology, All India Institute of Medical Science, New Delhi
[2]Department of Translational and Clinical Research, School of Chemical and Life Sciences, Jamia Hamdard, New Delhi

6.1 INTRODUCTION

Informed consent is a process that ensures conscious decision-making and voluntary participation of an individual in a research study. Its genesis over time has been based on a series of unethical practices in medicine and research. One of the oldest recorded medical cases was Slater v. Baker and Stapleton (1767), where the patient's leg was re-broken without consent to re-set it using experimental methods. During World War II, the Nazi doctors performed several inhumane experiments on prisoners of war to study survival techniques, such as exposing prisoners to extremes of temperature, testing experimental drugs, and sterilization methods. Another unethical series of trials was conducted in Tuskegee from 1932 to 1972, where the effects of untreated syphilis were studied in African American men. The known treatment for syphilis at that time, penicillin, was withheld, and patients were allowed to suffer serious health complications and even death. Yet another series of unethical experiments took place at Willow Brook State School (Lynch 2024) in New York, where disabled children were infected with hepatitis for nearly 15 years, to study disease progression. Even the parents of such children were forced to give consent (Schmidt 2023). These cases led to the establishment of legal and ethical frameworks, such as the Nuremberg Code (1947), Declaration of Helsinki adopted by the World Medical Association (1964), and the Belmont Report (1979), which reinforce the importance of obtaining informed consent in both medical and research practices (Pritchard 2021). The informed consent process ensures that participants provide voluntary and unbiased choice to participate in a study or procedure. It outlines clear, comprehensive, and truthful information about the research, which prevents exploitation and promotes autonomy. The ethics committees play a vital role in reviewing and approving informed consent documents to ensure compliance with ethical standards (Bazzano et al. 2021).

6.2 ETHICAL PRINCIPLES AND CONSENT

The principle of informed consent is governed by a combination of ethical guidelines and legal considerations that emphasize autonomy, transparency, and voluntariness of participation. The Nuremberg Code (1947) emphasized the importance of voluntary consent as an absolute requirement for medical research. It led to the formation of Institutional Review Board to review and approve research before initiation. The Declaration of Helsinki (1964 and amendments) details the guidelines for ethical conduct of research. The Belmont Report (1979) was issued by the U.S. National Commission for the Protection of Human Subjects of Biomedical and Behavioral Research. It laid down three fundamental ethical principles: respect for person (ensuring autonomy and informed decision-making); beneficence (minimizing harm and maximizing benefits); and justice (fair selection and treatment of research participants). The CIOMS Guidelines (Council for

 DOI: 10.1201/9781003533085-6

International Organizations of Medical Sciences, 1982, Revised 2016) (CIOMS & WHO 2016) were developed in collaboration with the World Health Organization (WHO), which provides internationally acceptable ethical standards for health-related research, with a focus on low-resource settings. Development of various national/regional guidelines led to the inception of the International Council of Harmonisation (ICH) in 1990, which came up with Good Clinical Practice (GCP) Guidelines in 1996 (Childress & Beauchamp 2022).

6.3 GUIDELINES AND LEGAL CONSIDERATIONS OF INFORMED CONSENT

6.3.1 ICH-GCP Guidelines

The ICH-GCP is an internationally accepted ethical and scientific quality standard for designing, conducting, recording, and reporting clinical trials involving human participants. These guidelines ensure the protection of human rights, safety, and well-being while ensuring the reliability of clinical trial data. Established in 1996 by the ICH, these guidelines standardize the conduct, design, monitoring, auditing, and reporting of clinical trials.

The primary goal of ICH-GCP is to ensure that clinical trials are conducted in compliance with ethical principles as documented in the Declaration of Helsinki, ensuring the rights, safety, and well-being of trial participants. The guidelines highlight the importance of obtaining informed consent from participants before enrolling them in the study, emphasizing transparency, voluntary participation, and disclosure of benefits and risks associated with the study. ICH-GCP has been adopted by major regulatory bodies, including the U.S. FDA, EMA (Europe), PMDA (Japan), and CDSCO (India), making it the global standard for ethical and scientifically valid clinical trials.

6.3.2 WHO-GCP Guidelines

The WHO-GCP guidelines provide an international ethical and scientific standard for design, conduct, and reporting of clinical trials, with a major focus on public health research in low- and middle-income countries. These guidelines also align with the Declaration of Helsinki and the CIOMS guidelines, emphasizing the importance of participant rights, risk minimization, and ethical integrity. Unlike ICH-GCP, which is designed mainly for regulatory-driven pharmaceutical trials, WHO-GCP guidelines are more flexible and adaptable to diverse research settings, including non-commercial, epidemiological, and disease-control studies. WHO-GCP also stresses capacity-building in developing countries for smooth and large-scale conduct of trials, promoting ethical research practices in regions with limited regulatory oversight. The most recent WHO-GCP updates focus on transparency of data, ethical review processes, and participant protection, particularly in global health emergencies, such as pandemics or infectious disease outbreaks (Idänpään-Heikkilä 1994).

6.3.3 UNESCO's Universal Declaration on Bioethics and Human Rights (2005)

The Universal Declaration on Bioethics and Human Rights was adopted by UNESCO in 2005 and serves as a comprehensive global framework guiding ethical decision-making in biomedical sciences and healthcare. This declaration was developed in response to the rapid advancements in biotechnology, genetic research, and medical interventions, ensuring that fundamental human rights and ethical principles are well protected. It emphasizes human dignity, autonomy, justice, and solidarity over science and research. A core aspect of the declaration is its focus on informed consent. It also stresses the importance of privacy and confidentiality, particularly concerning genetic and personal health data, to protect individuals from discrimination or misuse of information. This declaration has been influential in shaping national and international regulatory frameworks, including guidelines on clinical trials, public health policies, and genetic research ethics.

The governance of informed consent relies on a combination of ethical principles and legal regulations to protect research participants and patients. While ethical guidelines provide the moral foundation, legal frameworks ensure compliance and enforceability. Together, these systems uphold ethical integrity in medical research.

6.4 LEGAL FRAMEWORKS GOVERNING INFORMED CONSENT

Informed consent is not only an ethical subject but also a legal requirement in several countries. Various national and international laws regulate the informed consent process.

6.4.1 The United States

The U.S. Common Rule (45 CFR 46) is a federal regulation that governs the ethical conduct of research involving human subjects in the United States. Enforced by the Office for Human Research Protections (OHRP) under the U.S. Department of Health and Human Services, it established the guidelines to ensure the safety, rights, and well-being of research subjects. The regulation mandates that all research projects involving human subjects should undergo institutional review board approval, which assesses the risks, benefits, and ethical considerations of the study. One of the most crucial aspects of the Common Rule is the informed consent process. In 2017, significant revisions were also introduced to improve clarity, reduce administrative burdens, and strengthen participant protections. Additionally, special protections for vulnerable populations, such as pregnant women, prisoners, children, elderly, are also considered in detail, ensuring additional ethical oversight. The Common Rule also emphasized the need for data privacy and confidentiality, requiring secure storage and de-identification of research data. These regulations also align with international ethical standards, such as the Declaration of Helsinki and CIOMS Ethical Guidelines. The 2017 revisions further enhanced participant protection while promoting efficiency and transparency in clinical and behavioral research (Office for Human Research Protections (OHRP) 2025).

6.4.2 The European Union

The General Data Protection Regulation (GDPR) was enacted in 2018 by the European Union (EU) and is designed to protect the privacy and personal data of individuals within the EU and European Economic Area. It introduced strict regulations on data collection, processing, and storage. GDPR applies not only to EU-based organizations but also to non-EU entities that process the personal data of individuals residing in the EU, thereby having a global impact on data protection laws. The regulation is built on seven key principles: lawfulness, fairness, and transparency; purpose limitation; data minimization; accuracy; storage limitation; integrity and confidentiality; and accountability. One of the most significant aspects of GDPR is its emphasis on informed consent, requiring that organizations obtain clear and explicit permission from individuals before processing their personal data. GDPR also grants subjects the right to access, rectify, or erase their data (right to be forgotten) (Ezez. 2025).

6.4.3 The Indian Clinical Trial Rules (2019)

The New Drugs and Clinical Trial (NDCT) Rules, 2019, were introduced by the Ministry of Health and Family Welfare, Government of India, and serve as a comprehensive regulatory framework governing clinical trials, new drug approvals, and ethics committee oversight in India. Implemented under the Drugs and Cosmetics Act, 1940, these rules aim to regulate the approval process, strengthen participant safety, and align Indian regulations with global standards of research, such as ICH-GCP. The NDCT rules empower institute ethics committees in India to conduct site inspection, approve non-regulatory (academic trials) directly, and evaluate and recommend compensation for serious adverse events in clinical trials. Overall, they represent a significant advancement in India's clinical research landscape (Directorate General of Health Services Ministry of Health & Family Welfare 2019).

6.5 COMPONENTS OF INFORMED CONSENT

The informed consent is not just a document but a process that has two parts—information disclosure in the form of a participant information sheet (PIS) and the decision making in the form of a written informed consent through the informed consent form (ICF), both playing specific roles (Table 6.1). Upon obtaining informed consent, participants should receive a copy of the PIS and signed ICF, unless they explicitly decline. The original PIS and ICF must be retained and archived in compliance with relevant guidelines and regulations.

The commonly followed ICH-GCP outlines the components of PIS-ICF. It is usually designed and explained in English, being the de facto language of global communication in science. However, it is also translated into regional/vernacular languages or the mother tongue of the participants so that they can read and easily understand the study.

A checklist of essential and additional elements to be included in PIS can be found in section 5 of the National Ethical Guidelines for Biomedical and Health Research involving Human Participants, 2017, as well as Table of the Third Schedule of the New Drugs and Clinical Trial Rules, 2019, and listed in Table 6.2. A structured format of consent form (Table 6.3) ensures compliance with ethical and legal standards while protecting the rights of the participants (CIOMS & WHO 2016).

TABLE 6.1
Difference between Participant Information Sheet (PIS) and Informed Consent Form (ICF)

	Patient Information Sheet (PIS)	Informed Consent Form (ICF)
Purpose	Provides vital information about the research	Documents the consent from subjects as evidenced by signature
Format	Written in easy-to-understand plain language	More formal in nature
Signature	Does not require a signature	Requires signature to confirm consent
Sequence	Provided before the ICF, to help participants understand the study	Presented after PIS to document the consent before enrollment

TABLE 6.2
Components of a Participant Information Sheet

S.No.	Essential Components
1.	Title of the study with study identification number
2.	Introduction, explanation of the purpose of the study, specific objectives, and expected outcomes
3.	Expected duration of study participation
4.	Detailed description of interventions, study procedures, and visits, including randomization, placebo, possibility of failure of intervention
5.	Possible risks and discomforts associated with study interventions/procedures and their management
6.	Possible benefits directly for the participant or for society
7.	Available alternatives for the patient in case they do not wish to participate *vis-à-vis* the study intervention
8.	Explanation on confidentiality of personal information and protection of data, along with compliance with the data protection laws
9.	Management of study-related injuries and compensation for participation and injury, if any
10.	Voluntariness of participation and right to withdraw without bias
11.	Whom to contact for queries and concerns
12.	A clear statement of participant's responsibilities, consent, and signature

(Continued)

TABLE 6.2 (Continued)
Components of a Participant Information Sheet

S.No.	Additional Components
1.	Conditions and consequences for termination of participation or withdrawal
2.	Additional costs for participants, if any
3.	Communication of new findings
4.	Number of participants

TABLE 6.3
Format for Informed Consent Form

Subject's Initials:.................... Subject's Name:........................
Date of Birth/Age: .... Address of the Subject: ....
Qualification: ....
Occupation: Student or Self-Employed or Service or Housewife or Others
Annual Income of the subject: ....
Name and address of the nominees and his relation to the subject (for the purpose of compensation in case of trial related death).
Place Initial box (Subject)

(i)	I confirm that I have read and understood the information Sheet dated .... for the above study and have had the opportunity to ask questions.	[ ]
(ii)	I understand that my participation in the study is voluntary and that I am free to withdraw at any time, without giving any reason, without my medical care or legal rights being affected.	[ ]
(iii)	I understand that the Sponsor of the clinical trial, others working on the Sponsor's behalf, the Ethics Committee and the regulatory authorities will not need my permission to look at my health records both in respect of the current study and any further research that may be conducted in relation to it, even if I withdraw from the trial. I agree to this access. However, I understand that my identity will not be revealed in any information released to third parties or published.	[ ]
(iv)	I agree not to restrict the use of any data or results that arise from this study provided such a use is only for scientific purposes.	[ ]
(v)	I agree to take part in the above study.	[ ]

Signature (or Thumb impression) of Subject/Legally Acceptable Representative:.............
Date: ..../........./........
Signatory's Name: ....
Signature of the Investigator: .... Date: ..../....../........
Study Investigator's Name: ....
Signature of the Witness... Date: ..../....../..........
Name of the Witness: ....
Copy of the Patient Information Sheet and duly filled Informed Consent Form shall be handed over to the subject his or her attendant.

6.6 PROCESS OF OBTAINING INFORMED CONSENT

The process of obtaining a written informed consent for clinical research is a structured procedure that ensures participants' unbiased opinion regarding participation in the study. This process should adhere to the international guidelines, such as GCP and applicable local regulations. The key steps in the informed consent process include information disclosure, comprehension, voluntariness, competence, and consent (Figure 6.1). Disclosure provides detailed information to the participant regarding purpose, risks, and benefits to society and the individual associated with the study. Comprehension ensures that participants understand the information related to the study. Voluntariness ensures that the participant has the free will to make the decision without being influenced or under pressure. Competence refers to an individual's ability to make a decision, and consent is an agreement, either in written or recorded verbal form, to proceed with the study. The important aspects of an informed consent include:

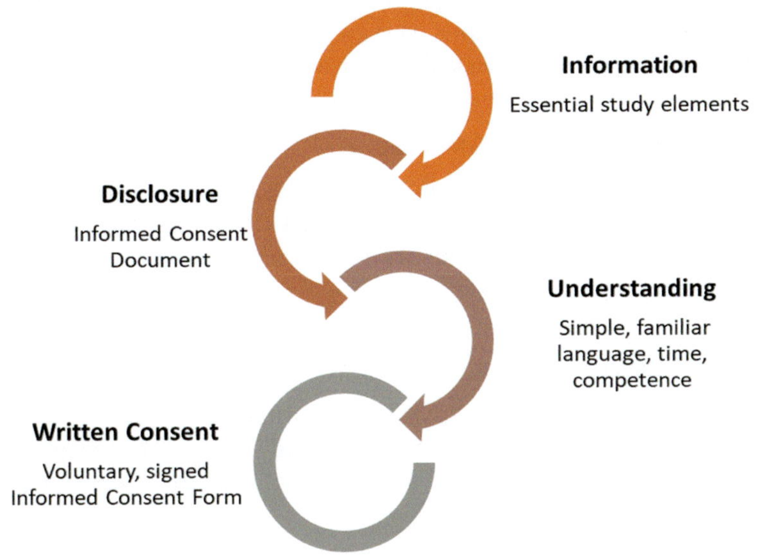

FIGURE 6.1 Key steps in informed consent process.

6.6.1 Stakeholders

According to the NDCT rules, 2019, informed consent can be obtained from a study participant or their legally acceptable representative (LAR refers to an individual who has the legal authority to act on behalf of another person) who is acceptable if the participant is incapacitated (e.g., unconsciousness/minor/has mental illness or disability). Additionally, if the subject or their LAR is unable to read or write, an impartial witness must be present throughout the informed consent process and sign the consent form as an attestation.

6.6.2 Language of Consent

The information about the study is to be presented in a clear, non-technical/layman's language that is easy to understand. If the person does not understand the language used in the ICD, a translated version of the document in their local language must be provided to ensure comprehension. Most people use translation software for this purpose. However, the software captures the literal meaning of words, which may lead to a change in the meaning. Therefore, back-translations are recommended, along with the use of colloquial language instead of literary translation.

It is generally recommended to keep ICD non-technical, simple, understandable, legible, and as short as possible. Studies suggest that longer documents are associated with poorer comprehension. Using lay terms (6–8th grade level), words <3 syllables, and sentences <10 words and restricting to about 1000 words (4 pages) are considered to improve comprehension. Writing the ICD in second person establishes a connection with the participants, for example, you are being asked . . ., you will need to do . . . etc. Using a template ensures that the important aspects are not missed out. Use of language indicating that the participant waives any of their rights must be avoided.

6.6.3 Providing Comprehensive Information

Once a potential study participant is identified based on the study eligibility criteria, they are provided with a detailed ICF as described earlier. The investigator is required to communicate study information to participants both verbally and in writing. They are given time to understand and discuss with their family/friends if required. However, it is the responsibility of the investigator to ensure that the written consent is also an understood consent.

6.6.4 Assessing Participant Understanding

Investigator must ensure that the participant fully understands the information provided. Methods such as discussions, question-answer sessions, simplified visual aids, and questionnaires may be used to enhance comprehension. Participants are encouraged to ask questions to clarify doubts and facilitate informed decision-making.

6.6.5 Voluntary Decision-Making

The participant must decide to participate or not to participate, freely without coercion, undue influence, or pressure. Special attention is given to the individuals in dependent relationships (e.g., students, employees, prisoners, patients) so that they are not pressured into participation.

6.6.6 Documenting Consent

In medicine, consent may be implied when the risk involved is minimal, for example, extending the arm for monitoring blood pressure, or it may be expressed (oral or written), depending upon the risk involved, for example, abdominal examination versus a surgical procedure. However, the consent is always written informed consent for research. The participant must sign and date the ICF, confirming that they have read and understood the study details and are agreeing voluntarily to participate. Furthermore, the ICF is signed and dated by the investigator as well. A witness, unrelated to the study, may be required for an illiterate or vulnerable person or in cases of verbal consent. The investigator also signs and dates the consent form.

6.6.7 Providing a Copy of the Consent Form

The participant receives a signed copy of the ICF for their records. This ensures they can refer to the study details and their rights at any time. One copy of the ICF goes in the site master file.

6.6.8 Re-Consenting

Any major modifications to the study or new risks identified, which may affect a participant's decision to participate in the study, must be duly informed to the participants, and a revised consent form needs to be signed. Re-consent may also be required in certain other conditions, like a change in participant age (minor becomes adult) or status (unconscious to conscious), planned extension of an ongoing study, or possibility of disclosure of identifiable information, for example, publication.

The participants retain the right to withdraw from the study at any point without any consequences. This structured approach ensures compliance with ethical and legal standards, protecting participant autonomy and rights as the study progresses.

6.6.9 Waiver of Consent

In certain situations, or types of studies, consent from the participant may not be required. However, this is to be decided and approved by the ethics committee and not the investigator. The conditions where the requirement for consent may be waived include less than minimal risk to the participant, where their rights/welfare are not affected. The types of studies for which consent may not be required include retrospective studies where de-identified data or anonymized biological samples are being collected and certain public health and program evaluation studies where data available in the public domain is being perused. During emergencies/disasters, the ethics committee may approve a waiver of consent on humanitarian grounds with the condition that consent is taken at the earliest possible time.

6.7 CHALLENGES AND ETHICAL DILEMMAS

In practice, several challenges and dilemmas are faced in the process of obtaining consent. These issues impact the validity and effectiveness of consent and may raise concerns about participant autonomy and research integrity.

6.7.1 Comprehension and Health Literacy

One of the major challenges in obtaining consent is ensuring that participants fully understand the study details. Many informed consent forms are complex, filled with medical and legal jargon that is not easily understandable by individuals with low health literacy. Studies suggest that even well-educated participants may struggle to grasp all elements of consent, leading to potentially uninformed decisions.

6.7.2 Language and Cultural Barriers

In multi-national or multi-ethnic studies, translating informed consent documents accurately into the local language of the participants while maintaining the legal and ethical integrity of the ICF is a challenge. Cultural differences in decision-making processes can also impact voluntary consent, as some individuals may feel obligated to participate due to familial or societal pressure.

6.7.3 Coercion and Undue Influence

Participants, especially in the presence of their treating doctor and those in vulnerable groups, may feel pressured to enroll in a study due to perceived benefits, such as free medical care or financial compensation. Use of misguiding or vague language also may be construed as coercion. This raises ethical concerns about whether consent is truly voluntary or influenced by external factors.

6.7.4 Therapeutic Misconception

In clinical trials, participants often misunderstand the difference between research and medical treatment, believing they will receive the best possible therapy rather than an experimental intervention. This misconception undermines true informed consent because participants may overestimate potential benefits while underestimating the risks.

6.7.5 Ongoing Consent and Withdrawal Issues

Informed consent is an ongoing process, but researchers often face challenges in keeping participants informed throughout long-term studies. Additionally, although participants can withdraw from the study at any time, logistical and ethical dilemmas arise when data collected before withdrawal remains in use, especially in genetic or biobank research.

6.7.6 Ethical Concerns in Emergency Research

In cases where research involves critically ill or unconscious patients, obtaining prior informed consent is nearly impossible. This creates an ethical dilemma between protecting patient rights and advancing life-saving research. Some regulations allow for deferred or surrogate consent, but these approaches remain controversial. Consent during epidemics, pandemics, and war casualties is another huge ethical dilemma, which is time sensitive as well. Addressing these challenges requires a multifaceted approach, including simplified consent forms, culturally sensitive communication, continuous education of participants, and the use of innovative methods such as audiovisual aids for better comprehension (Ezez. 2019).

6.8 SPECIAL CONSIDERATIONS IN INFORMED CONSENT

6.8.1 Pediatric Age Group

According to page 143 of the NDCT Rules, 2019, written informed consent can be obtained from a parent or legal guardian for minors participating in research. However, researchers should also ensure that children are informed about the study in a way they can understand, using language and terms suitable for their age and maturity level. When appropriate, mature children should also sign and date an additional assent form to participate in the study (Cotrim et al. 2021). The details of the assent form are given in **Table 6.4**.

6.8.2 Other Vulnerable Groups

Vulnerable, by definition, is a person who is weak or easy to hurt. With respect to clinical research, people who may be easily influenced to participate in a study, and therefore are at risk of exploitation and harm, are considered vulnerable subjects. Most guidelines and regulations give a list of groups considered vulnerable. Broadly, apart from children, women (especially pregnant or lactating); members of a group with hierarchical structure (e.g., prisoners, armed forces personnel, staff and students of medical, nursing and pharmacy institutions); unemployed or impoverished persons; minority groups, homeless persons, nomads, refugees; patients with incurable diseases; and patients in emergency situations are considered vulnerable.

As per the NDCT Rules, 2019, for vulnerable subjects participating in clinical trials of new chemical or molecular entities, an audio-visual recording of the informed consent process is mandatory.

TABLE 6.4
Difference between Consent and Assent

	Informed Consent	Assent
Mental capacity	Given by a competent individual with full mental capacity to make decisions	Given by an individual with limited mental capacity
Age group	Typically given by adults or legally acceptable representatives	Often given by mature minors and adolescents (7–18 years old)
Requirement	Always required before enrolling in the trial	Is preferred in addition to informed consent document, in case of mature children

This recording should capture the entire process, including the procedure of giving information and the subject's understanding of the same. However, the rules state that for clinical trials involving anti-HIV and anti-leprosy drugs, only an audio recording is required (Biros 2018).

6.8.3 Genetic Research and Biobanking

The ICF in genetic testing and biobanking ensures ethical collection, storage, and use of biological samples while protecting the rights of the participant. To obtain consent, participants are informed about the purpose of the study, types of samples collected, potential risks and benefits, confidentiality measures, and their right to withdraw consent at any time. Consent obtained can either be specific, that is, limited to a particular study, or broad (allowing future research use), and it must be documented with the participant's signature. In cases involving minors or individuals who are unable to provide consent, a legal guardian must provide approval. Special considerations include keeping data anonymous to protect privacy, ethical concerns regarding genetic discrimination, and transparency about potential commercial applications. Participants should also receive post-test genetic counseling, particularly if results indicate serious genetic risks. Hence, compliance with ICMR's National Ethical Guidelines is mandatory to ensure adherence to legal and ethical standards.

If samples are obtained directly from labs, consent may be waived under ICMR ethical guidelines, provided that the study poses minimal risk. The original purpose of sample collection, nature of research, confidentiality measures, and possible commercial applications must be transparently documented in the biobank's governance policies. Institutions must also adhere to data protection laws and biomedical research regulations to ensure ethical and lawful use of laboratory-sourced samples in biobanking (Beskow et al. 2015).

6.8.4 Electronic Consent in Research

Electronic informed consent (eConsent) is a digital alternative to traditional paper-based consent processes in clinical research. eConsenting utilizes electronic systems to improve comprehension by incorporating visual aids, videos, multimedia presentations, interactive websites, questionnaires, and quizzes to ensure that participants fully understand the study before consenting. It allows for remote identity verification of the participant and enables them to review, sign, and submit consent forms from home, thereby increasing accessibility and convenience.

The flexibility of eConsent also allows researchers to update consent forms in real time, ensuring that participants receive the most current study information promptly. However, it must meet the same legal and ethical requirements as traditional informed consent. The process must be secure, protect participant confidentiality, and provide an electronic copy of the consent document. While eConsent offers numerous benefits, it also presents several challenges in its implementation and ethical considerations.

6.8.5 Digital Literacy and Acceptability

Not all participants have equal access to digital devices or the internet, particularly in low-resource settings. Individuals with limited experience using technology may struggle to navigate eConsent platforms, leading to potential exclusion of certain populations and selection bias.

6.8.6 Data Privacy

Storing sensitive health information electronically increases the risk of cyberattacks and unauthorized access, necessitating appropriate steps to mitigate the risk.

6.8.7 Verification of Participant Identity

Unlike traditional consent, where the identity can be verified physically, digital consent requires additional verification, such as biometrics, digital signatures, and a two-step verification process.

6.8.8 True Comprehension

Although eConsent includes audiovisual aids, it is still difficult to know whether the patient fully understood the study in detail. Ensuring a question-and-answer session or a discussion before consenting will minimize this risk.

6.8.9 Regulatory Compliance and Legal Challenges

In case of multi-national studies, it becomes very difficult to cooperate with all the rules and regulations of different countries as some countries may follow the wet-ink or physical consent method. Hence, it becomes difficult to fully adopt digital consenting for such studies.

6.8.10 Technical Issues and System Reliability

Technical failure, bugs, computer viruses, compatibility issues, and difficulty in navigating the consent form are barriers to fully adopting eConsent (Jose Pablo Morales 2024).

6.9 CONCLUSION

Informed consent process is a cornerstone of ethical health research, which ensures participants' voluntary engagement in studies with a clear understanding of potential risks, benefits, and their rights and responsibilities. It upholds the fundamental ethical principle of autonomy, as outlined in key ethical frameworks like the Nuremberg Code, the Declaration of Helsinki, and ICH-GCP guidelines.

Informed consent not only safeguards the participants from potential harm but also strengthens their rights and the credibility and integrity of scientific research by fostering trust and transparency between researchers and society. In a rapidly evolving research landscape, particularly with advancements in digital health, personalized medicine, and eConsent, continuous efforts are needed to ensure that consent processes remain clear, accessible, and culturally appropriate.

Challenges such as language barriers, digital literacy issues, and ethical dilemmas in emergency research highlight the need for ongoing improvements in consent frameworks. Strengthening regulatory compliance, encouraging active participant involvement, and innovative consent methodologies will be essential to ensuring ethical and responsible health research in the future. Ultimately, informed consent is not just a legal obligation but a fundamental ethical commitment to respecting human dignity in scientific advancements.

REFERENCES

Bazzano, Lydia A., Durant, Jaquail & Brantley, Paula Rhode. 2021. "A Modern History of Informed Consent and the Role of Key Information". *Ochsner Journal* 21 (1) (martxoak 15): 81–85. https://doi.org/10.31486/toj.19.0105.

Beskow, Laura M. et al. 2015. "Informed Consent for Biobanking: Consensus-based Guidelines for Adequate Comprehension". *Genetics in Medicine* 17 (3) (martxoak): 226–233. https://doi.org/10.1038/gim.2014.102.

Biros, Michelle. 2018. "Capacity, Vulnerability, and Informed Consent for Research." *The Journal of Law, Medicine & Ethics: A Journal of the American Society of Law, Medicine & Ethics* 46 (1) (martxoak): 72–78. https://doi.org/10.1177/1073110518766021.

Childress, James F. & Beauchamp, Tom L. 2022. "Common Morality Principles in Biomedical Ethics: Responses to Critics". *Cambridge Quarterly of Healthcare Ethics* 31 (2) (apirilak 13): 164–176. https://doi.org/10.1017/S0963180121000566.

CIOMS & WHO. 2016. "International Ethical Guidelines for Health-related Research Involving Humans". Geneva, Switzerland. https://doi.org/10.56759/rgxl7405.

Cotrim, Hortense et al. 2021. "Children's Understanding of Informed Assents in Research Studies." *Healthcare (Basel, Switzerland)* 9 (7) (uztailak 10). https://doi.org/10.3390/healthcare9070871.

Directorate General of Health Services Ministry of Health & Family Welfare, CDSCO. 2019. "New Drugs and Clinical Trials Rules, 2019."

Ezez. 2019. "ICMR Guidelines".

Ezez. 2025. "Rules for the Protection of Personal Data Inside and Outside the EU."

Idänpään-Heikkilä, J. E. 1994. "WHO Guidelines for Good Clinical Practice (GCP) for Trials on Pharmaceutical Products: Responsibilities of the Investigator." *Annals of Medicine* 26 (2) (apirilak): 89–94. https://doi.org/10.3109/07853899409147334.

Jose Pablo Morales. 2024. "Informed Consent, Electronic Informed Consent & Key Information: An Overview". USA.

Lynch, John. 2024. "To Know Me Is to Exonerate Me: Appeals to Character in Defense of the Willowbrook Hepatitis Study". *The Journal of Medicine and Philosophy: A Forum for Bioethics and Philosophy of Medicine* 49 (5) (Irailak 3): 499–511. https://doi.org/10.1093/jmp/jhae024.

Office for Human Research Protections (OHRP). 2025. "US Department of Health and Human Services 45 CFR 46."

Pritchard, Ivor A. 2021. "Framework for the Ethical Conduct of Research: The Ethical Principles of the Belmont Report." in. *Handbook of Research Ethics in Psychological Science.*, 3–21. Washington: American Psychological Association. https://doi.org/10.1037/0000258-001.

Schmidt, Ulf. 2023. "From Nuremberg to Helsinki: Historicizing the Codification of Post-War Research Ethics" in. *Ethical Innovation for Global Health*, 149–174. Singapore: Springer Nature Singapore. https://doi.org/10.1007/978-981-99-6163-4_9.

7 Case Report Form

Shadan Hussain[1], *Mansi Dahalia*[2], *and Kamlesh Garg*[3]
[1] Department of Translational and Clinical Research, School of Chemical and Life Sciences, Jamia Hamdard, New Delhi, India
[2] Department of Pharmacology, School of Pharmaceutical Education and Research, Jamia Hamdard, New Delhi, India
[3] Department of Pharmacology, Vardhman Mahavir Medical College & Safdarjung Hospital, Ansari Nagar West, New Delhi, India

7.1 INTRODUCTION

Clinical trials depend on the Case Report Form (CRF) as their essential tool for systematic patient data recording. The development of CRFs represents an essential trial component that determines how successful the study will become. The International Council for Harmonisation (ICH) Guidelines for Good Clinical Practice (GCP) define the CRF as a printed, optical, or electronic document designed to record all protocol-required information to be reported to the sponsor for each trial subject. Investigators and site personnel are responsible for completing CRFs accurately from source data in accordance with the protocol (*9 Tips to Design Better Case Report Forms (CRFs) for Clinical Trials - Klindat*, n.d.; Bellary et al., 2014; Dixon, 1998).

A properly designed CRF plays a critical role by minimizing data omissions while enabling effective data management, together with statistical analysis, as well as reporting functions. The system follows the trial protocol design to convert complex clinical data into structured formats usable for planned analytical purposes. CRFs are created by sponsors and sponsor-investigators for maintenance at investigator sites using information from source documentation (*Case Report Form (CRF) Binder/Electronic Case Report Form (eCRF) | Social Science Research Institute*, n.d.).

CRFs capture data about adverse events (AEs) and serious adverse events (SAEs), together with data regarding concomitant therapies and intercurrent illnesses, dropout reports and reasons, as well as clinical laboratory tests (such as electrocardiograms (ECGs) and X-rays) and inclusion/exclusion criteria (*Case Report Form - Clinical Research Explained | VIARES*, n.d.; *What is a Case Report Form? | Novotech CRO*, n.d.). The CRFs should be reviewed and signed by the investigator prior to submission. Data-modifying entries become transparent when investigators draw a line through inaccurate fields and date and sign their corrections. The CRF serves a critical function in clinical trials because it helps maintain data consistency and enables regulatory compliance, which ensures reliable investigation outcomes(Bellary et al., 2014; *Case Report Form (CRF) Binder/Electronic Case Report Form (eCRF) | Social Science Research Institute*, n.d.).

7.2 REGULATORY FRAMEWORK AND GUIDELINES

Trial data collection depends primarily on CRFs as essential clinical research tools. The ICH, United States (U.S.) Food and Drug Administration (FDA), and the European Medicines Agency (EMA) enforce strict guidelines to establish data integrity while assuring patient security and maintaining regulatory compliance. This report delivers an exhaustive analysis of the regulatory requirements controlling CRF design procedures while describing the specifications for preparation and completion and error remediation methods alongside storage protocols, archival procedures, and inspection protocols (Bellary et al., 2014; Richesson & Nadkarni, 2011).

DOI: 10.1201/9781003533085-7

- ICH E6(R2) GCP: The CRFs are required to capture all protocol-specified data points essential for evaluating study endpoints and objectives (ICH E6(R2) 1.11, 4.9). Modern eCRFs often employ conditional formatting and skip logic to streamline data collection while maintaining protocol fidelity.
- 21 CFR Part 11 & EU Annex 11: Electronic CRFs (eCRFs) must be governed by requirements to validate fields, enable audit trails, and protect user access through secure controls.

7.2.1 Key Design Principles

A CRF relies on a protocol-guided approach. The way in which data is collected must be consistent with the study plan and track outcomes important for safety and treatment effectiveness. As a result, you collect only the data needed, so you reduce the risk of including unnecessary information. Categorizing the CRF into modules that review different features of the study allows easier and more reliable data to be entered.

Thinking about the needs of the end user plays an equal role in preparing the CRF. Using consistent fonts, giving clear steps, and including symbols like checkmarks help reduce the possibility of mistakes while entering data. Placing all related modules from a form onto the same page ensures that information is entered smoothly, which helps ensure the process is both accurate and efficient.

Data is kept consistent by having all participants respond in the same way, for instance, with pre-set yes/no and scale options. Using the same format for dates (like dd/mm/yyyy) and similar measurement units on every sheet helps keep data accurate. Carrying out pilot trials lets users show any parts they found challenging, so the CRF can be improved and different modules' workflows can be fine-tuned. Every module, together with those about AEs, should be conveniently placed on a single page.

Implementing eCRFs means that data quality is improved and rules are checked automatically. Users are notified right away if their blood pressure goes higher than 200 mmHg, which is the threshold set in the system. To ensure safety and track who makes changes, only the proper people are allowed to do so, and this is monitored using role-based permissions. Because the data is checked right away and access is secure, it remains both reliable and protected. The key guidelines related to CRF preparation, data entry procedures, and error management in clinical trials are summarized in Table 7.1.

7.3 ROLE AND IMPORTANCE OF CRFs IN CLINICAL TRIALS

The primary roles and applications of CRFs in clinical trials are summarized in Table 7.2.

7.4 PRINCIPLES OF CRF DESIGN

Developing a CRF involves an exacting methodology that merges research methodologies with interface-design practices for users. The main purpose focuses on acquiring accurate and detailed information through systems that prevent duplication and simplify the process of document transcription. Study design for CRF starts with the creation of structured data collection systems that support main study endpoints to achieve maximum operational efficiency and data quality. The key principles involved in the design of CRFs are summarized in Table 7.3 (Bellary et al., 2014; *Case Form Report Design SOP - King's Health Partners Clinical Trials Office*, n.d.; *Case Report Form - Clinical Research Explained | VIARES*, n.d.; *Case Report Form (CRF) Binder/Electronic Case Report Form (eCRF) | Social Science Research Institute*, n.d.; *Tips to Design an Optimal Case Report Form*, n.d.).

TABLE 7.1
Key Guidelines for CRF Preparation, Data Entry, and Error Management

Category	Description
Documentation & Training	Sponsors are responsible for providing clear instructions on data entry, document verification, and procedures for managing missing information. Training ensures that all users understand how to accurately complete the CRF
Stakeholder Collaboration	A multidisciplinary team, including statisticians, clinicians, and data managers, reviews the CRF to ensure alignment with the analysis plan. Regulatory approval processes are also coordinated at this stage
Ethics Committee Review	Before a CRF can be used in a clinical trial, it must be reviewed and approved by an Institutional Review Board (IRB) or equivalent ethics committee
Version Control	Each update or revision of the CRF is tracked with a specific date to maintain a clear version history and ensure all parties are using the correct form
Data Entry Standard	All data entries must be directly traceable to original source documents, such as laboratory reports or medical records. Data should be entered promptly, ideally during or immediately after a patient visit, to reduce recall errors.
Error Handling (Paper CRFs)	Corrections are made by drawing a single line through the error, entering the correct data nearby, and adding the corrector's name and date. The use of white-out or erasers is prohibited to preserve a clear audit trail
Error Handling (eCRFs)	Electronic systems automatically record the identity of the user and the time of any changes. Electronic signatures are used to authenticate corrections, ensuring data integrity and traceability

TABLE 7.2
Primary Uses of CRF

Uses	Description
Data Collection	CRFs are the main instruments for systematically recording all protocol-required data for each participant, including demographics, medical history, trial procedures, outcomes, and AEs. This ensures consistency and completeness in data acquisition across all study sites
Data Management	The structured format of CRFs enables efficient data entry, processing, and management, supporting accurate database creation for subsequent statistical analysis and reporting
Safety Monitoring	CRFs capture all AEs and SAEs experienced by participants, allowing for continuous monitoring of participant safety and rapid identification of potential risks associated with the investigational product
Protocol Compliance	By aligning with the clinical trial protocol, CRFs ensure that only relevant data required for hypothesis testing and regulatory submissions are collected, reducing unnecessary data and supporting protocol adherence
Regulatory Documentation	CRFs provide the essential documentation required by regulatory authorities (e.g., FDA, EMA) for trial audits, inspections, and approvals. Accurate and complete CRFs are necessary for demonstrating trial conduct and data integrity
Data De-Identification	CRFs facilitate the de-identification of patient data by assigning unique study numbers and omitting personal identifiers, thereby protecting participant privacy and meeting ethical standards
Statistical Analysis	The data collected in CRFs forms the basis for statistical evaluation of trial outcomes, enabling researchers to assess the safety and efficacy of the investigational product
Audit Trail and Traceability	eCRFs offer audit trails, tracking all data entries and modifications, which enhances traceability and accountability in the data management process
Communication Tool	CRFs serve as a communication bridge between research sites and sponsors, standardizing the reporting of study data and facilitating timely resolution of data queries

TABLE 7.3
Summarizes the Key Principles of CRF Design

Principle	Description	Purpose
User-Centric Approach	The design process must focus on meeting requirements of end-users	To create simple functions and prevent mistakes
Standardization	Standard operating procedures (SOPs) for CRF preparation must be established	To promote consistent data collection throughout multiple studies
Data Quality	The CRF must provide data collection at a detailed level	Avoids both confusing ambiguities and avoidable repetitions
Avoiding Duplication	A single piece of information must not be recorded more than once in different sections of the data collection form	To prevent informational pitfalls
Clear Instructions	The provision of straightforward instructions is essential to the process of CRF design	Avoid deviations
Layout and Organization	Only keep each module on one page while using a consistent page numbering system that avoids splitting sections across different pages	Makes reading and data entry processes easier for users

7.5 ESSENTIAL COMPONENTS OF A CRF

The foundation of accurate and effective data collection in clinical trials is a well-structured CRF. To guarantee both data quality and ease of analysis, a CRF's design should include a number of essential components and adhere to best practices.

Usually, the CRF starts with user-defined header and footer sections. Important identifying information like the protocol ID, site code, subject ID, and patient initials are included in the header. The investigator's signature, date stamp, version information, and page count, on the other hand, are all found in the footer and are necessary for accurate documentation and traceability (Bellary et al., 2014; *Case Report Form - Clinical Research Explained | VIARES*, n.d.; *What is a Case Report Form? | Novotech CRO*, n.d.)

Specialized safety and efficacy modules are included in the CRF body to collect important study data. Because they gather data on AEs, efficacy evaluations, and all related treatment protocols, the safety and efficacy sections are especially crucial. This guarantees that all pertinent clinical information is methodically documented and accessible for examination.

A collaborative approach is emphasized in best practices for CRF design. Involving stakeholders during the design phase, such as statisticians, data managers, and investigators, aids in determining user needs and guarantees the CRF is appropriate for its intended use. Before being finalized, a draft should be tested using pilot procedures to identify and fix any possible problems.

The quality of the data gathered is further improved by adherence to established standards. This includes utilizing pre-formatted answer choices whenever feasible, which simplifies data entry and reduces errors, and consistent data formats (for example, dd/mm/yyyy for dates).

The reliability and effectiveness of data collection in clinical trial operations will be greatly increased by a CRF that incorporates these elements and adheres to these best practices (*9 Tips to Design Better Case Report Forms (CRFs) for Clinical Trials - Klindat*, n.d.; *Case Report Form - Clinical Research Explained | VIARES*, n.d.; *Tips to Design an Optimal Case Report Form*, n.d.; Bellary et al., 2014).

7.6 COMPARISON OF WELL-DESIGNED AND POORLY DESIGNED CRFs

The major differences between well-designed and poorly designed CRFs are summarized in Table 7.4.

TABLE 7.4
Key Differences between Well-Designed and Poorly Designed CRFs

Characteristics	Well-Designed CRF	Poorly Designed CRF
Protocol Alignment and Data Relevance	• Strict adherence to study protocol: The protocol records only necessary data points needed for hypothesis testing without including data that is irrelevant to the analysis. • Avoids duplication: Research data collection will remove duplicated information by keeping only one of age or date of birth. • Structured endpoints: The data collection points should match the study endpoints so that analysis can use the collected information effectively. • Protocol deviations: Protocol-mandated information outside of standard parameters results in unnecessary resource consumption.	• Protocol deviations: Protocol-mandated information outside of standard parameters results in unnecessary resource consumption. • Redundant fields: The duplication of data collection points leads to higher analysis errors and more complicated analysis procedures. • Unclear objectives: The failure to establish safety and effectiveness parameters generates fragmented datasets with possible inconsistencies in research results.
Data Integrity and Standardization	• Predefined answer options: Utilizes checkboxes and drop-down menus and coded responses as response methods to limit the number of free-text entries. • Consistent formatting: All pages adopt consistent layouts and display font styles together with date formats formatted as dd/mm/yyyy. • Units and decimal points: The document includes standard measurement units such as mmHg for blood pressure measurements to prevent misunderstandings.	• Excessive free-text fields: Unstructured answers in these data sets create difficulties during interpretation and analytical stages. • Inconsistent layouts: Formats that merge portrait and landscape orientations and change font styles end up creating user confusion. • Missing units: Data entry errors occur when the system fails to specify the expected measurement units (kg or lbs) in weight data fields.
User Interface and Accessibility	• Visual cues: Uses boxes, lines, or shaded areas to guide data entry (e.g., date fields marked as dd/mm/yyyy. • Clear instructions: Provides prompts like "Enter values to one decimal place" to ensure uniformity. • Pilot testing: Validated through user feedback to identify ambiguities or usability issues before deployment	• Ambiguous questions: Uses vague terms like "frequent" or "severe" without operational definitions. • Lack of guidance: Omits instructions, forcing site personnel to make subjective judgments. • Untested design: Skips pilot phases, resulting in frequent post-deployment revisions and database modifications
Regulatory Compliance and Error Management	• ICH GCP compliance: Follows regulatory guidelines for data traceability and audit readiness. • Transparent corrections: Allows edits via strikethroughs with dates and initials, preserving an audit trail. • eCRFs Leverages real-time validation checks to flag discrepancies during data entry	• Non-compliance risks: Deviates from ICH GCP standards, potentially invalidating trial results during audits. • Opaque corrections: Permits undocumented changes, compromising data authenticity. • Paper-based limitations: Lacks automated checks, allowing errors to persist until manual query resolution.

TABLE 7.4 (Continued)
Key Differences between Well-Designed and Poorly Designed CRFs

Characteristics	Well-Designed CRF	Poorly Designed CRF
Impact on Clinical Trial Outcomes	• Reduced query rates: Minimizes discrepancies through standardized data collection, accelerating database lock. • Cost efficiency: Lowers resource waste by avoiding redundant data processing. • Enhanced reliability: Supports robust statistical analysis with high-quality, consistent datasets.	• Increased queries: Generates frequent data clarifications, delaying study timelines. • Higher costs: Wastes resources on non-essential data collection and error correction. • Compromised validity: Introduces bias or inaccuracies, undermining trial conclusions.

7.7 TRANSITION FROM PAPER-BASED SYSTEM TO eCRFs

Clinical trial data management has seen a revolution through eCRFs, which now replace paper-based systems to provide enhanced accuracy and efficiency alongside compliance benefits. This report examines eCRFs, starting with their design structure before delving into research applications and discussing their technological benefits and implementation frameworks. eCRFs perform essential functions, which include data collection through real-time validation from a centralized platform.

7.7.1 Real-Time Data Validation and Centralized Data Collection Are the Two Main Capabilities of eCRFs

Secure electronic platforms use eCRFs as digital questionnaires, which enable real-time patient data entry. The system validates patient data in real-time by applying predefined checks to electronic CRFs without the need for labor-intensive manual transcription. A systolic blood pressure value exceeding 300 mmHg would immediately trigger the system to show an alert that forces the clinician to review and fix the entry before continuing. Secure platforms implement eCRFs, which decrease the need for additional data cleanup work and maintain improved data quality throughout analytical processes.

7.7.2 Enhanced Accessibility and Collaboration

The use of eCRFs enables access to trial data globally through 24/7 availability on cloud-based platforms. The system enables investigators at different sites to process and view data at exactly the same time instead of waiting for physical document transportation. Sponsors receive real-time visibility of trial progress through platform transparency, which speeds up their decision-making abilities and makes it possible to create adaptive trial designs.

7.7.3 Regulatory Compliance and Audit Readiness

Today's eCRF systems integrate ICH GCP and 21 CFR Part 11 standards into their operation. System features, including audit trails along with electronic signatures and role-based access controls, enable both data integrity and traceability. Events of eCRF data entry modifications get recorded alongside timestamp information and user identification details, which enables simpler regulatory investigation processes.

7.8 ADVANTAGES OF eCRFs IN MODERN CLINICAL TRIALS

Efficiency and Cost Reduction: The elimination of transcription processes alongside time-reduced query responses and faster database lock speeds characterize this format. Electronic Data Capture (EDC) systems use automated workflows that streamline operations to eliminate unnecessary manual data handling, thus reducing expenses.

Improved Data Quality and Security: The implementation of eCRFs uses defined terminology like McdDRA codes with recognized structured formats like dd/mm/yyyy to decrease entry inconsistencies. Cloud storage systems backed by encryption protocols and multi-factor authentication methods create strong defense against data breaches and loss because they protect better than traditional paper record storage.

Regulatory and Industry Shifts: Regulatory agencies now demand electronic submissions, which favor eCRFs because they meet both audit requirements and adhere to FAIR (Findable, Accessible, Interoperable, Reusable) data principles. Both the FDA's Digital Health Center of Excellence and EMA's Data Integrity Guidelines specifically support the use of eCRFs for creating reproducible research outcomes.

7.9 OVERVIEW OF eCRF PLATFORMS AND THEIR CAPABILITIES

Medidata Rave: As an EDC system, Medidata Rave serves a wide range of clinical trial teams to collect and efficiently manage study data. Their realistic custom eCRFs can be adjusted to meet the needs of a particular study, and are especially valuable for a complicated trial like oncology, where the need to track biomarkers and manage complicated dosing schedules is needed. Rave's real-time analytics and low disruption with clinical trial management systems (CTMS) allow teams to see workflows and study development, along with site performance, on a real-time basis. The flexibility enables rapid mid-study adjustment and guarantees that even large-scale trials can be modified fast to adhere to the evolving requirements. Users value the simplicity of the platform due to its single sign-on feature, together with accessible on-demand training and full trial dataset extraction capability at all times. This auto-centric practice has made Rave a well-trusted tool in thousands of studies around the world.

Viedoc: It provides a contemporary, user-friendly interface for clinical data management. Its drag-and-drop form builder makes study setup easy, and offline data entry means that teams do not have to stop working with studies in cases of no stable internet. Viedoc also uses AI for identifying discrepancies in data, ensuring teams are upholding high data quality. The platform is validated on both General Data Protection Regulation (GDPR) and Health Insurance Portability and Accountability Act (HIPAA) compliance, which makes it a good option for multinational trials, where the aspect of data privacy and security is important.

Castor EDC: It is thought out with user-friendliness in mind, thus proving to be especially attractive to academic researchers. It is compatible with REDCap, which is a widely used data management solution in research, and it enables low-code customization options, allowing teams to customize the system to their workflows without knowing much about programming. Castor distinguishes itself with its unique application of natural language processing (NLP), allowing it to obtain the relevant information from the unstructured clinician notes, leading to easy data ingestion, and less manual labor.

OpenClinica: It is an open-source EDC platform that provides a cost-effective solution for smaller biotech companies and academic groups. Its open-source model allows organizations to customize and extend the system as needed. OpenClinica supports exports in the Standard Data Tabulation Model (SDTM), which facilitates regulatory submissions and ensures that data is formatted according to industry standards.

7.10 STORAGE AND ARCHIVING OF PAPER-BASED SYSTEM AND eCRFs (*CLINICAL DATA ARCHIVING*, 2023; EMA, 2017; FDA 21 CFR 312.62, n.d.; FDA 21 CFR PART 11, n.d.; ICH E6(R2), 2016)

7.10.1 Regulatory Guidelines for Storing and Archiving CRFs

Storing and archiving CRFs is critical for ensuring data integrity, regulatory compliance, and audit readiness in clinical trials. Guidelines vary across countries but align with core principles from the ICH GCP. The following is a detailed breakdown of regional regulations. The major regulatory requirements for the storage and archiving of CRFs across different regions are summarized in Table 7.5.

7.10.2 Global Best Practices

The recommended best practices for the storage and archiving of CRFs are summarized in Table 7.6.

TABLE 7.5
Summarizes the Guidelines for CRF Storage and Archiving

Region/Authority	Key Regulations	Storage & Archiving Requirements
United States (FDA)	- 21 CFR Part 11: Requires validation of eCRF systems, audit trails, and electronic signatures. - FDA Guidance on Computerized Systems: Mandates regular backups, role-based access, and verifiable data retrieval from archives.	- Retention period: 2 years after marketing application approval for the investigated indication, or 2 years after investigation discontinuation with FDA notification. - Physical CRFs: Must be stored in secure, climate-controlled facilities with restricted access; original signed documents must be preserved. - eCRFs: Should be archived in non-editable formats (e.g., PDF/A) with metadata (timestamps, user IDs); stored on secure, encrypted platforms compliant with HIPAA. - All changes must be tracked via audit trails.
European Union (EMA)	- EU Annex 11: Requires validation of eCRF systems, audit trails, and periodic backups. - EMA TMF Guideline: Mandates archiving of Trial Master Files (TMFs) for at least 25 years.	- eTMF Systems: Must use role-based permissions and prevent any changes after archiving; metadata and audit trails must be stored as usable datasets. - Physical CRFs: Labeled and stored in secure, environmentally controlled locations. - Third-Party Archiving: Sponsors are responsible for data integrity, even if storage is outsourced to clinical research organizations (CROs).

TABLE 7.6
Recommended Best Practices for the Storage and Archiving of CRFs

Practice	Details
Standardization	Use coded answer sets (e.g., MedDRA for AEs) and consistent date formats (dd/mm/yyyy) to ensure uniformity and facilitate data retrieval.
Third-Party Archiving	Engage reputable storage providers (such as Grace Records Management) to ensure compliance with local regulations (e.g., Australia's 10 kg box limit for physical records).
Migration Protocols	Convert dynamic files (like Excel spreadsheets) to static, long-term formats (such as PDF/A) to preserve data integrity and facilitate future access.

7.10.3 Best Practices for eCRF Implementation

The recommended strategies for effective implementation of eCRFs in clinical trials are summarized in Table 7.7.

TABLE 7.7
Recommended Strategies for Effective Electronic eCRF Implementation

Category	Best Practice	Description
Design and Validation	Protocol Alignment	Ensure eCRF fields are directly mapped to study endpoints to avoid redundant data collection.
	Pilot Testing	Test the eCRF with site staff to evaluate the effectiveness of skip logic and clarity of instructions.
Training and Compliance	Role-Based Training	Provide tailored training for different roles, such as data managers (validation rules) and site coordinators (data entry).
	Continuous Monitoring	Use real-time dashboards to track missing data, query rates, and protocol deviations.
Data Correction	Error Handling	Implement edit checks to prevent invalid entries and allow corrections within the system, maintaining a complete audit trail.

7.11 REGULATORY GUIDELINES FOR eCRFs IN CLINICAL TRIALS

The data, safety, and readiness of using eCRFs are overseen by the U.S. FDA, EMA, and International Council for Harmonisation (ICH), which create strict rules for their use.

Several significant rules oversee how eCRFs are built. In the US, 21 CFR Part 11 requires that systems be validated, audits leave solid trails, and electronic signatures guarantee data is real. According to the EU's Annex 11, all changes important to Good Manufacturing Practice (GMP) must be logged in an audit trail, and it is required to document the rationale for deleting data. The guideline E6(R2) as part of the ICH GCP provides that eCRF must be consistent with the study protocol and automatically check the accuracy of the data. Overall, these rules demand that eCRFs are built to correspond with the protocol endpoints, and this significantly cuts down on entering more data than necessary and helps to use standard modules where possible.

The website/software also needs to be arranged to suit users' needs. The rules for compliance suggest that UIs be easy to understand, entry fields be organized logically, and data re-entry through skip logic should be reduced. With checkboxes and date pickers helping, along with responses that are set in advance (for instance, yes/no), users are more likely to complete the form with accurate data. It is necessary to have real-time validation so that outliers and missing details, such as unusually high systolic blood pressure, are spotted, and changes are made before data is submitted. Any updates to the eCRF should be tagged with the person making the changes, when it happened, and the reason, so a full audit trail is there.

Developing rules for finishing eCRF forms, checking entered information against original data, and dealing with data gaps are all part of the preparation process. Working as a team, clinicians, data managers, and statisticians ensure that the eCRFs fulfill analysis needs and meet regulations. Validating computer system validation (CSV) is required to demonstrate that eCRF systems meet the standards in FDA 21 CFR Part 11 and EU Annex 11.

When data is entered, SDV checks that the eCRF entries agree with the original laboratory or medical records. All team members must learn to handle the eCRF systems, knowledge of standard terms and methods for handling errors. All important fields should be shown in bold or otherwise highlighted, and there should be a clear progression for data entry. Both automated reminders and verified data during the process minimize long waits and missing information.

Error correction protocols have very strict regulations. Any change made to the system should be recorded using an audit trail that adds the time, who made the changes, and the reason. All post-submission updates must have an electronic signature, which helps ensure no one changes the records without being noticed. Changing or deleting entries is not permitted; ensure mistakes are identified and fixed clearly while still saving the original details for audit reasons.

Data in eCRFs should be ensured through encryption and validated access, just as the laws GDPR and HIPAA demand. Backups should be stored in different places and uneditable formats (PDF/A), while analysis is done with files that can be edited (ODM XML). Depending on therapy and location, most records are kept for 25 to 30 years. Sometimes, sponsors can use third-party ecosystems to archive data, though they are still responsible for its security and compliance with laws.

These auditing and inspection processes are based on the ALCOA (Attributable, Legible, Contemporaneous, Original, and Accurate) guidelines, which set rules for data to be attributable, legible, contemporaneous, original, and accurate. Any discrepancies have to be sorted before the database lock, and both audit trails and relevant source documents should be available within 48 hours for inspection by regulators. Continual review of errors and delays in the system helps monitor its performance and always ensures the site stays in compliance.

7.12 FUTURE TRENDS

CRF's future trends are being driven very strongly by technology advances and changing clinical trial ways. An even more exciting prospect for CRF processes is the integration of artificial intelligence (AI) and machine learning in CRF processes, expected to reduce the study duration by as much as 30% of the initial timeline and reduce the required operational costs by 20% (enhancing the accuracy of data and efficiency). Defining trends include the expansion of decentralized clinical trials (DCTs) that promote the use of digital platforms and wearable devices, more efficient remote data capture, and better patient access and diversity of participant compositions in trial populations. Adaptive trial designs, enabled by the use of eCRFs to collect real-time data, allow a more adaptable and individualized study protocol. In addition, blockchain technology is becoming a tool to maintain data integrity and transparency during the CRF lifecycle. These innovations as a whole encourage streamlined, standardized, and patient-focused data capture techniques, which in turn expedite drug development and enhance clinical trial results.

REFERENCES

9 Tips to Design Better Case Report Forms (CRFs) for Clinical Trials - Klindat. n.d. Retrieved March 16, 2026, from https://www.klindat.com/9-tips-to-design-better-case-report-forms-crfs-for-clinical-trials/.

Bellary, S.; Krishnankutty, B. & Latha, M. 2014. "Basics of case report form designing in clinical research". *Perspectives in Clinical Research* 5 (4): 159. https://doi.org/10.4103/2229-3485.140555.

Case Form Report Design SOP - King's Health Partners Clinical Trials Office. n.d. Retrieved March 16, 2026, from https://khpcto.co.uk/standard-operating-procedures/case-report-form-design/.

Case Report Form - Clinical Research Explained | VIARES. n.d. Retrieved March 16, 2026, from https://viares.com/blog/clinical-research-explained/case-report-form/.

Case Report Form (CRF) Binder/Electronic Case Report Form (eCRF) | Social Science Research Institute. n.d. Retrieved March 16, 2026, from https://ssri.psu.edu/clinicalresearchguidebook/case-report-form-crf-binderelectronic-case-report-form-ecrf.

Clinical Data Archiving. 2023. https://doi.org/10.47912/jscdm.323.

Dixon, J. R. 1998. "The international conference on harmonization good clinical practice guideline". *Quality Assurance* 6 (2): 65–74. https://doi.org/10.1080/105294199277860.

EMA. 2017. *Guideline on the content, management and archiving of the clinical trial master file*. www.ema.europa.eu/contact.

FDA 21 CFR 312.62. n.d. *eCFR :: 21 CFR 312.62 -- Investigator recordkeeping and record retention*. Retrieved March 16, 2026, from https://www.ecfr.gov/current/title-21/chapter-I/subchapter-D/part-312/subpart-D/section-312.62.

FDA 21 CFR Part 11. n.d. *eCFR :: 21 CFR Part 11 -- Electronic Records; Electronic Signatures*. Retrieved March 16, 2026, from https://www.ecfr.gov/current/title-21/chapter-I/subchapter-A/part-11

ICH E6(R2). 2016. International council for harmonisation of technical requirements for pharmaceuticals for human use (ICH) ICH harmonised guideline integrated addendum to ICH E6(R1): Guideline for good clinical practice E6(R2).

Richesson, R. L. & Nadkarni, P. 2011. "Data standards for clinical research data collection forms: current status and challenges". *Journal of the American Medical Informatics Association : JAMIA* 18 (3): 341. https://doi.org/10.1136/amiajnl-2011-000107.

Tips to Design an Optimal Case Report Form. n.d. Retrieved March 16, 2026, from https://www.linical.com/articles-research/tips-to-design-an-optimal-crf.

What is a Case Report Form? | Novotech CRO. n.d. Retrieved March 16, 2026, from https://novotech-cro.com/faq/what-case-report-form.

8 Study Designs Used in Clinical Research

Haya Majid[1] *and Seema Jain*[2]
[1]Department of Translational and Clinical Research, School of Chemical and Life Sciences, Jamia Hamdard, New Delhi, India
[2]Department of Pharmacology, University College of Medical Sciences & GTB Hospital, New Delhi, India

8.1 INTRODUCTION

A study design is a structured framework that outlines how a clinical or scientific study is conducted to address a specific research question. A well-structured study design is essential for ensuring that research is conducted systematically, ethically, and efficiently. The selection of an appropriate study design depends on factors such as the research question, ethical considerations, resource availability, and feasibility. It serves as a blueprint for guiding researchers in data collection, analysis, and interpretation, ultimately determining the reliability and validity of study findings.

Choosing the right study design is crucial for effectively answering research questions, minimizing bias, ensuring reproducibility, and maximizing the research impact. A robust design enhances the credibility of findings by providing a structured methodology, enabling systematic data collection, and ensuring accurate measurement of variables. Without a well-defined design, research outcomes may be inconsistent, leading to unreliable conclusions.

Ethical considerations are particularly vital in clinical research, especially when human participants are involved. A well-planned study design ensures adherence to ethical guidelines, including obtaining informed consent, minimizing risks to participants, and ensuring fair treatment allocation. Institutional Review Boards (IRBs) and Ethics Committees review study designs to ensure compliance with ethical standards before granting approval. Poor study design can expose participants to unnecessary risks and lead to ethical violations (Chidambaram and Josephson 2019).

8.2 STUDY DESIGNS INVOLVED IN CLINICAL RESEARCH

8.2.1 Observational Study Design

Observational study design is a fundamental approach in clinical and epidemiological research where researchers observe and analyze data without intervening in the participants' exposures or treatments. These studies are used to understand disease patterns, identify risk factors, and generate hypotheses for further experimental research. Observational studies are particularly useful when ethical or practical constraints make experimental studies unfeasible. Observational study designs can be broadly classified into descriptive studies and analytical studies (Lu 2009).

8.2.2 Descriptive Observational Studies

Descriptive observational study designs aim to characterize the distribution, patterns, and prevalence of diseases or exposures within a specific population. Unlike analytical studies, they do not establish causal relationships but provide foundational data for hypothesis generation and further

DOI: 10.1201/9781003533085-8

research. These studies are particularly useful for identifying trends, assessing healthcare needs, and informing policy decisions. They focus on the "what," "who," "where," and "when" aspects of health-related phenomena, providing a detailed account of disease frequency and distribution without manipulating variables or determining causality. Descriptive studies help researchers and healthcare professionals understand disease burden, track outbreaks, and identify at-risk populations. For example, during an infectious disease outbreak, these studies served as the initial step in gathering data on case numbers, geographic spread, affected demographics, and potential transmission sources. The data gained can then guide more rigorous analytical studies to explore risk factors and interventions. Descriptive observational studies can be categorized into case reports, case series, cross-sectional studies, and ecological studies, each serving a distinct role in clinical and epidemiological research. While they do not establish causality, they provide essential preliminary data that generate hypotheses for further investigation, ultimately contributing to a deeper understanding of public health concerns (Aggarwal and Ranganathan 2019b).

8.2.3 Case Reports

A case report is a detailed account of a single patient presenting with an unusual or novel condition. It is commonly used to highlight rare diseases, unexpected complications, or unique treatment responses. Case reports provide critical clinical information and contribute to the early identification of emerging health issues. For instance, during the early stages of the COVID-19 pandemic, several case reports documented atypical symptoms such as loss of taste and smell, which later became hallmark features of the disease. While case reports are limited by their reliance on a single observation and lack of generalizability, they play a crucial role in medical literature by alerting the healthcare community to new or rare conditions, potentially guiding further research and clinical practice (Sayre et al. 2017).

8.2.4 Case Series

A case series builds upon the case report model by describing multiple patients with similar conditions or characteristics. It offers more comprehensive information than a single case report and can help identify potential patterns or emerging trends in clinical practice. For example, a case series documenting adverse reactions to a newly approved drug can serve as an early warning signal for regulatory agencies, prompting further investigation. However, since case series lack a control group, it cannot establish causal relationships or determine the true incidence of a condition. Despite this limitation, it plays a crucial role in generating hypotheses for future analytical studies (Sayre et al. 2017).

8.2.5 Cross-Sectional Studies

A cross-sectional study, also known as a prevalence study, collects data at a single point in time to assess the frequency of a disease or exposure within a population. It provides a snapshot of health status, behaviors, and risk factors at a given moment. For example, a cross-sectional study on diabetes prevalence might survey a population to determine the percentage of individuals with high blood glucose levels. These studies are widely used in public health to monitor disease prevalence, assess healthcare needs, and inform policy decisions. However, since cross-sectional studies do not track changes over time, they cannot establish cause-and-effect relationships between exposure and outcome (X. Wang and Cheng 2020).

8.2.6 Ecological Studies

An ecological study examines the relationship between exposures and health outcomes at a population or group level rather than at an individual level. These studies use aggregated data, such as national health records, census data, or environmental exposure levels, to identify potential associations. For instance, an ecological study might explore the relationship between air pollution levels and asthma prevalence across different cities. While these studies can generate important hypotheses, they are prone to ecological fallacy, where assumptions about individuals are incorrectly derived from population-level data ("Chapter 6. Ecological Studies" 2025; Morgenstern 1995).

8.3 STRENGTHS OF DESCRIPTIVE STUDY DESIGN

One of the primary strengths of this study design is its ability to generate hypotheses for future research. Since descriptive studies focus on documenting patterns, trends, and frequencies of diseases or health-related conditions, they serve as a foundation for analytical studies that seek to identify causes and associations. For example, a cross-sectional study that identifies a high prevalence of obesity in a particular demographic group can lead to further research on lifestyle, diet, and genetic factors contributing to obesity.

Another major advantage of descriptive studies is that they are relatively quick and cost-effective compared to analytical or experimental study designs. Since they often rely on existing medical records, surveys, or public health data, they do not require long follow-up periods or extensive resources. This makes them particularly useful for public health monitoring, such as tracking disease outbreaks or assessing vaccination coverage in a community. For instance, case reports and case series provide immediate information about rare diseases or adverse drug reactions, allowing healthcare professionals to respond quickly.

Additionally, descriptive studies are useful for public health planning and policy-making because they help identify high-risk populations, geographic disease patterns, and emerging health threats. Government agencies and health organizations frequently use these studies to design targeted interventions. For example, if a cross-sectional study identifies high rates of smoking among teenagers in a specific region, public health officials can develop anti-smoking campaigns tailored to that group.

Descriptive studies also have the advantage of being ethically less complex compared to experimental studies. Since these studies do not involve active interventions, they do not pose direct risks to participants. This makes them particularly useful for studying vulnerable populations, such as children, pregnant women, or individuals with chronic diseases, where experimental studies might be ethically challenging.

8.3.1 Limitations of Descriptive Study Design

Despite their many strengths, descriptive studies have several limitations that affect their ability to provide definitive conclusions. The most significant limitation is their inability to establish causality between an exposure and an outcome. Since these studies do not involve manipulation of variables or long-term follow-up, they can only describe associations but cannot determine whether one factor causes another. For example, a cross-sectional study may show that people who consume high amounts of sugar have a higher prevalence of diabetes, but it cannot prove that sugar consumption directly leads to diabetes. Other factors, such as genetics or lack of physical activity, may contribute to the observed association.

Another major drawback is the risk of bias, particularly selection bias and reporting bias. In case reports and case series, researchers may choose to document only unusual or severe cases, leading to a distorted representation of a disease. Similarly, in survey-based descriptive studies, participants may provide inaccurate or socially desirable responses, affecting data accuracy. For example, self-reported studies on alcohol consumption often underestimate actual drinking habits due to social stigma.

Descriptive studies also suffer from limited generalizability because they often focus on specific populations or settings. Findings from a case series conducted in a single hospital may not be applicable to the general population. Likewise, an ecological study that examines disease trends at a national level may not reflect individual-level risks accurately, leading to what is known as the ecological fallacy—where associations observed at the group level are incorrectly assumed to apply to individuals.

Furthermore, cross-sectional studies, which are commonly used in descriptive research, provide only a snapshot in time and do not account for changes over time. This limits their ability to track disease progression or long-term outcomes. For example, a cross-sectional study on mental health during a pandemic may indicate high levels of anxiety and depression, but it cannot determine whether these conditions are temporary or persistent. Longitudinal studies are needed to assess how mental health evolves over time.

Lastly, descriptive studies lack control groups, making it difficult to distinguish between real associations and random occurrences. Without a comparative group, it is challenging to determine whether an observed health trend is due to a specific factor or simply part of natural variation. For instance, an increase in flu cases in a city might be attributed to a new virus strain, but without comparing data from other regions, researchers cannot rule out other factors like seasonal variation or increased testing (Aggarwal and Ranganathan 2019b).

8.4 ANALYTICAL OBSERVATIONAL STUDIES

Analytical study designs determine associations and possible causal relationships between exposures (such as risk factors, treatments, or environmental conditions) and health outcomes (such as diseases or adverse events). Unlike descriptive studies, which focus on describing disease patterns and health conditions without investigating relationships, analytical studies seek to establish statistical associations between variables and evaluate the strength of these relationships. These study designs are essential in understanding disease etiology, assessing treatment effectiveness, and shaping healthcare policies. Analytical studies are broadly classified into observational and experimental (interventional) studies (Ranganathan and Aggarwal 2019).

8.4.1 Case-Control Studies

A case-control study is an observational study that compares individuals with a specific disease or outcome (cases) to individuals without the disease (controls) to determine differences in past exposures. Unlike cohort studies, which follow participants over time to observe disease development, case-control studies work in reverse by identifying disease cases first and then looking at previous risk factors. The primary measure of association in case-control studies is the odds ratio (OR), which estimates the likelihood of disease in exposed versus unexposed individuals. For example, a case-control study investigating the association between smoking and lung cancer would compare the smoking history of lung cancer patients (cases) with that of individuals without lung cancer (controls). If smoking is significantly more prevalent among cases, it suggests an association between smoking and lung cancer.

8.4.1.1 Study Design and Methodology

The first step in a case-control study is selecting appropriate cases and controls. Cases should be individuals who have been accurately diagnosed with the disease under investigation, often selected from hospitals, clinics, or disease registries. Proper diagnostic criteria must be established to ensure all cases truly have the condition being studied. Controls should represent the population from which the cases arose but should not have the disease. The selection of controls can be hospital-based, population-based, or matched (one-to-one matching based on specific characteristics).

Data collection in case-control studies is primarily retrospective but may also be performed in prospective settings, involving medical records, patient interviews, surveys, or laboratory tests. Since data relies majorly on past exposures, recall bias—differences in how cases and controls remember past exposures—is a major concern. Statistical analysis is conducted using odds ratios

(ORs) to determine the strength of the association between an exposure and an outcome. If OR > 1, the exposure is positively associated with the disease (i.e., it may be a risk factor). If OR < 1, the exposure is negatively associated with the disease (i.e., it may be protective). If OR = 1, there is no association between the exposure and the disease. Advanced statistical techniques like logistic regression are often used to adjust for confounding factors that might distort the results.

8.4.1.2 Strengths of Case-Control Studies

One of the biggest advantages of case-control studies is that they are efficient for studying rare diseases or conditions with long latency periods. Since researchers start with cases, they do not need to follow a large population over time, making the study more feasible. Another advantage is that case-control studies are relatively quick and cost-effective compared to cohort studies or randomized controlled trials (RCTs). They require fewer participants, less time, and lower costs since they often rely on existing records or recall data, avoiding lengthy follow-up periods. Additionally, these studies allow researchers to examine multiple risk factors for a single disease, making them highly versatile. For example, a study on breast cancer can assess diet, genetic factors, hormone therapy, and lifestyle habits simultaneously. Ethically, case-control studies are less complex than experimental studies since they do not require researchers to expose individuals to harmful conditions, making them particularly useful in scenarios where experimental studies would be unethical.

8.4.1.3 Limitations of Case-Control Studies

Despite their advantages, case-control studies have several limitations. One major drawback is the potential for bias, particularly recall bias (cases may overestimate or underestimate past exposures) and selection bias (if controls are not properly selected, they may not accurately represent the general population). Another limitation is that case-control studies cannot establish causality—they can only suggest associations. Because the exposure data is collected after disease development, it is often unclear whether the exposure preceded the disease or was a consequence of it. Additionally, unlike cohort studies that allow researchers to track multiple outcomes from a single exposure, case-control studies are limited to investigating one disease at a time. These studies are particularly useful for investigating rare diseases or conditions with long latency periods, such as cancer (Tenny et al. 2023).

8.4.2 Cohort Studies

A cohort study follows groups of people over time to assess how different exposures influence health outcomes. Cohort study design is one of the most widely used observational analytical study designs in clinical and epidemiological research. Unlike case-control studies, which start with an outcome and look back at exposures, cohort studies begin with an exposure and follow participants over time to observe the development of outcomes. This design allows researchers to establish temporal relationships between risk factors and diseases, making cohort studies one of the strongest observational methods for inferring causality. Cohort studies are particularly useful for studying disease incidence, natural history, risk factors, and long-term health effects of exposures. Cohort studies can be classified into two main types based on the direction of data collection: prospective cohort studies and retrospective cohort studies.

In prospective cohort studies, researchers may start by selecting a group of individuals who are initially disease-free and then follow them over time to record exposures and subsequent health outcomes. These studies collect real-time data as events unfold, allowing for precise measurement of exposures and reducing recall bias. A classic example of a prospective cohort study is the Framingham Heart Study, which began in 1948 and followed thousands of participants over decades to assess risk factors for cardiovascular disease. While prospective studies provide stronger evidence for causality, they are expensive, time-consuming, and require long-term follow-up (Mahmood et al. 2013).

In retrospective cohort studies, researchers use historical data to classify participants based on past exposures and then analyze their health outcomes. These studies rely on pre-existing records, such as hospital databases, medical charts, or employment records, to reconstruct exposure histories. An example is a study examining the long-term effects of radiation exposure in nuclear power plant workers by analyzing their medical records over the past 20 years. Retrospective cohort studies are faster and less expensive than prospective studies, but they are prone to recall bias, incomplete records, and less control over data quality (Kitamura et al. 2022).

8.4.2.1 Study Design and Methodology

The first step in a cohort study is selecting the study population. Ideally, the cohort should be representative of the population at risk and should include individuals who are free from the outcome of interest at the start of the study, or they may be the population that are diseased or under intervention, based on what the researcher wants to check. The cohort is then divided into exposed and unexposed groups. To minimize bias, researchers often use matching techniques to ensure the exposed and unexposed groups are comparable in terms of age, gender, socioeconomic status, and other confounding variables.

Cohort studies collect longitudinal data on participants, including their exposure levels, health behaviors, disease, and intervention outcomes. Data collection methods include medical records, direct measurements (e.g., blood pressure, cholesterol levels), questionnaires, interviews, and environmental assessments.

Cohort studies use statistical measures such as Relative Risk (RR) to determine the strength of the association between an exposure and an outcome. If $RR > 1$, the exposure is associated with increased disease risk, whereas if $RR < 1$, the exposure may have a protective effect. Attributable Risk (AR) measures the excess risk of disease due to exposure, and survival analysis is often used to assess the time until an event (e.g., disease diagnosis) occurs. Advanced statistical techniques like Cox proportional hazards models are commonly employed to adjust for confounding factors and strengthen causal inferences.

8.4.2.2 Advantages of Cohort Studies

One of the biggest advantages of cohort studies is that they establish temporal relationships since exposures are measured before disease onset. This makes them stronger than case-control studies for inferring causality. Additionally, cohort studies allow the study of multiple outcomes from a single exposure. For example, a cohort of smokers can be studied not only for lung cancer but also for cardiovascular disease and chronic obstructive pulmonary disease (COPD). Another advantage is that recall bias is minimized in prospective cohort studies since data is collected in real-time rather than relying on participants' memories. These studies also directly measure disease incidence and provide absolute risk estimates, making them valuable for public health planning.

8.4.2.3 Limitations of Cohort Studies

They are expensive and time-consuming, requiring large sample sizes and long-term follow-up. Loss to follow-up (attrition bias) is a common issue, as participants may drop out due to relocation, loss of interest, or death, potentially affecting the validity of results. Cohort studies are also not ideal for rare diseases because they require a large population to detect sufficient cases, making them inefficient for studying conditions with very low incidence. Another limitation is confounding, where other variables may influence the association between exposure and outcome. Even with statistical adjustments, unmeasured confounders can still affect results. Retrospective cohort studies, in particular, face data quality issues, as they rely on pre-existing records that may be incomplete or inconsistent (Capili and Anastasi 2021).

8.4.3 Interventional (Experimental) Study Designs

Interventional, or experimental, study designs are considered the gold standard in clinical research for establishing causal relationships between an exposure (such as a drug, medical procedure, or lifestyle intervention) and a health outcome. Unlike observational studies (such as cohort or case-control studies), where researchers passively observe participants, interventional studies involve actively assigning interventions to study participants. These studies are primarily used in clinical trials to assess the safety and efficacy of new treatments, drugs, vaccines, or medical devices before they are approved for widespread use.

The fundamental feature of experimental studies is the manipulation of independent variables under controlled conditions, allowing researchers to isolate the effects of the intervention from other confounding factors. Experimental studies also employ randomization, blinding, and control groups to minimize bias and increase the validity of results. These characteristics make interventional study designs the most reliable form of evidence for making clinical and public health decisions (Aggarwal and Ranganathan 2019a, 2019c).

8.4.4 Randomized Controlled Trials

Randomized Controlled Trials (RCTs) are considered the gold standard in clinical and medical research for evaluating the safety and effectiveness of interventions such as drugs, vaccines, medical devices, surgical procedures, and behavioral therapies. Unlike observational studies, which rely on natural exposure to risk factors or treatments, RCTs involve deliberate intervention where participants are assigned to different treatment groups in a controlled manner. The key feature of RCTs is randomization, which ensures that the groups being compared are similar in all respects except for the intervention received.

RCTs play a crucial role in evidence-based medicine and are essential for obtaining regulatory approval for new treatments by agencies such as the U.S. Food and Drug Administration (FDA), European Medicines Agency (EMA), and Central Drugs Standard Control Organisation (CDSCO) in India. These trials are structured to minimize bias, control for confounding variables, and establish causality, making them the most reliable type of clinical research for determining treatment efficacy.

It is an experimental study in which participants are randomly assigned to two or more groups to receive different treatments. Typically, there is an intervention group, which receives the treatment under investigation, and a control group, which may receive a placebo, standard treatment, or no intervention. The primary goal of an RCT is to compare outcomes between these groups to determine whether the new treatment is superior, equivalent, or inferior to the current standard of care.

Key features of RCTs include randomization, blinding, control groups, and pre-specified outcomes. Randomization ensures that participants are assigned to groups without bias, preventing systematic differences between groups at the start of the study. Blinding (or masking) is used to prevent biases by ensuring that participants, healthcare providers, or researchers do not know which treatment is being administered. Control groups serve as a benchmark for evaluating the intervention's true effect, and pre-specified outcomes ensure that researchers measure relevant health changes systematically (Hariton and Locascio 2018).

8.4.4.1 Parallel-Group RCTs

In a parallel-group RCT, participants are randomly assigned to separate groups, and each group receives a specific intervention throughout the study. The key characteristic of this design is that each participant remains in their assigned group for the entire duration of the trial, allowing for direct comparison between different treatment arms. This design is particularly useful for studying conditions that require long-term treatment, such as chronic diseases (e.g., diabetes, hypertension, and cancer), where measuring sustained effects is crucial.

The first step in the study design is the selection of participants, where eligible individuals meeting specific inclusion and exclusion criteria are recruited. These criteria help define the study population and ensure that the results are applicable to a broader clinical setting. Once participants are enrolled, they are randomly assigned to different groups, ensuring that each participant has an equal chance of being allocated to any treatment arm. Randomization helps eliminate selection bias and ensures that known and unknown confounding factors are evenly distributed between groups. After randomization, each group receives one specific intervention. For example, in a two-group parallel RCT evaluating a new antihypertensive drug, one group would receive the new drug while the other group receives a placebo or standard treatment. Participants remain in their assigned groups for the entire duration of the study, and the researchers monitor the effects of the treatment at pre-specified intervals. The primary and secondary outcomes, such as changes in blood pressure, adverse effects, and overall health improvements, are recorded and analyzed to determine the effectiveness of the intervention. To improve the reliability of the results, blinding (masking) is often incorporated into parallel-group RCTs. Single-blind studies conceal treatment allocation from participants to reduce psychological biases, while double-blind studies conceal allocation from both participants and researchers to prevent observer bias. In some cases, triple-blind trials ensure that data analysts are also unaware of group assignments, further eliminating bias during statistical analysis ("Parallel Design/Parallel Group Study—Statistics How To" 2025; Hariton and Locascio 2018; Aggarwal and Ranganathan 2019c, 2019a).

8.4.4.2 Crossover RCTs

Unlike parallel-group RCTs, where participants remain in one assigned treatment group for the entire study, crossover RCTs allow each participant to receive multiple treatments at different time points. This means that every participant serves as their own control, improving the precision of comparisons between interventions. Crossover RCTs are particularly useful in studying chronic conditions, pharmacological treatments, and behavioral interventions where the effects of treatment are reversible and do not result in permanent changes. By minimizing between-subject variability, these trials provide more statistically powerful results with a smaller sample size compared to traditional parallel-group RCTs. However, their design requires careful planning, as they are vulnerable to issues such as carryover effects and period effects, which can influence study outcomes.

The defining feature of a crossover RCT is that each participant undergoes multiple treatment conditions, typically in a randomized sequence. The trial is conducted in distinct phases, with a washout period between treatments to allow for the effects of the first intervention to dissipate before administering the next. This washout period is critical in ensuring that residual effects from the first treatment do not influence the outcomes of the second treatment. Participants are randomly assigned to different treatment sequences to avoid selection bias. A break between treatment periods ensures that residual effects do not interfere with subsequent treatments.

A standard crossover RCT consists of two periods where:

- Half of the participants receive Treatment A first, followed by Treatment B after a washout period.
- The other half receives Treatment B first, followed by Treatment A after a washout period.

For example, in a study evaluating two pain medications, Drug X and Drug Y, patients would be randomized into two sequences:

- Sequence 1: Drug X → Washout → Drug Y
- Sequence 2: Drug Y → Washout → Drug X

Since each participant receives both treatments, comparisons between interventions are within-subject, eliminating inter-individual variability that often affects parallel-group trials. This means that the study can detect smaller differences between treatments with fewer participants, making crossover RCTs more efficient and statistically significant.

One of the biggest advantages of crossover RCTs is their increased statistical power. Since participants act as their own controls, variability between subjects is reduced, making it easier to detect treatment differences with a smaller sample size. This makes crossover trials particularly useful in studies with limited patient populations, such as rare diseases or personalized medicine research. Another key benefit is greater efficiency in treatment comparisons because each participant receives multiple treatments; fewer individuals are required to achieve meaningful results, reducing the overall cost and duration of the trial. Additionally, since all participants receive both interventions, ethical concerns regarding placebo use are minimized, as every participant is guaranteed access to an active treatment at some point during the study. Crossover RCTs are also ideal for evaluating pharmacological treatments, particularly in dose-response studies where researchers need to compare different drug dosages within the same individuals. These studies provide valuable insights into optimal dosing regimens, drug interactions, and personalized medicine approaches.

Despite their advantages, crossover RCTs have several limitations that must be carefully managed. One major challenge is the carryover effect, where residual effects from the first treatment influence responses to the second treatment. If the washout period is not long enough, lingering drug effects or physiological adaptations can bias the results. For example, in a trial studying the effects of a long-acting diabetes medication, an insufficient washout period might result in the second treatment being affected by the first, leading to misleading conclusions.

Another limitation is the period effect, where changes in a participant's health or external conditions over time can influence treatment responses. For example, in a study assessing treatments for seasonal allergies, symptoms might naturally improve or worsen due to changes in environmental pollen levels, making it difficult to attribute differences to the intervention alone.

Crossover trials are also not suitable for all medical conditions, particularly those involving permanent or long-term effects. If a treatment leads to irreversible changes (such as surgery, vaccination, or gene therapy), a crossover design is inappropriate, as participants cannot "switch back" to their original state. Similarly, conditions that have a progressive course, such as Alzheimer's disease or cancer, are not ideal for crossover trials, as disease progression over time can confound treatment effects. Another practical limitation is longer trial duration. Since each participant receives multiple treatments with washout periods in between, crossover trials take more time to complete than parallel-group trials. This can lead to increased patient dropout rates, particularly in studies involving lengthy follow-up periods (Sambandan and Turcu-Stiolica 2018; "Crossover Study—an Overview | ScienceDirect Topics" 2025).

8.4.4.3 Cluster-Randomized Trials

Cluster-randomized trials (CRTs), also known as group-randomized trials, are a unique type of RCT in which entire groups, rather than individual participants, are randomly assigned to different interventions. This design is commonly used in public health, epidemiology, education, and healthcare system research, where interventions are naturally delivered at the community or institutional level rather than to individuals. CRTs are particularly useful for evaluating behavioral interventions, policy changes, health education programs, and vaccination strategies, where it is impractical or inefficient to randomize individuals within a population. The defining characteristic of CRTs is that randomization occurs at the cluster level—such as schools, hospitals, villages, workplaces, or entire communities—instead of at the individual level. This approach reduces contamination, which occurs when individuals in different treatment groups interact and inadvertently receive parts of each other's interventions. However, CRTs also introduce statistical challenges, such as intra-cluster correlation, which must be accounted for during study design and analysis.

The design of a cluster-randomized trial follows the same fundamental principles as an individual-level RCT but differs in how participants are grouped and assigned to interventions. The first step in a CRT is the selection of clusters, which are often naturally occurring groups. Once clusters are identified, they are randomly assigned to receive either the intervention or control condition. This means that all individuals within a given cluster receive the same intervention, ensuring that the effects of the intervention are evaluated at a group level.

For example, in a school-based nutrition program, entire schools may be randomized to receive either a new dietary intervention or the standard school meal program. This allows researchers to evaluate whether changes in school meal policies lead to improved student health outcomes without the risk of contamination between students in the same school. Similarly, in community vaccination programs, villages may be assigned to different vaccine rollout strategies, allowing researchers to compare coverage rates, disease prevention, and public acceptance across different groups. After cluster randomization, researchers collect data at both the cluster and individual levels to measure outcomes. Since individuals within the same cluster tend to be more similar to each other than to individuals in other clusters, statistical adjustments are required to account for intra-cluster correlation (ICC). The ICC represents the degree of similarity among individuals within a cluster and affects the required sample size—higher ICC values mean that more clusters are needed to achieve statistical significance.

In standard RCTs, individuals in different treatment groups may interact, leading to unintended exposure to the intervention. This is especially problematic in behavioral or educational studies, where participants in the control group might learn about the intervention and modify their behavior. CRTs eliminate this issue by ensuring that everyone within a cluster experiences the same intervention conditions. CRTs are also ethically favorable in certain situations. In interventions that require system-wide changes, such as improving access to mental health care or modifying food supply chains in schools, it would be unfair or impractical to provide the intervention to only some individuals while withholding it from others in the same setting. Cluster randomization ensures that all individuals within a given institution or community receive the same treatment, preventing ethical concerns related to selective treatment access.

Another strength of CRTs is their cost-effectiveness. Since interventions are administered to groups rather than individuals, CRTs often require fewer resources per participant than individual-level RCTs. This makes them particularly useful for large-scale public health research, vaccine trials, and policy evaluations, where conducting individual-level randomization would be impractical.

Despite their advantages, CRTs come with several challenges that must be carefully addressed. One of the biggest concerns is intra-cluster correlation (ICC), which arises because individuals within the same cluster tend to be more similar to each other than to individuals in other clusters. This reduces the statistical independence of observations, requiring larger sample sizes compared to individual-level RCTs. Researchers must account for ICC during study design, sample size calculation, and statistical analysis to avoid misleading results. Another challenge is the loss of statistical power due to cluster randomization. Because randomization occurs at the group level rather than the individual level, there are fewer units of randomization, which reduces the ability to detect small but meaningful effects. To compensate for this, researchers often need to increase the number of clusters, which can make CRTs logistically complex and expensive. CRTs also face challenges related to cluster variability. Differences between clusters, such as geographical location, socioeconomic factors, healthcare access, and cultural practices, can introduce bias and affect study outcomes. This is particularly relevant in multi-site or multi-country trials, where external factors may vary significantly across clusters. Stratified randomization or adjusting for baseline differences using statistical models can help mitigate these effects, but these adjustments add complexity to data analysis. Finally, CRTs may encounter ethical challenges related to consent. In some cases, interventions affect an entire population within a cluster, meaning individuals may not have a choice in whether they participate in the study. For example, if a hospital implements a new infection control protocol as part of a CRT, all patients and healthcare workers within that hospital are affected, regardless of whether they consented to be part of the research. Ensuring transparent ethical oversight, community engagement, and institutional approvals is essential to conducting ethical CRTs (Dron et al. 2021).

8.4.4.4 Factorial RCT

Factorial RCTs are an advanced type of experimental study design that allows researchers to evaluate the effects of multiple interventions simultaneously within the same study. Unlike traditional

RCTs, factorial RCTs test the independent and combined effects of two or more interventions in a structured manner. This design enhances the efficiency of clinical trials by maximizing the information gained from a single study, making it particularly useful in drug development, public health interventions, and behavioral research. Factorial RCTs are widely used when researchers suspect that two treatments may interact with each other, meaning that the combination of both treatments may produce different effects than each treatment alone. By allowing for the simultaneous assessment of multiple interventions, factorial RCTs help identify synergistic, additive, or antagonistic interactions between treatments, leading to more precise and informative conclusions.

The defining characteristic of a factorial RCT is that participants are randomly assigned to multiple treatment combinations, creating different study arms that allow researchers to assess both individual and combined treatment effects. The most common type is the 2×2 factorial design, in which two interventions (A and B) are tested, leading to four groups:

Group 1: Receives neither intervention (control group).
Group 2: Receives only Intervention A.
Group 3: Receives only Intervention B.
Group 4: Receives both Interventions A and B.

For example, in a study assessing the effects of aspirin and omega-3 fatty acids on cardiovascular disease, researchers might assign participants into four groups: (1) no treatment, (2) aspirin alone, (3) omega-3 alone, and (4) both aspirin and omega-3 together. This setup allows researchers to evaluate whether each treatment independently reduces cardiovascular risk and whether the combination of both treatments leads to an enhanced or diminished effect compared to individual treatments. Factorial RCTs can also be extended to higher-order designs, such as 2×3 factorial designs (testing two interventions with three levels each) or even 3×3 designs (testing three interventions with three levels each), but these require significantly larger sample sizes to maintain statistical power.

One of the biggest advantages of factorial RCTs is their efficiency in evaluating multiple interventions simultaneously. Instead of conducting two or more separate trials to test different treatments, researchers can combine these investigations into a single study, reducing costs, time, and logistical complexity. This approach is particularly valuable in large-scale public health studies, where testing multiple interventions within the same population saves resources and increases generalizability. Another major benefit is the ability to detect interactions between treatments. In many cases, medical interventions are used together in clinical practice, and understanding how they interact is crucial for optimizing patient care. Factorial RCTs allow researchers to determine whether combining treatments enhances effectiveness (synergistic effect), has no added benefit (additive effect), or reduces effectiveness (antagonistic effect). This is especially important in pharmacology, where drug-drug interactions can significantly impact therapeutic outcomes. Factorial RCTs also improve statistical efficiency by allowing multiple comparisons within the same dataset. Since all participants contribute data to multiple treatment comparisons, factorial trials often require fewer participants than conducting multiple separate RCTs, making them more resource-efficient. Additionally, factorial designs reduce selection bias because all treatment comparisons occur within the same study population, ensuring a more uniform distribution of baseline characteristics.

Despite their advantages, factorial RCTs also present significant challenges that must be carefully managed. One of the biggest concerns is the need for larger sample sizes, particularly when assessing interaction effects. If researchers want to detect whether the combination of two interventions has a unique effect beyond their individual effects, they must include a sufficient number of participants in each study arm. This requirement can make factorial trials more expensive and logistically demanding. Another challenge is treatment interaction complexity. If two interventions interact in unexpected ways, the results can be difficult to interpret. For example, if one treatment alters the absorption, metabolism, or effectiveness of another, it may complicate statistical analysis and lead to misleading conclusions. This issue is particularly relevant in drug trials, where pharmacokinetic interactions can significantly impact study outcomes.

Factorial RCTs are also more susceptible to dropouts and adherence issues, as participants must adhere to multiple treatments throughout the study. If a participant stops taking one treatment but continues another, it can introduce bias and affect the validity of the findings. Researchers must carefully design compliance strategies, follow-up assessments, and statistical adjustments to account for such challenges. Additionally, factorial designs may not always be ethically feasible, especially when testing interventions with potential adverse effects. If one intervention is already known to be beneficial, it may be unethical to randomize participants to a group that does not receive that treatment. This issue is commonly encountered in life-threatening diseases or clinical settings where withholding treatment could cause harm (Cipriani and Barbui 2013).

8.4.4.5 Adaptive RCTs

Unlike traditional RCTs, where all aspects of the trial remain fixed from start to finish, adaptive RCTs provide flexibility to refine key trial elements while maintaining the integrity and scientific rigor of the study. This adaptability makes them particularly useful in drug development, personalized medicine, and complex interventions, where early insights can help optimize the study for better efficiency and patient outcomes. Adaptive trials have gained increasing popularity, especially in oncology, rare disease research, and pandemic response trials, such as those conducted during the COVID-19 pandemic. By incorporating real-time data monitoring, adaptive RCTs enhance efficiency, reduce trial duration, and maximize patient benefit, making them a crucial advancement in evidence-based medicine. However, they also require advanced statistical methods, careful planning, and regulatory oversight to ensure that modifications do not introduce bias or compromise the validity of results.

The key feature of an adaptive RCT is that it allows for pre-planned modifications to various aspects of the study based on ongoing data analysis. These modifications can include adjusting sample size, changing treatment arms, modifying patient eligibility criteria, or stopping ineffective treatments early. However, all adaptations must be specified before the trial begins, ensuring that changes are driven by data and not by bias or convenience.

The study design typically involves predefined interim analyses, where data is periodically reviewed by an independent data monitoring committee (DMC). The DMC evaluates whether modifications should be made based on the accumulated evidence while maintaining trial integrity. These interim analyses ensure that adjustments are statistically justified, ethical, and scientifically valid. For example, in an adaptive cancer trial, researchers may start with multiple drug candidates but eliminate ineffective ones early in the study, allowing resources to focus on promising treatments. Similarly, in a vaccine trial, an adaptive design might increase the sample size if early results indicate that more participants are needed to confirm effectiveness.

Adaptive RCTs can include several types of modifications, each designed to improve trial efficiency and relevance. The following are some of the most commonly used adaptations:

i. Sample Size Re-Estimation: If interim results suggest that the initial sample size is too small to detect a meaningful effect, the trial can increase the number of participants to maintain statistical power.
ii. Adaptive Dose-Finding: Allows for adjustments in drug dosage based on early safety and efficacy data, ensuring that participants receive the most effective and tolerable dose.
iii. Treatment Arm Modification: If an experimental treatment shows strong early benefits, additional treatment groups may be added, or ineffective treatment arms may be dropped.
iv. Biomarker-Guided Adaptation: Enables personalized medicine approaches by modifying the trial to focus on specific patient subgroups who are more likely to respond to the treatment.

v. Early Stopping for Efficacy or Futility: Trials can be stopped early if a treatment is overwhelmingly effective, allowing faster approval, or terminated if a treatment is clearly ineffective, preventing unnecessary exposure to ineffective therapies.
vi. Response-Adaptive Randomization: As more data becomes available, the probability of assigning participants to more effective treatments increases, improving patient outcomes within the trial.

Each of these adaptations helps ensure that the trial remains efficient, ethical, and responsive to emerging data, making adaptive RCTs a preferred choice in fields where treatment responses can vary widely across patient populations.

One of the most significant advantages of adaptive RCTs is their efficiency in drug development and clinical decision-making. Traditional RCTs often require years of data collection before meaningful conclusions can be drawn, but adaptive designs allow researchers to make informed adjustments during the trial, potentially accelerating the approval of effective treatments. This is particularly beneficial in life-threatening conditions such as cancer, rare diseases, and infectious disease outbreaks, where time-sensitive decisions are crucial. Another key benefit is that adaptive RCTs reduce patient exposure to ineffective or harmful treatments. By allowing early stopping for futility, researchers can prevent unnecessary risks and reallocate resources to more promising interventions. This approach is highly ethical, as it prioritizes patient safety and ensures that participants receive the most beneficial treatments possible.

Adaptive designs also support personalized medicine, as they enable researchers to refine patient selection criteria based on emerging biomarker data. This ensures that treatments are tested on the most relevant patient populations, leading to more targeted and effective therapies. For example, an adaptive trial in oncology might identify genetic markers that predict better treatment responses and modify the trial to focus on those subgroups, improving overall success rates. Additionally, adaptive trials are cost-effective, as they optimize resource allocation by eliminating ineffective treatments early. This reduces wasted funding and allows for more efficient drug development pipelines, benefiting pharmaceutical companies, regulatory agencies, and healthcare systems.

Despite their many advantages, adaptive RCTs also pose several challenges that must be carefully managed. One of the biggest concerns is the increased complexity of trial design and statistical analysis. Since adaptations require real-time decision-making, researchers must use sophisticated statistical models and rigorous pre-planning to ensure that modifications do not introduce bias. This complexity often requires the involvement of specialized biostatisticians and regulatory experts throughout the trial. Another challenge is the risk of operational bias. If trial modifications are not properly blinded, knowledge of early results might influence decision-making or patient recruitment, leading to unintended biases. To mitigate this, adaptive trials typically require independent data monitoring committees to oversee interim analyses and make unbiased recommendations. Regulatory approval can also be more challenging for adaptive trials, as agencies like the FDA and EMA require clear justification for all planned adaptations. Regulatory guidelines emphasize that modifications must be pre-specified in the trial protocol to prevent researchers from making arbitrary changes that could skew results. This requires extensive documentation, transparency, and adherence to strict ethical standards.

Another limitation is that adaptive trials may require larger initial sample sizes compared to traditional RCTs. Since certain adaptations, such as reallocating participants to more effective treatment arms, require maintaining statistical power across different study phases, researchers often need to enroll more participants upfront to accommodate potential adjustments. This can increase early-phase costs, although the long-term efficiency of the trial may offset these expenses. Finally, interpretation of results can be more complex in adaptive RCTs, as multiple modifications during the trial may affect outcome comparisons. Advanced Bayesian statistical methods or adaptive frequentist approaches are often required to ensure that results remain valid despite trial adjustments (Pallmann et al. 2018).

8.4.5 Non-Randomized Trials (Quasi-Experimental Studies)

Non-randomized trials, also known as quasi-experimental studies, are a category of experimental research where participants are not assigned to treatment groups using a random process. Instead, the allocation of interventions is determined by natural occurrences, pre-existing conditions, or researcher discretion. These studies are widely used in clinical and public health research when randomization is unethical, impractical, or infeasible, such as when evaluating the effectiveness of policy changes, public health interventions, or rare medical treatments. Although non-randomized trials lack the rigor of RCTs in eliminating confounding factors, they remain valuable for real-world evidence generation, especially in situations where controlled trials are impossible. However, because participants in these studies are not randomly assigned, they are more susceptible to selection bias, confounding, and measurement bias, requiring careful statistical adjustments to ensure validity.

Non-randomized trials follow similar methodologies as RCTs but differ in how participants receive their treatment assignments. In these studies, groups are typically pre-existing or assigned based on external factors, rather than through randomization. This results in a comparison between a treatment group and a control group, where researchers analyze outcomes based on natural variations rather than random allocation. For example, in a study evaluating a new hospital infection control protocol, one hospital might implement the new procedure while another hospital continues with standard care. Since hospitals cannot be randomly assigned due to logistical constraints, researchers must adjust for differences in patient demographics, hospital resources, and baseline infection rates when analyzing the results.

To address potential biases, researchers in non-randomized trials often use matching techniques (e.g., propensity score matching), statistical adjustments (e.g., regression analysis), or historical controls to ensure that differences between groups are minimized. These approaches help improve the study's internal validity while acknowledging that some level of bias is unavoidable (Bärnighausen et al. 2017). There are several common types of non-randomized trials, each with different methodologies and applications:

8.4.5.1 Before-and-After Studies

Before-and-after studies compare outcomes before and after the introduction of an intervention in the same population. These studies are widely used in policy evaluations, hospital quality improvement programs, and public health interventions. For example, a study evaluating the effectiveness of a new hand hygiene protocol in reducing hospital-acquired infections by comparing infection rates before and after implementing the protocol (Bagul and Rajhans 2024).

8.4.5.2 Interrupted Time Series Studies

Interrupted time series (ITS) studies involve multiple measurements before and after an intervention, allowing researchers to observe trends over time. These studies help determine whether changes in an outcome are truly due to the intervention or part of a natural trend. For example, a study measuring the impact of a nationwide smoking ban on hospitalization rates for heart attacks over a 10-year period (Ewusie et al. 2020).

8.4.5.3 Propensity Score Matched Studies

Propensity score matching (PSM) is a statistical technique used in non-randomized trials to match participants in treatment and control groups based on similar characteristics. This method helps reduce selection bias and improve comparability between groups. For example, a study evaluating the impact of physical therapy on stroke recovery, where patients receiving therapy are matched to non-therapy patients with similar baseline conditions.

One of the main advantages of non-randomized trials is their practicality and feasibility in real-world settings. Many medical and public health interventions cannot be randomly assigned due to ethical, logistical, or financial constraints. Non-randomized trials allow researchers to study these interventions while still providing valuable insights into their effectiveness. These studies also allow for faster implementation of interventions, particularly in emergency or public health crisis settings. For example, during the COVID-19 pandemic, many treatments and policies (e.g., lockdowns, mask mandates) were evaluated through non-randomized studies because conducting large RCTs was impractical. Additionally, non-randomized trials often have higher external validity than RCTs, meaning that their findings may be more generalizable to real-world populations. Because these studies occur in routine clinical settings rather than tightly controlled environments, their results reflect how interventions perform in everyday medical practice.

Despite their advantages, non-randomized trials have several limitations, the most significant being their susceptibility to bias and confounding variables. Without randomization, treatment groups may differ in ways that influence outcomes, making it difficult to determine whether observed effects are truly due to the intervention or other external factors. For example, in a study assessing a new cancer drug, if younger and healthier patients are more likely to receive the drug while older, sicker patients receive standard care, differences in survival rates may reflect baseline differences rather than drug effectiveness. Researchers must use statistical methods, such as multivariable regression analysis and propensity score matching, to adjust for these imbalances, but residual confounding may still exist.

Another limitation is the risk of selection bias, where patients who receive an intervention differ systematically from those who do not. This is particularly problematic in studies where treatment choice is influenced by physician discretion, patient preferences, or healthcare access. Selection bias can distort study results and lead to overestimation or underestimation of treatment effects. Additionally, non-randomized trials may suffer from measurement bias, particularly if data is collected retrospectively. In before-and-after studies, for example, changes in outcome measurement methods or patient reporting over time may introduce inconsistencies, affecting study validity.

Non-randomized trials are commonly used in health policy evaluations, medical device assessments, and clinical interventions where RCTs are impractical. For example, they have been widely used to:

i. Evaluate public health initiatives, such as smoking bans, vaccination programs, and health education campaigns.
ii. Assess hospital quality improvement programs, such as new infection control procedures or electronic health record implementation.
iii. Study long-term treatment effects, particularly for rare diseases where large RCTs are not feasible.
iv. Investigate surgical and procedural outcomes, where patient selection and surgical expertise influence results (Wan 2025).

8.4.6 Other Study Designs Used in Clinical Trials

8.4.6.1 Single-Arm Trials

A single-arm trial is a type of clinical study that evaluates the safety and efficacy of an intervention without using a control group. Instead of comparing the new treatment against a placebo or an existing standard therapy, all participants in the trial receive the same intervention. These trials are commonly used in situations where it may be unethical or impractical to include a control group, such as when testing life-saving treatments for serious conditions that lack effective therapies. Single-arm trials are particularly valuable in early-phase clinical research, where the primary goal is to assess the treatment's safety, tolerability, and preliminary efficacy before advancing to larger, more rigorous comparative studies.

In a single-arm trial, researchers define clear inclusion and exclusion criteria to select participants who meet the study requirements. Once enrolled, all participants receive the investigational treatment, and various clinical outcomes, such as disease progression, survival rates, or biomarker changes, are measured over time. Since there is no control group, comparisons are often made against historical data, previous clinical studies, or expected disease progression based on epidemiological evidence. The primary endpoints in these trials typically include response rates, overall survival, progression-free survival, and changes in laboratory markers indicative of disease improvement or treatment effects.

To strengthen the reliability of findings, single-arm trials often incorporate objective response criteria and blinded assessments to minimize bias. In some cases, researchers use advanced statistical techniques, such as propensity score matching or Bayesian modeling, to estimate how the observed effects might compare to a control group derived from historical or real-world data. Despite these measures, the absence of a control group remains a major limitation that can affect the study's validity (M. Wang et al. 2025).

8.4.6.2 Pragmatic Clinical Trials

Pragmatic Clinical Trials (PCTs) are a type of clinical research designed to evaluate the effectiveness of interventions in real-world settings. Unlike traditional randomized controlled trials (RCTs), which focus on internal validity by conducting studies in highly controlled environments, PCTs prioritize external validity by testing interventions under routine clinical conditions. These trials are particularly valuable in assessing how well treatments work across diverse patient populations, healthcare settings, and everyday medical practices. PCTs differ from traditional RCTs in several ways. One of their defining characteristics is the broad eligibility criteria, which allow the inclusion of a diverse patient population representative of real-world settings. This ensures that findings are more generalizable and applicable to everyday clinical practice. Another critical feature is that interventions are typically delivered as they would be in routine healthcare settings, without strict adherence to rigid protocols. This approach helps assess how treatments perform outside the confines of controlled research environments.

Additionally, PCTs often utilize existing healthcare infrastructure for data collection, reducing the need for extensive additional resources. Electronic health records (EHRs), administrative databases, and patient registries are commonly leveraged to track patient outcomes efficiently. Moreover, these trials emphasize patient-centered outcomes, focusing on measures that matter most to patients, such as quality of life, treatment adherence, and functional health improvements. The flexibility in trial design makes PCTs a powerful tool for evaluating comparative effectiveness, optimizing treatment strategies, and improving healthcare delivery (Dave and Ling 2024).

8.4.6.3 Platform Trials

Platform trials are ongoing clinical trials that allow multiple treatments to be tested within the same study framework. New treatments can be added, modified, or removed based on interim results, making platform trials highly flexible and efficient. One of the defining characteristics of platform trials is their adaptive design. Traditional clinical trials often require a fixed protocol, making modifications difficult once the study is underway. In contrast, platform trials utilize pre-specified rules that allow for dynamic changes based on accumulating data. This includes adding new treatment arms, adjusting patient allocation, and discontinuing interventions that show inadequate efficacy or safety concerns.

Another crucial aspect is the use of a common control group. In many traditional trials, each new treatment requires a separate control group, leading to redundancy and inefficiencies. Platform trials, however, employ a shared control arm, reducing the number of participants required and increasing statistical power. This approach not only conserves resources but also enhances the comparability of results across multiple treatment arms (Burki 2023).

8.4.6.4 Umbrella Trials

Umbrella trials evaluate multiple targeted therapies within a single disease type by stratifying patients based on biomarkers or genetic mutations. This trial design is particularly useful in diseases with significant heterogeneity, such as cancer, where different subtypes respond differently to various treatments. By tailoring therapies to individual patient profiles, umbrella trials help identify the most effective treatment for each subgroup, enhancing therapeutic precision and improving patient outcomes. The goal is to accelerate drug development, reduce trial costs, and generate clinically meaningful data that can be directly applied to personalized treatment strategies.

One of the defining characteristics of umbrella trials is the use of a centralized master protocol that governs multiple treatment arms, each assigned to a specific patient subgroup. Instead of conducting separate trials for each molecular subtype, umbrella trials allow for concurrent evaluation of different targeted therapies within a single disease framework. This not only streamlines research efforts but also reduces the time and resources required to identify effective treatments.

Patients enrolled in an umbrella trial undergo comprehensive biomarker screening, often through next-generation sequencing (NGS) or other advanced diagnostic techniques. Based on their molecular or genetic profile, they are assigned to the most appropriate treatment arm. This adaptive stratification ensures that patients receive the therapy most likely to benefit them, rather than a one-size-fits-all approach commonly used in conventional trials.

Another essential feature of umbrella trials is their flexibility. Unlike traditional trials with fixed treatment protocols, umbrella trials allow for modifications based on interim analyses. Ineffective treatments can be discontinued, and new therapies can be introduced as scientific knowledge evolves. This adaptive nature ensures that the trial remains relevant and continues to generate valuable clinical insights over time (Park et al. 2020).

8.4.6.5 Basket Trials

Basket trials test a single drug across multiple different diseases that share a common genetic mutation or molecular target. This approach is useful when a therapy is believed to work across various tumor types or disease conditions.

One of the defining characteristics of basket trials is their molecular-driven approach to patient selection. Instead of enrolling patients based on the location of their cancer or disease, participants are grouped according to specific genetic mutations, protein expressions, or molecular pathways that are hypothesized to be responsive to the experimental treatment. This allows researchers to evaluate whether a single drug can be effective across multiple disease types that share a common molecular profile.

Another critical feature is the multi-disease structure of the trial. In a traditional clinical trial, a drug is tested in a single disease population, requiring multiple separate trials for different conditions. Basket trials, however, include multiple "baskets" or disease cohorts within a single study. Each basket represents a different disease type that shares the targeted molecular alteration. This structure enables simultaneous testing of the drug's efficacy across multiple conditions, significantly reducing the time and cost of drug development.

Additionally, basket trials often employ adaptive trial designs, allowing researchers to modify the study as new data emerge. If a drug shows promising results in a particular basket, that cohort can be expanded to include more patients. Conversely, if a treatment proves ineffective in a certain group, that basket can be closed without affecting the overall trial. This flexibility enhances efficiency and ensures that resources are allocated toward the most promising therapeutic strategies (Park et al. 2020).

8.4.6.6 Stepped-Wedge Trials

Stepped-wedge trials involve gradual implementation of an intervention across different groups over time, allowing each group to serve as its own control before receiving the intervention. Unlike traditional randomized controlled trials (RCTs), where participants are randomly assigned to intervention or control groups at the start, a stepped-wedge trial gradually introduces the intervention to all clusters in a phased manner. This means that, by the end of the trial, all participants will have received the intervention, but at different time points. The staggered implementation allows for comparisons between those who have received the intervention and those who have not yet received it, creating a natural control group at each step. Stepped-wedge trials are commonly employed when an intervention is expected to be beneficial, but its implementation needs to be phased due to logistical, financial, or ethical reasons. They are widely used in fields such as infectious disease control, maternal and child health programs, vaccine rollouts, and hospital-based quality improvement initiatives. One of the defining features of stepped-wedge trials is their progressive implementation of an intervention. Participants or clusters (such as hospitals, schools, or communities) are randomly assigned to different rollout periods. At each time step, one or more clusters cross over from the control condition to the intervention, while others remain in the control phase until their assigned time arrives. This continues until all clusters have received the intervention. The staggered approach allows researchers to collect longitudinal data, analyzing both pre-intervention and post-intervention outcomes within each cluster. Another critical feature is the use of repeated measurements. Data are collected continuously throughout the study, allowing researchers to assess how the intervention impacts outcomes over time. This enables the evaluation of both immediate and long-term effects, providing a more comprehensive understanding of the intervention's effectiveness. Additionally, the stepped-wedge design accounts for temporal trends, meaning it can distinguish between changes due to the intervention and external factors, such as seasonal variations or policy shifts. A unique advantage of stepped-wedge trials is their practical feasibility in large-scale implementation studies. Because interventions are introduced gradually, they are easier to integrate into real-world settings, particularly when resources or trained personnel are limited. This phased rollout approach is especially valuable in evaluating national health programs or large organizational changes where an immediate, simultaneous implementation is not possible (Copas et al. 2015).

8.4.6.7 N-of-1 Trials

N-of-1 trials are a unique clinical trial design that focuses on evaluating the effectiveness of an intervention in a single individual over time. Unlike traditional RCTs, which assess treatments across large populations, N-of-1 trials use a repeated crossover design where a single participant alternates between treatment and control (or alternative treatment) conditions multiple times. This approach allows for individualized assessment of treatment effects, helping to determine whether a particular therapy is beneficial for a specific patient.

One of the defining characteristics of N-of-1 trials is their crossover design, where a participant is exposed to multiple treatment phases in a randomized order. This could involve alternating between an active drug and a placebo, two competing medications, or different lifestyle interventions. Each phase is followed by a washout period to minimize carryover effects from the previous treatment. By repeating this cycle multiple times, researchers can assess whether observed improvements are due to the intervention or natural fluctuations in the patient's condition.

Another essential feature is blinded and randomized treatment allocation. Whenever feasible, N-of-1 trials are conducted in a double-blind manner, meaning neither the patient nor the healthcare provider knows which treatment is being administered at any given time. This reduces bias and enhances the reliability of findings. Additionally, randomizing the order of treatment phases ensures that the observed effects are not simply due to external factors such as disease progression or psychological expectations. N-of-1 trials also rely on frequent and precise outcome measurements. Patients typically record their symptoms, functional status, or biomarker levels using diaries, wearable devices, or laboratory tests. The continuous collection of individualized data allows researchers to generate highly detailed treatment response profiles, enabling tailored adjustments to the patient's therapeutic plan. This makes N-of-1 trials particularly valuable in conditions with subjective symptoms, such as chronic pain, where patient-reported outcomes are critical (Lillie et al. 2011; "Introduction to N-of-1 Trials: Indications and Barriers (Chapter 1) | Effective Health Care (EHC) Program" 2025).

8.5 CONCLUSION

Selecting the appropriate study design is fundamental to the success of clinical research, as it directly influences the validity, reliability, and applicability of study findings. This chapter has provided a comprehensive overview of both observational and interventional study designs, highlighting their respective strengths, limitations, and applications in clinical research. Observational studies, including descriptive and analytical designs, play a crucial role in identifying disease patterns, risk factors, and associations, while interventional studies, particularly RCTs, provide the highest level of evidence for evaluating new treatments and interventions. Beyond traditional study designs, emerging methodologies such as pragmatic trials, platform trials, umbrella trials, basket trials, stepped-wedge trials, and N-of-1 trials have revolutionized clinical research by offering greater flexibility, efficiency, and personalized treatment strategies. These innovative designs are particularly valuable in precision medicine, public health interventions, and rare disease research. Ultimately, no single study design is universally superior; the choice depends on the research question, ethical considerations, feasibility, and available resources. A well-structured study design ensures systematic data collection, minimizes bias, and enhances the credibility of research findings. By understanding and selecting the most suitable study design, researchers can contribute to high-quality clinical evidence, ultimately improving patient care and public health outcomes.

REFERENCES

Aggarwal, Rakesh, and Priya Ranganathan. 2019a. "Study Designs: Part 4—Interventional Studies." *Perspectives in Clinical Research* 10 (3). Medknow: 137. https://doi.org/10.4103/PICR.PICR_91_19.

Aggarwal, Rakesh, and Priya Ranganathan. 2019b. "Study Designs: Part 2—Descriptive Studies." *Perspectives in Clinical Research* 10 (1). Wolters Kluwer Medknow Publications: 34. https://doi.org/10.4103/PICR.PICR_154_18.

Aggarwal, Rakesh, and Priya Ranganathan. 2019c. "Study Designs: Part 5—Interventional Studies (II)." *Perspectives in Clinical Research* 10 (4). Wolters Kluwer Medknow Publications: 183. https://doi.org/10.4103/PICR.PICR_138_19.

Bagul, Avinash, and Rajni Kant Rajhans. 2024. "How to Conduct Before-and-after Studies." *How to Conduct Before-and-after Studies*, January. SAGE Publications Ltd. https://doi.org/10.4135/9781529685626.

Bärnighausen, Till, John Arne Røttingen, Peter Rockers, Ian Shemilt, and Peter Tugwell. 2017. "Quasi-Experimental Study Designs Series—Paper 1: Introduction: Two Historical Lineages." *Journal of Clinical Epidemiology* 89 (September). Elsevier USA: 4–11. https://doi.org/10.1016/J.JCLINEPI.2017.02.020.

Burki, Talha. 2023. "Platform Trials: The Future of Medical Research?" *The Lancet Respiratory Medicine* 11 (3). Elsevier Ltd: 232–3. https://doi.org/10.1016/S2213-2600(23)00052-8.

Capili, Bernadette, and Joyce K. Anastasi. 2021. "Overview: Cohort Study Designs." *The American Journal of Nursing* 121 (12). Lippincott Williams and Wilkins: 45. https://doi.org/10.1097/01.NAJ.0000803196.49507.08.

"Chapter 6. Ecological Studies." 2025. Accessed February 27. https://www.bmj.com/about-bmj/resources-readers/publications/epidemiology-uninitiated/6-ecological-studies.

Chidambaram, Ambika G., and Maureen Josephson. 2019. "Clinical Research Study Designs: The Essentials." *Pediatric Investigation* 3 (4). Blackwell Publishing Ltd: 245. https://doi.org/10.1002/PED4.12166.

Cipriani, A., and C. Barbui. 2013. "What Is a Factorial Trial?" *Epidemiology and Psychiatric Sciences* 22 (3): 213. https://doi.org/10.1017/S2045796013000231.

Copas, Andrew J., James J. Lewis, Jennifer A. Thompson, Calum Davey, Gianluca Baio, and James R. Hargreaves. 2015. "Designing a Stepped Wedge Trial: Three Main Designs, Carry-over Effects and Randomisation Approaches." *Trials* 16 (1). BioMed Central Ltd.: 1–12. https://doi.org/10.1186/S13063-015-0842-7/FIGURES/3.

"Crossover Study—An Overview | ScienceDirect Topics." 2025. Accessed February 27. https://www.sciencedirect.com/topics/neuroscience/crossover-study.

Dave, Udit, and Daphne I. Ling. 2024. "Pragmatic Trials." *Introduction to Surgical Trials*. Cham: Springer Nature Switzerland, 185–91. https://doi.org/10.1007/978-3-031-77563-5_21.

Dron, Louis, Monica Taljaard, Yin Bun Cheung, Rebecca Grais, Nathan Ford, Kristian Thorlund, Fyezah Jahan, et al. 2021. "The Role and Challenges of Cluster Randomised Trials for Global Health." *The*

Lancet Global Health 9 (5). Elsevier Ltd: e701–10. https://doi.org/10.1016/S2214-109X(20)30541-6/ATTACHMENT/8845AFC1-8673-484C-AEF1-AC7B5EDC7FBC/MMC1.PDF.

Ewusie, Joycelyne E., Charlene Soobiah, Erik Blondal, Joseph Beyene, Lehana Thabane, and Jemila S. Hamid. 2020. "Methods, Applications and Challenges in the Analysis of Interrupted Time Series Data: A Scoping Review." *Journal of Multidisciplinary Healthcare* 13. Dove Medical Press Ltd.: 411. https://doi.org/10.2147/JMDH.S241085.

Hariton, Eduardo, and Joseph J. Locascio. 2018. "Randomised Controlled Trials—The Gold Standard for Effectiveness Research." *BJOG: An International Journal of Obstetrics and Gynaecology* 125 (13). Blackwell Publishing Ltd: 1716. https://doi.org/10.1111/1471-0528.15199.

"Introduction to N-of-1 Trials: Indications and Barriers (Chapter 1) | Effective Health Care (EHC) Program." 2025. Accessed February 27. https://effectivehealthcare.ahrq.gov/products/n-1-trials/research-2014-4.

Kitamura, Hiroko, Waka Ohishi, Kazunori Kodama, and Toshiteru Ohkubo. 2022. "Epidemiological Study of Health Effects in Fukushima Emergency Workers: Progress Report on the Health Examination Study, 2016–2019." *Environmental Advances* 9 (October). Elsevier: 100275. https://doi.org/10.1016/J.ENVADV.2022.100275.

Lillie, Elizabeth O., Bradley Patay, Joel Diamant, Brian Issell, Eric J. Topol, and Nicholas J. Schork. 2011. "The N-of-1 Clinical Trial: The Ultimate Strategy for Individualizing Medicine?" *Personalized Medicine* 8 (2): 161. https://doi.org/10.2217/PME.11.7.

Lu, C. Y. 2009. "Observational Studies: A Review of Study Designs, Challenges and Strategies to Reduce Confounding." *International Journal of Clinical Practice* 63 (5): 691–7. https://doi.org/10.1111/J.1742-1241.2009.02056.X.

Mahmood, Syed S., Daniel Levy, Ramachandran S. Vasan, and Thomas J. Wang. 2013. "The Framingham Heart Study and the Epidemiology of Cardiovascular Diseases: A Historical Perspective." *Lancet* 383 (9921). Elsevier B.V.: 999. https://doi.org/10.1016/S0140-6736(13)61752-3.

Morgenstern, H. 1995. "Ecologic Studies in Epidemiology: Concepts, Principles, and Methods." *Annual Review of Public Health* 16 (Volume 16, 1995). Annual Reviews Inc.: 61–81. https://doi.org/10.1146/ANNUREV.PU.16.050195.000425/CITE/REFWORKS.

Pallmann, Philip, Alun W. Bedding, Babak Choodari-Oskooei, Munyaradzi Dimairo, Laura Flight, Lisa V. Hampson, Jane Holmes, et al. 2018. "Adaptive Designs in Clinical Trials: Why Use Them, and How to Run and Report Them." *BMC Medicine 2018 16:1* 16 (1). BioMed Central: 1–15. https://doi.org/10.1186/S12916-018-1017-7.

"Parallel Design/Parallel Group Study—Statistics How To." 2025. Accessed February 27. https://www.statisticshowto.com/parallel-design-parallel-group-study/.

Park, Jay J. H., Grace Hsu, Ellie G. Siden, Kristian Thorlund, and Edward J. Mills. 2020. "An Overview of Precision Oncology Basket and Umbrella Trials for Clinicians." *CA: A Cancer Journal for Clinicians* 70 (2). American Cancer Society: 125–37. https://doi.org/10.3322/CAAC.21600.

Ranganathan, Priya, and Rakesh Aggarwal. 2019. "Study Designs: Part 3—Analytical Observational Studies." *Perspectives in Clinical Research* 10 (2). Wolters Kluwer Medknow Publications: 91. https://doi.org/10.4103/PICR.PICR_35_19.

Sambandan, Gunasakaran, and Adina Turcu-Stiolica. 2018. "Clinical Trials." *Clinical Pharmacy Education, Practice and Research: Clinical Pharmacy, Drug Information, Pharmacovigilance, Pharmacoeconomics and Clinical Research*, January. Elsevier: 323–44. https://doi.org/10.1016/B978-0-12-814276-9.00023-4.

Sayre, Jerry W, Hale Z Toklu, Fan Ye, Joseph Mazza, and Steven Yale. 2017. "Case Reports, Case Series—From Clinical Practice to Evidence-Based Medicine in Graduate Medical Education." *Cureus* 9 (8). Springer Science and Business Media LLC: e1546. https://doi.org/10.7759/CUREUS.1546.

Tenny, Steven, Connor C. Kerndt, and Mary R. Hoffman. 2023. "Case Control Studies." *Textbook of Clinical Epidemiology: For Medical Students*, March. StatPearls Publishing: 83–104. https://doi.org/10.1007/978-981-99-3622-9_5.

Wan, Fei. 2025. "Propensity Score Matching: Should We Use It in Designing Observational Studies?" *BMC Medical Research Methodology* 25 (1). BioMed Central: 25. https://doi.org/10.1186/S12874-025-02481-W/FIGURES/4.

Wang, Minyan, Huan Ma, Yun Shi, Haojie Ni, Chu Qin, and Conghua Ji. 2025. "Single-Arm Clinical Trials: Design, Ethics, Principles." *BMJ Supportive & Palliative Care* 15 (1). British Medical Journal Publishing Group: 46–54. https://doi.org/10.1136/SPCARE-2024-004984.

Wang, Xiaofeng, and Zhenshun Cheng. 2020. "Cross-Sectional Studies: Strengths, Weaknesses, and Recommendations." *Chest* 158 (1). Elsevier: S65–71. https://doi.org/10.1016/J.CHEST.2020.03.012.

9 Regulatory Frameworks in India

Divya Sahu, Lokendra Singh Rathor, Manju Rawat Singh, and Deependra Singh
University Institute of Pharmacy, Pt. Ravishankar Shukla University, Raipur, Chhattisgarh, India

9.1 INTRODUCTION

In recent years, the pharmaceutical industry has experienced rapid transformation, creating new expectations and challenges for manufacturers, healthcare providers, and payers (1). Pharmaceutical regulatory authorities ensure that medicines are safe and effective to use, meeting regulatory standards. Moreover, these authorities also ensure that accurate information about their use is made available to the public (2). As the global pharmaceutical sector becomes increasingly competitive, many nations have established or restructured their regulatory bodies to better align with evolving industry demands (3). Within life science organizations, the regulatory agencies also play an important role in ensuring that companies operate in full compliance with relevant laws and regulations. It serves as a key component of a pharmaceutical company's organizational framework, linking product development, manufacturing, and legal compliance (4). In the Indian context, growing global collaboration, the rise of outsourcing opportunities, and the gradual integration of domestic firms with the international pharmaceutical market have led to the formation of a new industrial ecosystem. Indian pharmaceutical companies have carved out unique positions through innovation while simultaneously adapting to pressures within the global research environment. Their strong domestic base enables them to supply medications addressing both local and international health needs (Figure 9.1).

However, deeper integration into global markets also makes Indian enterprises more susceptible to fluctuations and policy changes in international regulatory systems. In India, pharmacy regulation is governed by a robust framework of laws, regulatory bodies, and professional councils to ensure a safe and ethical practice of pharmaceutical sciences (5). Key legislations include the Drugs and Cosmetics Act, 1940 (6), and the Pharmacy Act, 1948, which regulates pharmacy education and professional standards through the Pharmacy Council of India (PCI) (7). The Central Drugs Standard Control Organisation (CDSCO) works as the national regulatory authority, while state-level drug control departments handle local licensing and enforcement (8). Additionally, bodies like the National Pharmaceutical Pricing Authority (NPPA) regulate drug cost to make sure that it is affordable by general public (9). Pharmacists are required to register with state councils and adhere to strict guidelines for dispensing prescription and over-the-counter drugs. As pharmacy practice evolves with advancements like e-pharmacies, regulatory frameworks are being updated to address emerging challenges, leading to continued therapeutic advancement of pharmaceutical services in India (Figure 9.1). The aim of this chapter is to signify the importance of regulatory affairs in the field of pharmacy (10).

DOI: 10.1201/9781003533085-9

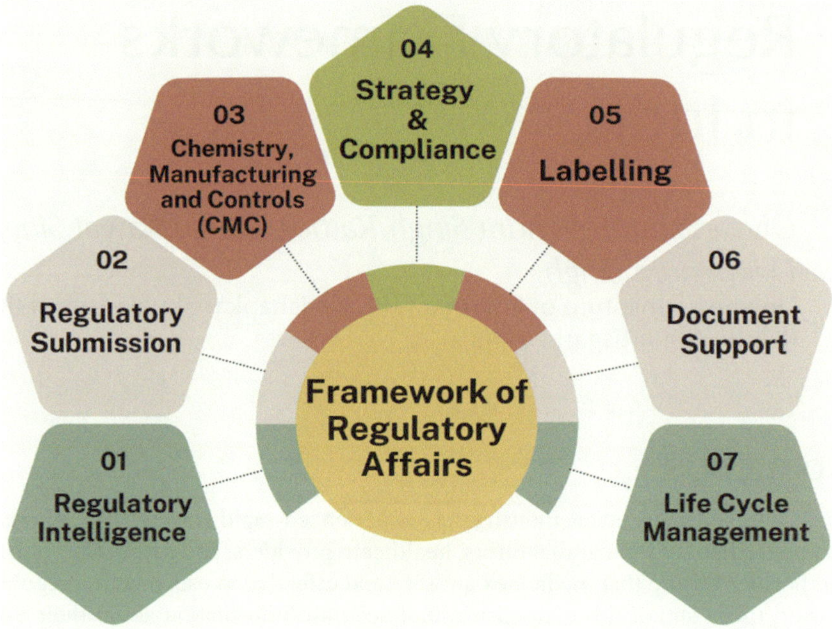

FIGURE 9.1 Emerging challenges of regulatory affairs.

9.2 REGULATORY BODIES

The most influential regulatory bodies worldwide that oversee the pharmaceutical industry, each ensuring a standardized therapeutic profile of medicines. The World Health Organization (WHO) plays an important role in global drug regulatory affairs, although it is not a direct regulatory authority like national agencies such as the FDA or EMA. Instead, WHO acts as a global health leader, setting standards, providing technical assistance, and promoting international cooperation in drug regulation. These standards, such as Good Manufacturing Practices (GMP) and Good Clinical Practice (GCP), provide a framework for national regulatory authorities to develop and implement their own regulations. It also encourages the alignment of regulatory standards and procedures across countries to support and streamline global trade in pharmaceuticals. Additionally, the World Trade Organization (WTO) facilitates trade at an international level and ensures that trade policies are fair and equitable. The WTO's Agreement on Trade-Related Aspects of Intellectual Property Rights (TRIPS) provides a protocol for the protection of patents, trademarks, and other forms of intellectual property rights. This includes pharmaceutical patents, which can significantly impact the pricing and availability of medicines. The TRIPS Agreement also allows for flexibilities, such as compulsory licensing, which can be used by countries to address public health crises, like HIV/AIDS, by allowing the production of generic medicines. Moreover, the International Council for Harmonisation (ICH) plays a significant role in aligning and standardizing scientific and regulatory requirements for the marketing of pharmaceuticals for clinical use. By developing and implementing common technical guidelines, ICH aims to facilitate and accelerate the drug development and approval process, reduce unnecessary duplication of studies and regulatory submissions, and ensure the development of safe and high-quality medicines (11) (Figure 9.2).

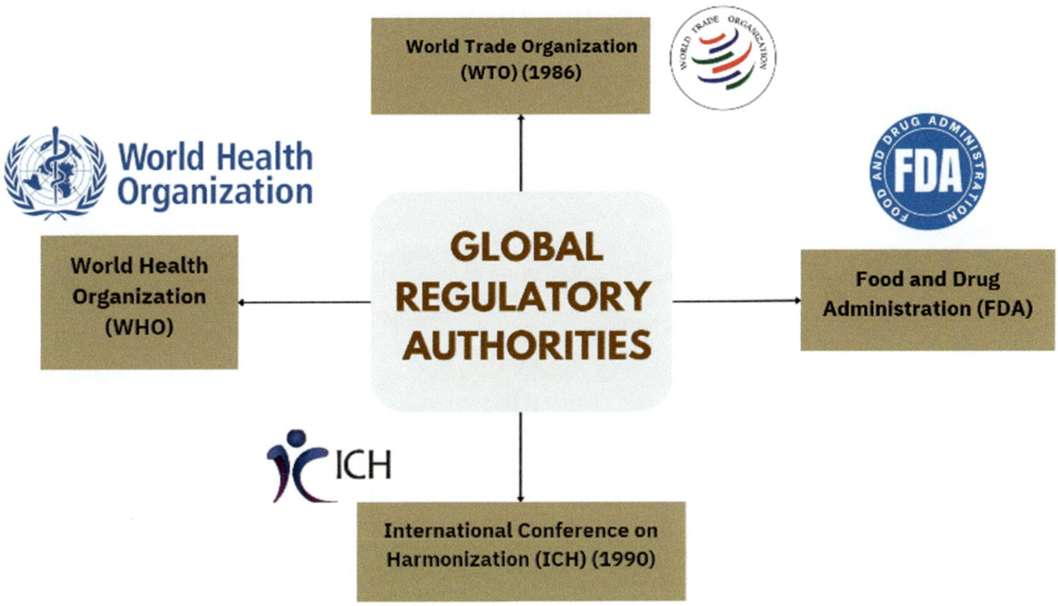

FIGURE 9.2 Authorities overseeing drug development.

9.3 WORLD REGULATORY AUTHORITY

Regulatory authorities in pharmaceutical industries play a significant role in ensuring the therapeutic performance and reliability of drugs and medical devices. These authorities are responsible for the entire drug development process, from initial research to post-market surveillance. Recently, significant developments in the pharmaceutical sector have been made to challenge producers, payers, and providers. A systematic approach in pharmaceutical research helps establish clear objectives and ensures a comprehensive assessment of preformulation parameters, which collectively support the protection of public health. Regulatory authorities in the pharmaceutical sector hold a key responsibility in supervising the processes of drug development and marketing to maintain safety and reliability. These organizations outline specific standards for production to guarantee uniformity and quality, including guidelines for infrastructure, equipment maintenance, personnel qualifications, and documentation practices. Strict compliance with GMP principles is fundamental to avoiding contamination, procedural errors, and other deviations during drug production. Furthermore, regulatory bodies design mechanisms for monitoring adverse drug reactions (ADRs) by thoroughly reviewing clinical trial findings, conducting post-marketing safety assessments, and ensuring continuous pharmacovigilance. They also regulate labeling and packaging to deliver precise and reliable information to both patients and healthcare providers. In addition, ongoing post-marketing monitoring systems enable the identification of unanticipated adverse effects, allowing timely action by the authorities to preserve drug safety and efficacy. Collaboration between regulatory bodies on an international level is another critical aspect of pharmaceutical regulation. World regulatory authority comes under the WHO, ICH (1990), WTO (1986), and the Food and Drug Administration (FDA) (Figure 9.3) (12).

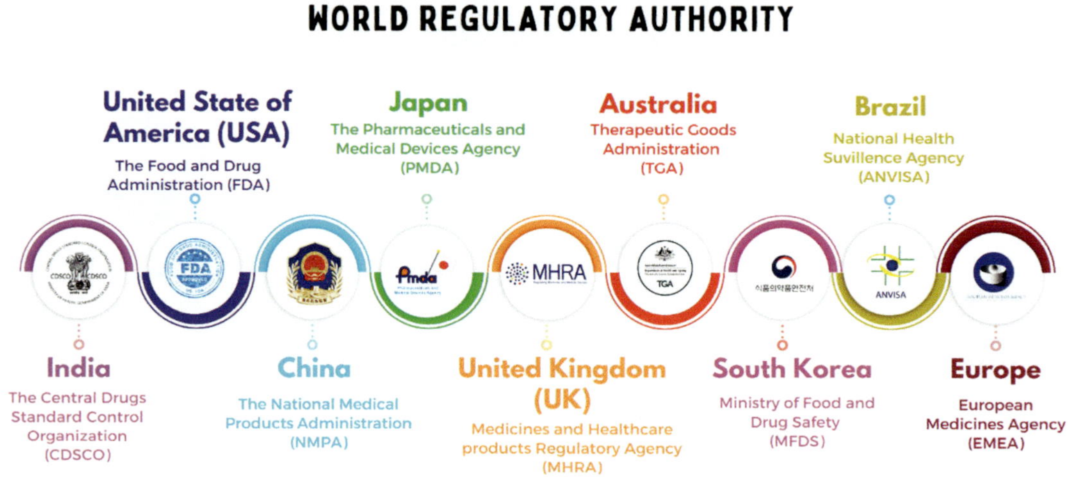

FIGURE 9.3 Overview of national regulatory bodies within country.

9.4 INDIAN REGULATORY AUTHORITY

Until the early 20th century, India's pharmaceutical industry was in its infancy, with most medicines being imported from abroad. The situation changed drastically after the First World War, when the demand for medicines was rising, which led to the circulation of numerous substandard and counterfeit drugs in the market. By 1947, the year India gained independence, the pharmaceutical sector was almost entirely dominated by Western multinational corporations. At that time, approximately 90% of the country's drug supply depended on imports, and nearly 99% of patented pharmaceutical products were owned by foreign companies. Consequently, domestic drug prices in India ranked among the highest in the world. In response, the Indian government began implementing policies in the 1960s that encouraged local production of medicines. However, this period also witnessed an influx of adulterated and fake drugs from unregulated foreign manufacturers. One of the major turning points was the "Gigantic Quinine Fraud," which prompted the government to appoint a Drug Inquiry Committee under the leadership of Sir Ram Nath Chopra. The recommendations of this "Chopra Committee" eventually formed the basis of the Drugs Bill, which later evolved into the Drugs and Cosmetics Act of 1940 and the accompanying Drugs and Cosmetics Rules of 1945. To ensure self-sufficiency in the supply of medicines, the Government of India subsequently established five state-owned pharmaceutical enterprises. Policy measures were also introduced to strengthen domestic capabilities—these included eliminating product patents on chemicals, food, and pharmaceuticals; limiting the equity participation of multinational corporations in Indian drug companies; introducing process patents; and enforcing price control regulations on selected formulations of drugs. The absence of strong legal protections for product patents led many foreign manufacturers to withdraw from the Indian market, paving the way for the growth of indigenous pharmaceutical enterprises.

Due to the policy interventions that promoted local manufacturing, the proportion of India's pharmaceutical market controlled by foreign companies steadily declined, falling to below 20% by 2005. These changes opened opportunities for domestic manufacturers, who rapidly expanded production to meet national needs. By the 1990s, India had achieved full self-reliance in the manufacture of finished formulations. At present, the nation is recognized as one of the largest global players in the pharmaceutical sector—ranking fifth in bulk drug production, third in total production volume, and 13th in terms of market value. Domestic manufacturers now

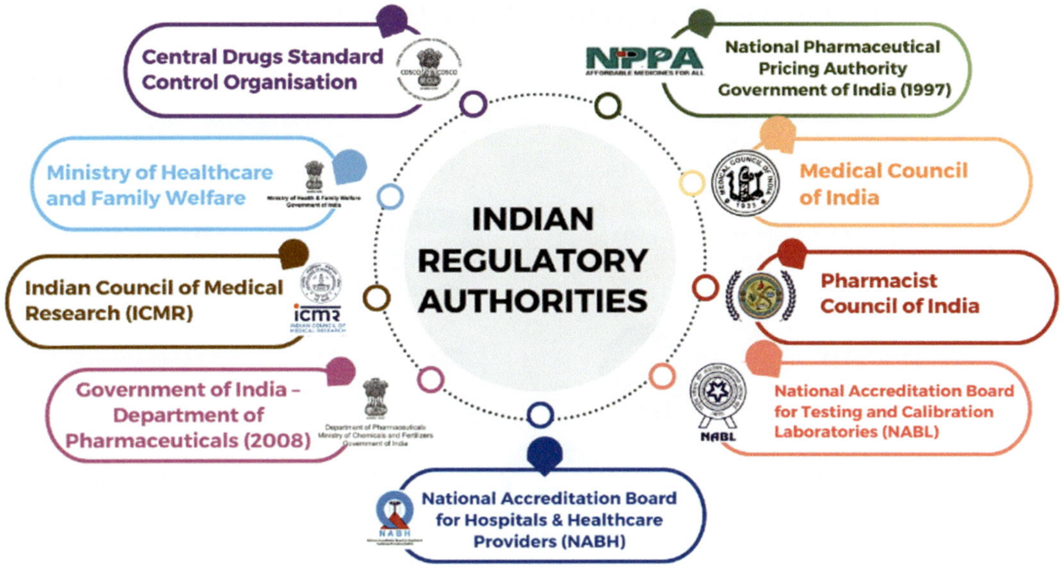

FIGURE 9.4 Schematic representation of Indian regulatory authorities.

supply around 95% of the country's total pharmaceutical demands, underscoring India's strong industrial capability.

The chapter further explores India's pharmaceutical regulatory framework, which is governed by multiple institutions and oversight bodies. Major authorities include the CDSCO, operating under the Ministry of Health and Family Welfare; the Indian Council of Medical Research (ICMR); and the Department of Pharmaceuticals, established in 2008. Price regulation and market control are managed by the National Pharmaceutical Pricing Authority (NPPA), created in 1997. Additionally, several professional and quality assurance bodies contribute to regulatory governance, including the Medical Council of India (MCI), the Pharmacy Council of India (PCI), the National Accreditation Board for Testing and Calibration Laboratories (NABL), and the National Accreditation Board for Hospitals & Healthcare Providers (NABH). Together, these organizations form the foundation of India's multifaceted drug regulation system (Figure 9.4) (13).

9.5 DEPARTMENT OF REGULATORY AFFAIRS

A Department of Regulatory Affairs (DRA) is a crucial body within organizations that is subjected to government regulations. This department helps the organization comply with all laws, rules, and regulations. The DRA is also responsible for the development and implementation of regulatory strategies, regulatory submissions, monitoring compliance with regulations, and managing post-market surveillance activities (Figure 9.5) (14).

9.6 MAJOR LEGISLATION

9.6.1 Drugs and Cosmetics Act, 1940, and Rules, 1945

The Drugs and Cosmetics Act, 1940, and its associated Rules, 1945, form the cornerstone of pharmaceutical regulation in India. The main objective of this act is (a) to ensure that drugs and cosmetics sold in India are safe, effective, and conform to prescribed quality standards; (b) to prevent

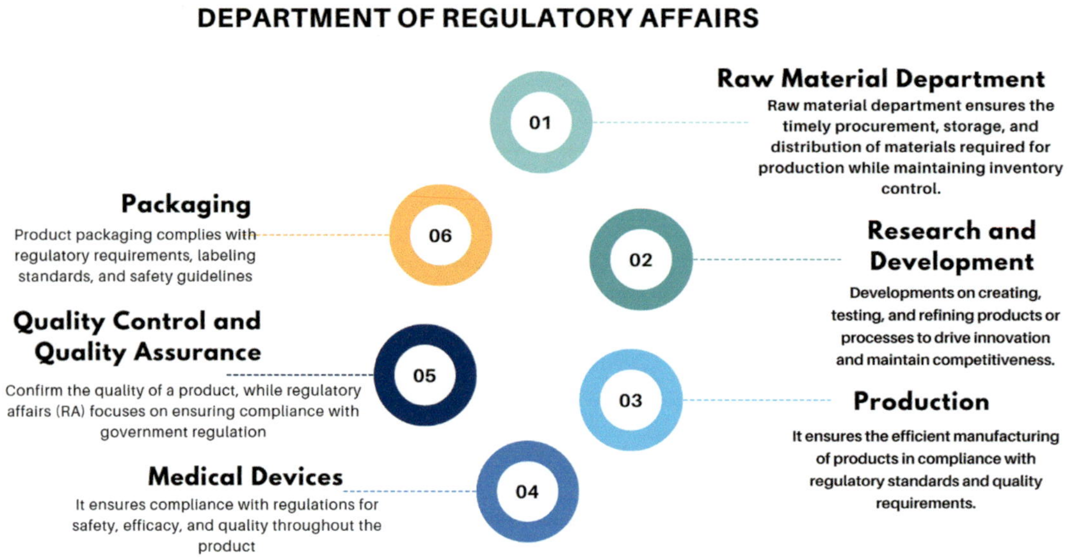

FIGURE 9.5 Illustration of various departments of drug regulatory affairs.

TABLE 9.1
Role and Framework of Indian Regulatory Authorities

S.No.	Indian Regulatory Authorities	Role & Functions	References
1.	Central Drugs Standard Control Organisation (CDSCO)	**a) Drug Approval and Regulation:** CDSCO is responsible for approving new drugs, including conducting clinical trials and evaluating their safety and efficacy. **b) Drug Licensing:** CDSCO grants licenses to drug manufacturers and importers. **c) Import Regulation:** CDSCO regulates the import of drugs to ensure they meet Indian quality standards. **d) Clinical Trials Regulation:** CDSCO ensures that clinical trials are conducted ethically and in compliance with international standards.	(15)
2.	Ministry of Healthcare and Family Welfare	**a) Policy Formulation:** The MoHFW provides CDSCO with the necessary financial resources, human resources, and infrastructure to carry out its regulatory activities effectively. **b) International Cooperation:** The MoHFW collaborates with international regulatory authorities to harmonize regulatory standards. Also implements programs to control and prevent the spread of infectious diseases.	(16)
3.	Indian Council of Medical Research	**a) Clinical Research Standards:** ICMR promotes adherence to GCP guidelines to ensure the quality, safety, and integrity of clinical trials. The Indian Council of Medical Research (ICMR) plays a crucial role in India's regulatory affairs, particularly in the areas of clinical research and biomedical research. While it's not directly a regulatory body like CDSCO, its guidelines and ethical standards significantly influence the regulatory landscape.	(17)

TABLE 9.1 (Continued)
Role and Framework of Indian Regulatory Authorities

S.No.	Indian Regulatory Authorities	Role & Functions	References
4.	National Accreditation Board for Hospitals and Healthcare Providers (NABH)	a) **Quality Standards and Accreditation:** NABH sets high standards for healthcare organizations, covering various aspects like patient care, infection control, medical records, and quality management. b) **Regulatory Compliance:** NABH standards often align with national and international regulations, helping healthcare facilities comply with regulatory requirements. c) **Patient Safety and Rights**	(18)
5.	National Accreditation Board for Testing and Calibration Laboratories (NABL)	a) **Setting Quality Standards:** NABL adopts and implements international standards like ISO/IEC 17025 for testing and calibration laboratories. It promotes a culture of quality assurance and continuous improvement in laboratories. b) **Accreditation Process:** It ensures rigorous assessment, third-party verification, & periodic reviews. c) **Regulatory Compliance:** NABL-accredited food testing laboratories must comply with the Food Safety and Standards Regulations, 2011, which regulate the food industry in India. By setting high standards and promoting best practices, NABL helps laboratories meet regulatory requirements and avoid penalties for non-compliance.	(19)
6.	Pharmacy Council of India	a) **Setting Standards for Pharmacy Education:** PCI develops and updates the curriculum for pharmacy courses, ensuring that future pharmacists are equipped with the necessary knowledge and skills to meet industry standards. b) **Collaboration with Regulatory Bodies:** Coordination with CDSCO and input on regulatory policies. PCI also actively participates in workshops, conferences, and other forums organized by CDSCO and other regulatory bodies to discuss issues related to pharmaceutical education and practice.	(20)
7.	Medical Council of India	a) **Setting Standards for Medical Education:** The MCI was responsible for developing and updating the curriculum for undergraduate and postgraduate medical courses.	(21)
8.	National Pharmaceutical Pricing Authority	a) **Price Control:** NPPA fixes or revises the prices of essential medicines, including bulk drugs and formulations. This involves a thorough analysis of various factors such as manufacturing costs, research and development expenses, and market dynamics. NPPA also considers the therapeutic value of the drug and its impact on public health. b) **Monitoring and Enforcement:** NPPA monitors the prices of decontrolled drugs to ensure they remain reasonable and takes action against manufacturers who overcharge consumers. The authority also enforces the provisions of the Drugs (Price Control) Order (DPCO) and other relevant regulations to ensure compliance. c) **Drug Availability:** NPPA plays a crucial role in ensuring the availability of essential medicines. It monitors the availability of drugs, identifies shortages, and takes necessary steps to address them. This may involve issuing directives to manufacturers or importers, or taking other regulatory actions to ensure that essential medicines are readily available to patients. NPPA also works with other stakeholders, such as state governments and healthcare providers, to coordinate efforts to address drug shortages and improve access to medicines.	(22)

substandard, adulterated, or spurious products from being marketed; and (c) to regulate clinical trials and ensure ethical practices (23). In this act, the Drug Technical Advisory Board consists of the following members:

(i) The Director General of Health Services, ex officio, who shall be Chairman
(ii) The Drugs Controller, India, ex officio
(iii) The Director of the Central Drugs Laboratory, Calcutta, ex officio
(iv) The Director of the Central Research Institute, Kasauli, ex officio
(v) The Director of Indian Veterinary Research Institute, Izatnagar, ex officio
(vi) The President of Medical Council of India, ex officio
(vii) The President of the Pharmacy Council of India, ex officio
(viii) The Director of Central Drug Research Institute, Lucknow, ex officio
(ix) Two persons to be nominated by the Central Government from among persons who are in charge of drug control in the states
(x) One person, to be elected by the Executive Committee of the Pharmacy Council of India, from among teachers in pharmacy or pharmaceutical chemistry or pharmacognosy on the staff of an Indian university or a college affiliated thereto
(xi) One person, to be elected by the Executive Committee of the Medical Council of India, from among teachers in medicine or therapeutics on the staff of an Indian university or a college affiliated thereto
(xii) One person to be nominated by the Central Government from the pharmaceutical industry
(xiii) One pharmacologist to be elected by the Governing Body of the Indian Council of Medical Research
(xiv) One person to be elected by the Central Council of the Indian Medical Association
(xv) One person to be elected by the Council of the Indian Pharmaceutical Association
(xvi) Two persons holding the appointment of Government Analyst under this Act, to be nominated

Additionally, the regulations help to prevent the sale of counterfeit or substandard drugs, which can have serious health consequences. The regulations also require that drugs are manufactured in clean and hygienic conditions and that they are stored and transported properly to prevent contamination or degradation.

9.6.2 Pharmacy Act, 1948

The Pharmacy Bill, 1947, having been passed by the legislature, received its assent on March 4, 1948. It came on the Statute Book as the Pharmacy Act, 1948 (8 of 1948). The purpose of this act is (a) to regulate the profession of pharmacy in India, (b) to establish educational standards and qualifications for pharmacists, (c) to create and maintain a register of qualified pharmacists, and (d) to oversee the professional conduct of pharmacists and promote public health. This act comprises 5 chapters and 45 sections. The chapters are as follows: (i) Chapter I: Preliminary, which defines the term "Pharmacist and Pharmacy Council, which applies to the whole of India; (ii) Chapter II: Pharmacy Council of India, which is the central authority for regulating pharmacy education and practice. And also, representatives from the central government, state governments, universities, and practicing pharmacists. It explains the education regulation and functions of PCI; (iii) Chapter III: State Pharmacy Council, which elaborates the establishment and functions of State Pharmacy Council; (iv) Chapter IV: Registration of Pharmacist: maintained by State Pharmacy Council and elucidated about details of qualified and registered pharmacist, their eligibility of registration and rights of registered pharmacists; and (v) Chapter V: Miscellaneous, which explicated penalties, inspection, and monitoring (24).

9.6.3 Drugs and Magic Remedies (Objectionable Advertisements) Act, 1954

In this Act, "advertisement" includes any notice, circular, label, wrapper, or other document, and any announcement made orally or by any means of producing or transmitting light, sound, or smoke; a "drug" includes a medicine for the internal or external use of human beings or animals; "magic remedy" includes a talisman, mantra, kavacha, and any other charm of any kind that is alleged to possess miraculous powers for or in the diagnosis, cure, mitigation, treatment, or prevention of any disease in human beings or animals or for affecting or influencing in any way the structure or any organic function of the body of human beings or animals. By preventing misleading and deceptive advertising, the Act helps to create a more informed and empowered consumer base. It also ensures that the pharmaceutical industry operates within ethical and legal boundaries, promoting the responsible use of medicines (25).

9.6.4 Narcotic Drugs and Psychotropic Substances (NDPS) Act, 1985

This Act is applicable throughout India and extends to Indian citizens residing abroad, as well as to individuals present on ships and aircraft registered in India. The term "addict" holds particular significance within the Act, referring to a person who is dependent on any narcotic drug or psychotropic substance. Substances such as charas, ganja, cannabis (hemp), coca derivatives including cocaine, ecgonine, and coca leaves, along with opium poppy, are classified under narcotic drugs and psychotropic substances.

Any activity related to the production, manufacture, possession, sale, purchase, transport, storage, concealment, use, consumption, inter-state import or export, import into India, export from India, or transshipment of these substances falls within the scope of this legislation. In accordance with the provisions of the Act, the Central Government is empowered to undertake all necessary or appropriate actions to prevent and control the misuse and illegal trade of narcotic drugs and psychotropic substances, while ensuring their utilization strictly for medical and scientific purposes (26).

9.6.5 Medical Devices Rules, 2017

Academic clinical studies are investigations conducted for educational or research purposes on medical devices. These studies may examine devices for approved or new applications, test new materials, improved designs, or assess their use in different patient populations. Active diagnostic medical devices are those that operate alone or alongside other devices to provide information for detecting, diagnosing, or monitoring health conditions, diseases, or congenital disorders, and to support treatment decisions. A medical device officer is a person appointed by the central or state government to oversee regulatory compliance, while a medical device testing laboratory is an organization approved to perform testing or evaluation of devices on behalf of licensed manufacturers. Medical devices, including in-vitro diagnostic devices, are classified based on risk into four categories: Class A (low risk), Class B (low-to-moderate risk), Class C (moderate-to-high risk), and Class D (high risk).

The Central Licensing Authority is responsible for regulating the import of all medical device classes, overseeing the manufacture of Class C and D devices, approving clinical trials, and evaluating new in-vitro diagnostic devices. It also coordinates with State Licensing Authorities. The State Licensing Authority, usually the State Drugs Controller, manages licensing for the manufacture, sale, and distribution of Class A and B devices and monitors the distribution and sale of devices across all classes within the state. These rules make sure that medical devices, such as insulin pumps and inhalers, are manufactured, tested, and supplied following strict quality standards to reduce risks of errors or adverse effects. Manufacturers are required to conduct detailed testing and clinical evaluations, including for device-drug combination products, to confirm their safety and effectiveness. The regulations also mandate post-market monitoring to track the ongoing safety and performance of devices, allowing prompt action if any issues are detected. By setting clear guidelines for traders, the Medical Devices Rules, 2017, contribute to safer, more reliable, and high-quality healthcare delivery in India (27).

9.6.6 Clinical Establishments Act, 2010

The term "clinical establishment" refers to any facility—such as a hospital, nursing home, maternity home, dispensary, clinic, or sanatorium, irrespective of the name by which it is known—that provides diagnostic, treatment, or care-related services for conditions including illness, injury, deformity, abnormality, or pregnancy. Such establishments may operate under any recognized system of medicine and may be managed, owned, or maintained by an individual, organization, or group of persons, whether incorporated or otherwise. Initially, the provisions of this Act extend to the States of Arunachal Pradesh, Himachal Pradesh, Mizoram, and Sikkim, as well as to all Union Territories. It may also be implemented in other states that choose to adopt the Act through a resolution passed in accordance with clause (1) of Article 252 of the Constitution of India.

The Act came into force at once in the states of Arunachal Pradesh, Himachal Pradesh, Mizoram, and Sikkim, and the Union territories, on such date as the Central Government may, by notification, appoint, and in any other state that adopts this Act under clause (1) of Article 252 of the Constitution. The Act also provided for the establishment of the National Council, State Councils, and the registration and regulation of clinical establishments. The Clinical Establishments Act is not directly a drug regulatory act. It plays a vital role in the overall regulatory framework for healthcare in India. By setting standards for healthcare facilities, promoting quality and safety, and ensuring ethical practices, the Act indirectly contributes to the safe and effective use of drugs (28).

9.7 CLINICAL ASPECT OF REGULATORY BODIES

Clinical manifestations, the observable signs and symptoms that patients experience due to a disease or medical condition, are multifaceted and cover a broad spectrum of physical, psychological, and physiological changes (29). In the context of drug regulatory affairs, clinical manifestations lead to the understanding of the therapeutic profile of new drugs, guiding clinical trial design, interpreting study results, and ensuring the appropriate use of medications (30). Regulatory bodies ensure that clinical trials are conducted with respect to the ethical guidelines issued by the Institutional Review Board (IRB). IRBs review protocols to protect the ethical rights of the trial participants (31). Regulatory bodies enforce national and international regulations and guidelines for governing clinical trials. This includes adherence to GCP standards, data quality standards, and reporting requirements. The roles of regulatory bodies include (i) ensuring safety and efficacy, (ii) protecting participant rights, and (iii) ensuring regulatory compliance. GCP refers to an internationally recognized set of ethical and scientific quality standards that guide the design, conduct, documentation, and reporting of clinical trials involving human participants. It is intended to protect the ethical rights of trial subjects. It includes (a) reviewing progress reports to assess the overall conduct of the trial and identify any deviations from the protocol, (b) monitoring safety data to identify any adverse events or safety signals that may require further investigation or intervention, (c) reviewing adverse event reports to ensure that they are reported accurately and completely, and that appropriate follow-up actions are taken, and (d) conducting site visits to assess the quality of data collection, storage, and analysis, as well as to verify compliance with regulatory requirements and ethical guidelines (31). Upon completion of a clinical trial, the collected data and final study report are carefully examined by regulatory authorities to determine the therapeutic profile of the investigational product. These agencies review whether the study objectives have been achieved and if the evidence supports the sponsor's intended claims. Through these evaluations, regulatory bodies serve a critical function in protecting public health, ensuring that new medical devices and drugs meet established therapeutic effectiveness before they become accessible to the general population.

Globally recognized regulatory authorities such as the Food and Drug Administration (FDA), the European Medicines Agency (EMA), the Medicines and Healthcare Products Regulatory Agency (MHRA), and India's Central Drugs Standard Control Organisation (CDSCO) oversee clinical research and approval processes in their respective jurisdictions. For example, during the COVID-19 pandemic, these organizations issued specific guidelines for the conduct of clinical trials in emergency situations. The guidance addressed exceptional circumstances, including participant self-isolation or quarantine, restricted access to hospitals due to infection risk, reassignment of healthcare personnel, communication procedures with national regulatory agencies, distribution of investigational drugs, remote verification of source data under social-distancing constraints, and prompt notification of authorities regarding urgent safety measures. It also provided direction for COVID-19-related clinical trials, emphasizing the importance of large, multinational study designs (32). This guidance was developed by the Clinical Trials Expert Group (CTEG) of the European Commission, with contributions from the European Medicines Agency (EMA), the Clinical Trials Facilitation and Coordination Group of the Heads of Medicines Agencies (HMA), and the GCP Inspectors' Working Group. Its principal objective was to ensure the protection of trial participants throughout the European Union while maintaining the credibility and trustworthiness of clinical data. The document was first released in March 2020 (33).

9.8 CONCLUSION

The regulatory landscape in India is complex and multifaceted, encompassing a wide range of sectors and industries. It is characterized by a mix of central- and state-level regulations, with various agencies responsible for overseeing different aspects of economic and social activity. The regulatory framework aims to ensure public safety, protect consumer interests, promote fair competition, and foster economic growth.

REFERENCES

1. Arden NS, Fisher AC, Tyner K, Yu LX, Lee SL, Kopcha M. Industry 4.0 for pharmaceutical manufacturing: Preparing for the smart factories of the future. Int J Pharm [Internet]. 2021;602:120554. Available from: https://doi.org/10.1016/j.ijpharm.2021.120554
2. Wang H, Chen Y, Wang L, Liu Q, Yang S, Wang C. Advancing herbal medicine: enhancing product quality and safety through robust quality control practices. Front Pharmacol. 2023;14(September):1–16.
3. Pimenta C, Bettiol V, Alencar-Silva T, Franco OL, Pogue R, Carvalho JL, et al. Advanced therapies and regulatory framework in different areas of the globe: Past, present, and future. Clin Ther [Internet]. 2021;43(5):e103–38. Available from: https://doi.org/10.1016/j.clinthera.2021.02.006
4. Praneeth P. Regulatory affairs and its role in pharmaceutical industry. Int J Pharm Biomed Eng. 2016,3(1):1–2.
5. Positioning India as a Pharmaceutical Innovation Hub. 2024;(September).
6. Biswal S. Drugs and cosmetics act, 1940 and interpretation of definitions. Res J Pharm Life Sci. 2020;1(1):1–9.
7. Sud S, Khyati S, Mahavidyalaya GA. An overview of laws governing pharmacy in India. Sushant al World J Pharm Res [Internet]. 2016;5(9):480. Available from: www.wjpr.net
8. Yadav P, Bahmani K, Jambheshwar G, Pawar N, Sharma A. A review on: Indian pharma regulatory system and list of new drugs approved by central drugs standard control organization in the year 2021 till date. Asian Pac J Heal Sci [Internet]. 2021;(January):2360–0964. Available from: https://en.wikipedia.org/
9. Management HR, Management F, Management M. Human resource management, financial management. ASM's International E-Journal on Ongoing Research in Management & IT. 2018.
10. Desai C. Online pharmacies: A boon or bane? Indian J Pharmacol. 2016; 48(6):615–616.
11. Rajput H, Raikwar MA. Regulatory authority and government policies. Cent Drug Eval Res . . . [Internet]. 2024;14(1):42–50. Available from: https://www.researchgate.net/profile/Ankita-Raikwar/publication/378856576_Regulatory_Authority_And_Goverment_Policies/links/65edb5b4aaf8d548dcbdff85/Regulatory-Authority-And-Goverment-Policies.pdf

12. Singam SLSR, Yetukuri K, Nadendla RR. Drug registration requirements for pharmaceuticals in emerging markets. Int J Drug Regul Aff. 2020;8(4):73–82.
13. Darade RB. Indian pharmaceutical regulatory authority: Review Indian pharmaceutical regulatory authority: Review. 2024;(May).
14. Pandiyan B, Dhanaraj R. Advanced analytical and bioanalytical estimation of Ertugliflozin: An overview. Int J Res Pharm Sci. 2018;10(1):339–45.
15. Chowdhury N, Joshi P, Patnaik A, Saraswathy B. Administrative Structure and Functions of Drug Regulatory Authorities in India. ICRIER Work Pap 309. 2015;(September).
16. Jain D. Regulation of digital healthcare in India: Ethical and legal challenges. Healthc. 2023;11(6).
17. Adolph R. 済無No Title No Title No Title. 2016;12(11):1–23.
18. Thiagesan R, Gopichandran V, Subramaniam S, Soundari H, Kosalram K. Prevalence of type 2 diabetes among persons with disabilities in the South – East Asian region: A systematic review and meta - analysis. Curr Med Issues. 2021;(19):185–7.
19. No I, Date I, No A, Date A. Board for Testing and Calibration Laboratories (NABL) General Information Brochure;2024.
20. Centre N. Regulations of the Pharmacy Council of India;1948;(2).
21. Medical I, Act C. The Indian Medical Council (professional conduct, etiquette and ethics) regulations, 2002. Issues Med Ethics. 2002;10(3):66–70.
22. Bhaskarabhatla A, Mahagaonkar A. Regulating Pharmaceutical Prices in India. Berlin: Springer, 2018.
23. Anonymous. The Drugs and Cosmetics Act and Rules as amended upto 30th June, 2005. Minist Heal Fam Welf. 2005;1940:268–95.
24. Миков В. No TitleПредисторическото селище до Криводол, Врачанско. Разкопки И Проучвания. 1948;(April 1946):26–62.
25. Gupta RN. Urgent amendment in the drugs and magic remedies (Objectionable Advertisements) Act, 1954. Pharma Times. 2014;46(10):48.
26. Malhotra N, Goel R, Goel S. The Narcotic Drugs and Psychotropic Substances Act, 1985. Man Dr Law. 2013;282.
27. Medical Devices Rules. Medical Devices Rules, 2017 india. Cent Drugs Stand Control Organ Minist Heal Fam Welfare, Govt India [Internet]. 2017;2017(2). Available from: https://cdsco.gov.in/opencms/resources/UploadCDSCOWeb/2022/m_device/Medical Devices Rules, 2017.pdf
28. Malhotra N, Goel R, Goel S. The clinical establishments (registration and regulation) ACT, 2010. Man Dr Law. 2013;217.
29. Paul S, Nath I, Zafar F. Regulatory affairs in clinical research: Present scenario. 2014;1(1):9–11. Available from: http://www.wma.net/
30. Framework R. Clinical Trials and Biomedical Research in India Clinical Trials and Biomedical Research in India Legal and Regulatory Framework;2023;(July).
31. Grady C. Institutional review boards purpose and challenges. Chest. 2015;148(5):1148–55.
32. Lythgoe MP, Middleton P. Ongoing clinical trials for the management of the COVID-19 pandemic. Trends Pharmacol Sci [Internet]. 2020;41(6):363–82. Available from: https://doi.org/10.1016/j.tips.2020.03.006
33. de Jong AJ, Santa-Ana-Tellez Y, van Thiel GJMW, Zuidgeest MGP, Siiskonen SJ, Mistry D, de Boer A, Gardarsdottir H, Trials@ Home Consortium. COVID-19 and the emerging regulatory guidance for ongoing clinical trials in the European Union. Clin Pharmacol Ther. 2021;109(6):1517–1527.

10 Regulatory Frameworks across the United States

Rizwana Parveen[1] *and Mansi Dahalia*[2]
[1]Department of Translational and Clinical Research, School of Chemical and Life Sciences, Jamia Hamdard, New Delhi, India
[2]Department of Pharmacology, School of Pharmaceutical Education and Research, Jamia Hamdard, New Delhi, India

10.1 INTRODUCTION

Clinical research is an aspect of patient-centered research that aims to generate knowledge that enhances the understanding of human disease, prevention, and treatment, thus promoting overall health. Clinical research comprises various stages that may involve patient participation and undertaking diagnostic clinical samples or data for understanding of disease mechanisms; detection, diagnosis, and study of natural history of the disease; development of therapeutic interventions; prevention of disease and health promotion; health outcome and cost effectiveness study; epidemiology; and community-based trials (Roundtable et al. 2002). The purpose of clinical trials is to investigate the efficacy and safety of drugs or medical devices for the diagnosis, prevention, or treatment of a certain disease. Clinical trials are conducted in sequential phases, ranging from Phase 0 through Phase IV. Phase 0, also called microdosing, is conducted on healthy human volunteers to study the pharmacokinetics of a drug. The first phase, Phase I, also referred to as the non-therapeutic phase, focuses on determining the safety and dose range of a drug. Phase II is also called the exploratory trial phase. In this phase, the efficacy of an experimental drug is determined for a specific disease. Phase III, referred to as the therapeutic confirmatory phase, is designed to confirm the drug's safety and effectiveness through large-scale studies in patients. Phase IV, also known as the post-marketing surveillance or the post-approval phase, takes place after the approval of the drug to be sold in the market and provides additional evidence regarding the risks and benefits (Kandi and Vadakedath 2023; McNair 2022; David and Kim 2023).

It is vital to uphold the ethical principles that form the foundation of research regulations while conducting clinical research. While various oversight bodies may be involved, the primary responsibility for protecting participants' rights and welfare ultimately rests with the researcher and study team. Therefore, researchers must have a thorough understanding of the history, principles, and objectives of human subject protection (McNair 2022).

10.2 REGULATORY BODIES ACROSS THE GLOBE

Ensuring public health by regulating safe and efficient medications is the foremost responsibility of regulatory authorities. This role becomes increasingly complex as pharmaceutical production, manufacturing processes, and medical technologies continue to evolve. Such developments are challenging but also generate opportunities for regulators in maintaining stringent oversight. Licensing, inspecting manufacturing plants and distribution networks, evaluating and registering pharmaceutical products, monitoring adverse drug reactions, ensuring quality control, regulating advertising and promotion, and overseeing clinical drug trials are all examples of core regulatory functions. Effectively executing these responsibilities requires a dynamic approach to adapt to the

DOI: 10.1201/9781003533085-10

ever-changing landscape of medicine and healthcare innovation (National Academies of Sciences, Engineering, and Medicine 2019).

10.3 KEY REGULATORY AGENCIES IN THE UNITED STATES

Key regulatory agencies in the United States overseeing clinical research include the Food and Drug Administration (FDA) and Office for Human Research Protections (OHRP) ("Clinical Research Regulation For United States | ClinRegs" 2025).

10.3.1 Food and Drug Administration (FDA)

The Food and Drug Administration (FDA), which operates under the U.S. Department of Health and Human Services as part of the Public Health Service, is responsible for overseeing clinical trials. Its role includes ensuring that these trials are designed, implemented, evaluated, and reported according to federal regulations and Good Clinical Practice (GCP) standards" ("Clinical Trials and Human Subject Protection | FDA" 2025).

10.3.1.1 Evolution of 1906 Pure Food and Drugs Act

The events that preceded the Pure Food and Drugs Act of 1906 reflect a critical turning point in consumer protection, driven by growing concerns over food and drug adulteration during the 18th and 19th centuries. Urbanization and industrialization exacerbated the practice of adulteration, with examples such as the substitution of brown sugar with ground-up lice and the use of plaster of Paris and chalk in flour. Advancements in chemistry played a dual role, enabling both sophisticated adulteration methods and more precise detection techniques.

Key figures like Frederick Accum and Lewis Caleb Beck highlighted the dangers of adulteration through seminal publications, influencing public and governmental awareness. The establishment of the Department of Agriculture's Division of Chemistry in 1862 marked the first scientific efforts to regulate food safety, with Harvey W. Wiley later spearheading these initiatives. Wiley's groundbreaking "Poison Squad" experiments in the early 1900s exposed the health risks of chemical preservatives, galvanizing public and media support for reform despite experimental limitations by today's standards.

The push for federal regulation faced numerous legislative failures until public outrage over exposés, including Upton Sinclair's *The Jungle*, and support from activist groups finally led to the 1906 enactment of the Meat Inspection Act and the Pure Food and Drugs Act. The Act, known as the Wiley Act, established federal oversight of food and drug commerce, requiring labeling for specific substances and prohibiting false claims about ingredients, though it fell short of addressing advertising claims or securing adequate enforcement mechanisms.

Despite these limitations, the Act laid the groundwork for the modern FDA and a federal role in safeguarding consumer health, demonstrating the transformative power of scientific advocacy and public pressure in regulatory advancements (Borchers et al. 2007).

10.3.1.2 Mission of FDA

To safeguard public's health, the Food and Drug Administration (FDA) ensures that pharmaceuticals for humans and animals, medical equipment, and biological products are secure, safe, and effective. Additionally, it regulates the safety of the country's food supply, cosmetics, and radiation-emitting products. The FDA also controls the manufacture, promotion, and distribution of tobacco products in order to safeguard the public's health and discourage youth use. By supporting innovation, the FDA helps improve the safety, effectiveness, and affordability of medical products. It also ensures the public has access to precise, scientifically supported information that is necessary for the safe use of food and medical supplies. Moreover, the FDA contributes to national security by safeguarding the food supply and helping develop medical responses to both natural and intentional public health threats ("What We Do I FDA" 2025).

The FDA fulfils its mission by premarket clearance monitoring; inspections, investigations, and surveillance; enforcement actions including corrections and penalties; development of regulations; and monitoring of bioresearch and good laboratory practices (Institute of Medicine 1988).

10.3.1.3 Organization of FDA

The FDA is a division of the Department of Health and Human Services and consists of 9 center-level organizations and 13 Headquarter (HQ) Offices. The following is a list of the centers along with their responsibilities ("FDA Organization Charts I FDA" 2025).

10.3.1.3.1 Center for Biologics Evaluation and Research (CBER)

The center utilizes strong scientific and regulatory knowledge to protect and enhance public health within the United States and, when possible, internationally. It aids in advancing, approving, and ensuring the availability of breakthrough technologies and safe, efficient medical products. Additionally, it works to shield the public from threats such as emerging infectious diseases and bioterrorism ("CBER Vision & Mission I FDA" 2025).

10.3.1.3.2 Center for Devices and Radiological Health (CDRH)

The CDRH is dedicated to protecting and promoting public health by ensuring that patients and healthcare professionals have timely and reliable access to medical devices that are safe, effective, and of high quality, as well as to radiation-emitting products that meet safety standards. The center also shares scientifically accurate information with consumers, patients, caregivers, and health-care providers about the products it regulates. Furthermore, CDRH supports innovation in medical devices by advancing regulatory science, providing the industry with clear and consistent regulatory pathways, and fostering public trust in the safety and effectiveness of devices available in the U.S. market ("CDRH Mission, Vision and Shared Values I FDA" 2025).

10.3.1.3.3 Center for Drug Evaluation and Research (CDER)

The center is responsible for both prescription and over-the-counter medications, encompassing biological therapies as well as generic drugs. Its responsibilities also cover a range of non-traditional products, including sunscreen, dandruff shampoos, antiperspirants, and fluoride toothpaste. The center emphasizes collaborative decision-making by ensuring the involvement of scientific and regulatory expertise for informing crucial drug approval choices. The center integrates initiatives for modernization of the drug review process, prioritizing efficiency and transparency to expedite access to safe and effective treatments for patients while maintaining the highest scientific standards ("Center for Drug Evaluation and Research (CDER) I FDA" 2025).

10.3.1.3.4 Human Foods Program (HFP)

The HFP manages all FDA initiatives related to food safety and nutrition. It is responsible for safe-guarding public health through science-based strategies aimed at preventing foodborne illnesses, minimizing diet-related chronic conditions, and ensuring the safe use of chemicals in food. Leadership and strategic oversight for HFP efforts—including food inspections and investigations—are provided by the Office of the Deputy Commissioner for Human Foods ("Human Foods Program I FDA" 2025).

10.3.1.3.5 Center for Tobacco Products (CTP)

The Family Smoking Prevention and Tobacco Control Act is enforced by the center. Its duties involve establishing product performance standards, reviewing premarket submissions for new and modified-risk tobacco products, requiring updated warning labels, and overseeing the advertising and promotion of tobacco products. ("Center for Tobacco Products I FDA" 2025).

10.3.1.3.6 Center for Veterinary Medicine (CVM)

The center aims at protecting human as well as animal health. For achieving this aim, the center enforces several activities such as ensuring safety and effectiveness of animal drugs; proper manufacturing and labeling of the drugs; ensuring food additives in animal food are safe; educating pet owners and veterinarians; monitoring and investigating side effects and quality issues reported for animal food, drugs, and devices; and carrying out research to support their policies and regulatory decisions about animal food, drugs, and devices ("Center for Veterinary Medicine | FDA" 2025).

10.3.1.3.7 Oncology Center of Excellence

The center unites FDA specialists to speed up the evaluation of medical products targeting cancer and blood-related diseases. Furthermore, the Office of Cancer Evaluation (OCE) leads multiple research projects and educational initiatives to enhance the development and regulation of cancer-related medical treatments. ("Oncology Center of Excellence | FDA" 2025).

10.3.1.3.8 Office of External Affairs

Serves as the central point for managing communication and educational activities related to the FDA's public health and regulatory programs. This position involves planning, organizing, and leading all outreach and communication initiatives aimed at media outlets, healthcare providers, patient groups, industry stakeholders, state agencies, consumer advocates, and the general public. In addition, the office manages speechwriting, editorial and creative support, and the adoption of leading practices in digital and web-based technologies ("Office of External Affairs | FDA" 2025).

10.3.1.3.9 Office of Operations

The mission is to deliver timely, efficient, high-quality, and cost-effective support services across the FDA and its centers, while also coordinating emergency preparedness and response activities concerning FDA-regulated products in collaboration with FDA and its stakeholders ("Office of Operations | FDA" 2025).

10.3.1.3.10 Office of Inspections and Investigations

The office directs field inspections, investigations, import monitoring, and emergency response operations. It partners with both internal and external agencies to collect, evaluate, and apply evidence that informs coordinated regulatory decisions. The office inspects regulated products and manufacturers and reviews imported items entering the United States. To fulfill its mission, it collaborates closely with state, local, tribal, territorial, and international authorities ("Office of Inspections and Investigations | FDA" 2025).

10.3.2 Office for Human Research Protections (OHRP) ("About OHRP | HHS.Gov" 2025)

The Office for Human Research Protections (OHRP) leads efforts to safeguard the rights, welfare, and safety of individuals participating in research funded or conducted by the U.S. Department of Health and Human Services. OHRP supports this mission by offering guidance and clarification, creating educational resources and programs, overseeing regulatory compliance, and advising on moral and legal issues pertaining to social-behavioral and biological research.

The Department of Health and Human Services' efforts to safeguard subjects involved in medical and human behavior research are spearheaded by the Office for Human Research Protections (OHRP), which was founded in June 2000. Additionally, it offers guidelines to all federal agencies doing research with human beings in accordance with the Common Rule, generally known as the Federal Policy for the Protection of Human Beings. The Office for Protection from Research Risks (OPRR), set up in 1972 as a division of the National Institutes of Health (NIH), was replaced by OHRP. The National Human Research Protections Advisory Committee (NHRPAC) was also created by HHS in June 2000 to offer expert advice and recommendations on issues related to the protection of human research participants.

OHRP, housed within HHS' Office of the Assistant Secretary for Health, provides direction and clarification, creates educational materials, monitors regulatory compliance, provides advice on ethical and regulatory issues in behavioral and biomedical research, and oversees assurance of compliance and IRB registration programs. It also supports the Secretary's Advisory Committee on Human Research Protections (SACHRP), which provides recommendations to the HHS Secretary on issues related to human subject protection. SACHRP, established on January 3, 2003, succeeded NHRPAC with similar duties. OHRP oversees more than 13,000 institutions—both in the United States and internationally—that conduct HHS-supported human subjects research that is not exempt from regulation.

10.3.2.1 Key Responsibilities of OHRP

a) Leadership in Human Research Protections: OHRP provides guidance and oversight for human research subject protections within HHS and collaborates with other federal agencies to ensure ethical standards are upheld across the U.S. government.
b) Regulatory Oversight: The office develops, monitors, and enforces compliance with HHS regulations concerning the protection of human subjects in research. This includes establishing criteria for approving assurances of compliance for both domestic and international institutions engaged in HHS-conducted or supported research.
c) Policy Development and Coordination: OHRP promotes and coordinates the development of appropriate regulations, policies, and procedures related to human subject protections, both within HHS and in collaboration with other federal departments and agencies.
d) Educational Initiatives: The office conducts programs to clarify and provide guidance on involving humans in research. It leads the development and implementation of educational programs and produces resource materials to inform both federal and non-federal sectors.
e) Evaluation of Effectiveness: OHRP assesses the effectiveness of HHS policies and programs dedicated to the protection of human subjects, ensuring that ethical standards are consistently applied and maintained.
f) Ethical Advisory Role: OHRP leads the identification and resolution of ethical issues in research and medicine by acting as a liaison to interagency, non-governmental, legislative, presidential, departmental, and international commissions and boards.
g) Promotion of Quality Improvement: The office advocates for the development of approaches that enhance and improve methods, particularly at the institutional level, to minimize risks to human subjects participating in research.

10.3.2.2 Organizational Structure ("Organization | HHS.Gov" 2025)

a) Office of the Director: Reporting to the Assistant Secretary for Health, the Director provides leadership on ethical and other issues associated with the protection of human subjects in research. The Director supervises the development and implementation of policies and advises HHS officials on matters related to human subject protections.
b) Division of Compliance Oversight: This division evaluates reports of noncompliance with HHS regulations, determining whether regulatory actions are necessary to protect human research subjects. It conducts both for-cause and not-for-cause evaluations to ensure adherence to ethical standards.
c) Division of Education and Development (DED): DED is responsible for educational outreach, hosting events, advising researchers, and disseminating educational materials about human research subject protections. It also provides online resources through the official OHRP website.

d) Division of Policy and Assurances: This division develops policies, guidelines, and standards for protecting human research participants and disseminates them to the research community. It manages Federal-wide Assurances of Compliance and supervises the registration process for Institutional Review Boards (IRBs).

10.4 KEY REGULATIONS AND GUIDELINES

The key regulations regarding clinical research include the Federal Food, Drug, and Cosmetic Act (FDCA), Common Rule (45 CFR 46), and ICH Guidelines ("Clinical Research Regulation For United States | ClinRegs" 2025).

10.4.1 Federal Food, Drug, and Cosmetic Act (FDCA)

The FDA's power to oversee medical devices and electronic products that emit radiation comes from the Federal Food, Drug, and Cosmetic Act (FD&C Act). This law sets forth the regulatory framework defining the FDA's authority over these items. To implement and enforce the FD&C Act's provisions concerning medical devices and radiation-emitting products, the FDA develops, issues, and enforces specific regulations. Enacted in 1938, the FD&C Act serves as a key piece of U.S. legislation, granting the FDA oversight of the manufacturing, marketing, and distribution of food, drugs, medical devices, and cosmetics. The law was enacted to safeguard consumers against unsafe or inaccurately labeled products. Its passage was prompted by a major public health disaster involving Elixir Sulfanilamide, a drug containing the toxic chemical diethylene glycol, which led to fatalities exceeding 100 persons across 15 states.

Prior to the enactment of the FDCA, drug makers were not required to prove their products were safe or effective before selling them. This changed on June 25, 1938, when President Franklin D. Roosevelt signed the FDCA into law, establishing a major breakthrough in consumer protection. The act, together with later amendments, formed the basis for broad public health reforms that continue to have a lasting impact.

The FDA, under the U.S. Department of Health and Human Services, enforces the FDCA. Its responsibilities include:

a) Requiring manufacturers to demonstrate the effectiveness and safety of novel medications before their public release.
b) Establishing and enforcing quality standards for food, drugs, medical devices, and cosmetics.
c) Conducting inspections of facilities involved in manufacturing, processing, packaging, and storing these products, including tobacco items.
d) Recalling or seizing unsafe or non-compliant products.
e) Regulating the advertising of prescription drugs and medical devices.
f) Setting labeling and claim standards, such as nutritional information, details about dietary supplement health claims, and food packaging.
g) Approving new drugs, medical devices, and additives for food and color.

Currently, the FDA is responsible for regulating products valued at over $1 trillion each year. The FDCA remains the foundation for the FDA's mission to safeguard public health by assuring the safety, efficacy, and security of food, pharmaceuticals, medical devices, and cosmetics. The agency also oversees other products such as tobacco and biologics, which include vaccines, blood products, and transplantable tissues. Furthermore, the FDA monitors radiation-emitting devices to ensure they do not endanger public safety (Lam and Patel 2023).

10.4.2 Common Rule (45 CFR 46)

Federal laws establish the standards that apply to businesses engaged in interstate commerce and designate the agencies responsible for enforcing those laws. The FDA develops regulations that explain how these laws should be implemented in practice. These rules also define the procedures required for the approval of various products. All regulations, updates, and official announcements from the FDA are published in the Federal Register, a daily publication issued by the U.S. government (Roundtable et al. 2002). Draft regulations are first published in the Federal Register to allow for public feedback. Once finalized, these regulations are included in the Code of Federal Regulations (CFR). Each year, the finalized rules from the Federal Register are compiled into the printed version of the CFR. The CFR is divided into 50 titles, each representing a broad regulatory area. The FDA's regulations appear primarily in Title 21, which interprets the Federal Food, Drug, and Cosmetic Act. This section outlines the legal responsibilities and procedures that sponsors must follow under federal law regarding food and drug regulation ("Federal Regulations for Clinical Investigators | FDA" 2025).

The Federal Policy for the Protection of Human Subjects, commonly called the "Common Rule," was enacted in 1991 and has been approved by 15 federal departments and agencies as distinct rules. The Department of Health and Human Services (HHS) outlines its version in 45 CFR Part 46, which is divided into four subparts: Subpart A—known as the Common Rule—sets general requirements; Subpart B includes added protections for pregnant women, fetuses, and newborns; Subpart C focuses on protections for prisoners; and Subpart D addresses safeguards for children. Each participating federal agency replicates the HHS language and section numbers from Subpart A within its portion of the Code of Federal Regulations (CFR). The Common Rule defines the basic standards for Institutional Review Boards (IRBs), informed consent procedures, and compliance assurances. Any human subjects research that is either supported or carried out by a federal department or agency must comply with that agency's specific regulations. The final authority for determining whether a particular activity falls under the Common Rule lies with the head of the relevant department or agency ("45 CFR 46 | HHS.Gov" 2025).

10.4.3 ICH Guidelines

The ICH topics are divided into four categories, with each topic assigned a code based on its classification.

10.4.3.1 Quality Guidelines

The International Council for Harmonisation (ICH) has established a series of Quality Guidelines aimed at promoting the safety, effectiveness, and quality of pharmaceutical products across member countries. These guidelines address key components of drug development and manufacturing, such as stability studies, validation of analytical methods, adherence to impurity control, and good manufacturing practices (GMP). By standardizing these practices, the ICH supports the acceptance of data by regulatory bodies across different regions, helping to simplify the drug approval process and maintain uniform product standards. Notable progress in the quality domain includes the standardization of stability testing, setting impurity thresholds, and the adoption of a more adaptable quality system based on GMP and risk management principles ("ICH Official Web Site: ICH" 2025a).

10.4.3.2 Efficacy Guidelines

The ICH has created Efficacy Guidelines to harmonize how clinical trials are designed, conducted, and reported, with a strong focus on participant safety. These guidelines help ensure that clinical research is carried out ethically and that the resulting data is trustworthy and can be accepted by regulatory authorities across various regions.

The ICH Efficacy Guidelines encompass various aspects of clinical research, including:

a) General Considerations for Clinical Studies (E8): Provides an overview of the principles and planning required for clinical trials.
b) Good Clinical Practice (E6): Provides a common framework for planning, carrying out, documenting, and disclosing human subjects' clinical experiments.
c) Statistical Principles for Clinical Trials (E9): Guides the application of statistical methods to guarantee the reliability and validity of trial results.
d) Clinical Safety Data Management (E2): Addresses the collection and reporting of safety information during clinical development.

A globally recognized standard known as Good Clinical Practice (GCP) directs the morality and scientific caliber of clinical trials that use human participants. In accordance with the moral principles outlined in the Declaration of Helsinki, it is intended to protect the participants' rights, safety, and welfare. Following GCP principles also helps ensure that the data and results collected during the study are credible as well as reliable. The term "trial conduct" represents the comprehensive management of a clinical trial—from its initial planning and setup through to its execution, monitoring, data collection, evaluation, analysis, and final reporting.

The main objective of the ICH GCP Guideline is to establish a universal standard that facilitates the mutual acceptance of clinical trial data by regulatory authorities in ICH member countries and regions. This guideline is based on the foundational principles outlined in ICH E8(R1) General Considerations for Clinical Studies, highlighting the need to promote a culture of quality in clinical trial design and execution. It reinforces proactive integration of quality into trial planning, identification of critical factors influencing trial outcomes, engagement of relevant stakeholders, and the adoption of a proportionate, risk-based approach to trial oversight.

Given the diversity in clinical trial scale, complexity, and cost, a thorough assessment of critical-to-quality factors and associated risks is essential for optimizing trial efficiency. By concentrating on activities that are vital for meeting trial objectives, sponsors and stakeholders can ensure that trials are both scientifically rigorous and operationally efficient ("ICH Official Web Site: ICH" 2025b).

10.4.3.3 Safety Guidelines

The International Council for Harmonisation (ICH) has developed a comprehensive set of Safety Guidelines aimed at identifying probable risks that are associated with the pharmaceuticals, including genotoxicity, carcinogenicity, and reproductive toxicity. These guidelines are designed to ensure that medicines are safe for human use by providing standardized testing protocols and assessment criteria. By following these guidelines, pharmaceutical developers can systematically evaluate and mitigate safety risks during drug development, thereby enhancing patient safety and facilitating regulatory approval across different regions ("ICH Official Web Site: ICH" 2025c).

10.4.3.4 Multidisciplinary Guidelines

The multidisciplinary guidelines cover areas such as Common Technical Document (CTD) and Medical Dictionary for Regulatory Activities (MedDRA). They aim to harmonize technical requirements and terminology across various aspects of pharmaceutical development and regulation ("ICH Official Web Site: ICH" 2025d).

REFERENCES

"45 CFR 46 | HHS.Gov." 2025. Accessed February 24. https://www.hhs.gov/ohrp/regulations-and-policy/regulations/45-cfr-46/index.html.

"About OHRP | HHS.Gov." 2025. Accessed February 24. https://www.hhs.gov/ohrp/about-ohrp/index.html.

Borchers, Andrea T., Frank Hagie, Carl L. Keen, and M. Eric Gershwin. 2007. "The History and Contemporary Challenges of the US Food and Drug Administration." *Clinical Therapeutics* 29 (1). Clin Ther: 1–16. https://doi.org/10.1016/J.CLINTHERA.2007.01.006.

"CBER Vision & Mission | FDA." 2025. Accessed February 24. https://www.fda.gov/about-fda/center-biologics-evaluation-and-research-cber/cber-vision-mission.

"CDRH Mission, Vision and Shared Values | FDA." 2025. Accessed February 24. https://www.fda.gov/about-fda/center-devices-and-radiological-health/cdrh-mission-vision-and-shared-values.

"Center for Drug Evaluation and Research (CDER) | FDA." 2025. Accessed February 24. https://www.fda.gov/about-fda/fda-organization/center-drug-evaluation-and-research-cder.

"Center for Tobacco Products | FDA." 2025. Accessed February 24. https://www.fda.gov/about-fda/fda-organization/center-tobacco-products.

"Center for Veterinary Medicine | FDA." 2025. Accessed February 24. https://www.fda.gov/about-fda/fda-organization/center-veterinary-medicine.

"Clinical Research Regulation For United States | ClinRegs." 2025. Accessed February 24. https://clinregs.niaid.nih.gov/country/united-states.

"Clinical Trials and Human Subject Protection | FDA." 2025. Accessed February 24. https://www.fda.gov/science-research/science-and-research-special-topics/clinical-trials-and-human-subject-protection.

David, Sharoon, and Peggy Y. Kim. 2023. "Drug Trials." *StatPearls*, June. StatPearls Publishing. https://www.ncbi.nlm.nih.gov/books/NBK546595/.

"FDA Organization Charts | FDA." 2025. Accessed February 24. https://www.fda.gov/about-fda/fda-organization/fda-organization-charts.

"Federal Regulations for Clinical Investigators | FDA." 2025. Accessed February 24. https://www.fda.gov/drugs/investigational-new-drug-ind-application/federal-regulations-clinical-investigators.

"Human Foods Program | FDA." 2025. Accessed February 24. https://www.fda.gov/about-fda/fda-organization/human-foods-program.

"ICH Official Web Site: ICH." 2025a. Accessed February 24. https://www.ich.org/page/quality-guidelines.

"ICH Official Web Site: ICH." 2025b. Accessed February 24. https://www.ich.org/page/safety-guidelines.

"ICH Official Web Site: ICH." 2025c. Accessed February 24. https://www.ich.org/page/efficacy-guidelines.

"ICH Official Web Site: ICH." 2025d. Accessed February 24. https://www.ich.org/page/multidisciplinary-guidelines.

Institute of Medicine (US) Council on Health Care Technology; C. Goodman, ed. 1988. *Medical Technology Assessment Directory: A Pilot Reference To Organizations, Assessments, and Information Resources*. Washington, DC: National Academies Press (US) & Food and Drug Administration.

Kandi, Venkataramana, and Sabitha Vadakedath. 2023. "Clinical Trials and Clinical Research: A Comprehensive Review." *Cureus* 15 (2). Springer Science and Business Media LLC: e35077. https://doi.org/10.7759/CUREUS.35077.

Lam, Clinton, and Preeti Patel. 2023. "Food, Drug, and Cosmetic Act." *Drugs in American Society: An Encyclopedia of History, Politics, Culture, and the Law: Volumes 1–3* 2 (July). StatPearls Publishing: 415–17. https://www.ncbi.nlm.nih.gov/books/NBK585046/.

McNair, Lindsay. 2022. "Ethical and Regulatory Oversight of Clinical Research: The Role of the Institutional Review Board." *Experimental Biology and Medicine (Maywood, N.J.)* 247 (7). Exp Biol Med (Maywood): 561–6. https://doi.org/10.1177/15353702221078216.

National Academies of Sciences, Engineering, and Medicine; Health and Medicine Division; Board on Global Health; Committee on Mutual Recognition Agreements and Reliance in the Regulation of Medicines, Patricia Cuff, and Alastair J. Wood. 2019. *Regulating Medicines in a Globalized World: The Need for Increased Reliance among Regulators*. Washington, DC: National Academies Press (US).

"Office of External Affairs | FDA." 2025. Accessed February 24. https://www.fda.gov/about-fda/office-commissioner/office-external-affairs.

"Office of Inspections and Investigations | FDA." 2025. Accessed February 24. https://www.fda.gov/about-fda/fda-organization/office-inspections-and-investigations.

"Office of Operations | FDA." 2025. Accessed February 24. https://www.fda.gov/about-fda/office-commissioner/office-operations.

"Oncology Center of Excellence | FDA." 2025. Accessed February 24. https://www.fda.gov/about-fda/fda-organization/oncology-center-excellence.

"Organization | HHS.Gov." 2025. Accessed February 24. https://www.hhs.gov/ohrp/about-ohrp/organization/index.html.

Roundtable, Institute of Medicine (US) Clinical Research, Sean Tunis, Allan Korn, and Alex Ommaya. 2002. "Definitions of Clinical Research and Components of the Enterprise." National Academies Press (US). https://www.ncbi.nlm.nih.gov/books/NBK220717/.

"What We Do | FDA." 2025. Accessed February 24. https://www.fda.gov/about-fda/what-we-do.

11 Placebo and Noceb

Sparsh Gupta
Professor and Head, Department of Pharmacology, Vardhman Mahavir Medical College and Safdarjung Hospital, New Delhi, India

11.1 INTRODUCTION

The term "placebo" originated from St. Jerome's mistranslation of Psalm 116, which in the Latin version is "Placebo Domino in regione vivorum," meaning "I shall please the Lord in the land of the living." In 1811, the Hooper's Medical Dictionary first defined the term "placebo" as "any medicine adapted more to please than benefit the patient" [1]. In modern medicine, placebos are defined by their inactive ingredients and are commonly used as control substances in clinical trials and treatments. Recent findings reveal that the effects of placebo are real psychobiological phenomena influenced by the overall therapeutic settings, often showing significant impact in both laboratory and clinical settings. Interestingly, research also demonstrates that these effects can emerge in a clinical context even without administering an actual placebo [2]. Recent studies have shown that the utilization of placebos in clinical practice is pervasive, with an estimated 40% of prescriptions serving a placebo function [3,4]. This occurs with varying degrees of physician awareness, as some are cognizant of the placebo nature of their prescriptions, while others are not [3–5].

Placebos are generally classified into two types: pure placebo and impure placebo. A pure placebo is an inert substance without direct physiologic effect, whereas an impure placebo contains active pharmacological ingredients that are known or expected to be ineffective for the condition being treated, yet it is administered to potentially achieve a psychological benefit [6]. The placebo has also been employed in the form of placebo surgery, or sham surgery, which entails mimicking the surgical environment, including the use of anaesthesia and making an incision, but without performing any actual intervention.

11.2 CHARACTERISTICS OF PLACEBO

A place should be like active treatment in terms of the following:

a. Shape
b. Size
c. Colour
d. Weight
e. Smell
f. Name

11.3 PLACEBO, PLACEBO EFFECT, AND PLACEBO RESPONSE

In medical terminology, clear distinctions have been established between the concepts of placebo, placebo effect, and placebo response. According to Mitsikostas et al. 2020, a substance or an intervention can be considered as placebos if its administration or application leads to a beneficial outcome even though its active ingredients have no inherent therapeutic power [7]. In contrast, the placebo effect denotes the specific beneficial outcomes resulting from the administration or application of a placebo, attributed solely to placebo-related processes such as expectation, conditioning,

 DOI: 10.1201/9781003533085-11

and observational learning [7]. The response to placebo, however, describes any overall improvement in health observed from before to after placebo administration.

11.4 MECHANISM OF PLACEBO EFFECTS

A genuine placebo effect is a psychobiological response that arises in the brain of patient after receiving a substance which is inert or a sham physical treatment, such as sham surgery, accompanied by verbal or contextual signals suggesting clinical improvements. Consequently, the observed effects following placebo administration cannot be due to an inert substance alone, because agents like sugar pills and saline solutions have no therapeutic properties. Rather, the response arises from the psychosocial environment surrounding the inert substance and patient's perception [8]. Furthermore, the real placebo response, psychobiological phenomenon, is relevant and has a substantial contribution to the clinical improvement as shown in an antidepressant trial by Kirsch and Sapirstein, 1998 [9]. There are various placebo effects, each having distinct processes across various diseases, systems, and therapeutic interventions, where a variety of mechanisms may be involved in the patient's brain depending on the specific condition [10]. These mechanisms include the following:

a. Expecting therapeutic benefit
b. Anxiety modulation by expectations
c. Execrating reward
d. Behavioural conditioning
e. Reinforced expectations
f. Social learning

11.5 EXPECTING THERAPEUTIC BENEFIT

As a principle of evolution, expectations play a major role in preparing the body to anticipate an event so that the person can cope with it in a much better way. This can result in a cognitive re-evaluation of proper conduct, where favourable expectations may encourage behaviours, such as going back to a regular daily routine, while unfavourable expectations may prevent such behaviours. Numerous mechanisms exist through which the anticipation of a future event can influence physiological processes. For instance, anticipating unfavourable outcome can heighten anxiety by preparing for a potential threat, while expecting a favourable outcome can lower anxiety and activate reward-related neural networks. Furthermore, both anxiety and reward mechanisms play significant roles in placebo responsiveness, and it operates simultaneously with memory and motivation [11].

11.5.1 Anxiety Modulation by Expectations

Patients receiving a placebo have expectations regarding future responses. Several studies have demonstrated that when a topical placebo cream is administered to a participant experiencing experimentally produced pain along with verbal indication that the cream is a potent analgesic, the patient's expectation is manipulated and the placebo analgesic effects are mediated [12,13]. Furthermore, implementing a conditioning protocol to enhance expectations leads to stronger analgesic reactions to placebo. This demonstrates how expectation may interact with other concepts like desire and emotions, as well as mediate and modulate placebo effects [14–16].

11.5.2 Execrating Reward

Reward systems are regulated by distinct neural pathways that integrate cognitive, emotional, and motor functions, producing physiological responses similar to those observed with reward, such as food, money, or drugs. In several animal studies, it is found that the dopaminergic neurons in the ventral tegmental area of the brainstem, which project to the nucleus accumbens within the ventral basal ganglia, are responsive to both the expected magnitude of the rewards and any deviations from those expectations, reflecting an adaptive mechanism that shapes behavioural responses [17,18]. Furthermore, strong research findings indicate that the mesolimbic dopaminergic system is triggered when a person expects clinical improvements from placebo treatment [19].

In a study by Scott et al. (2007), using an experimental pain model in healthy participants, placebo responsiveness was found to correlate with dopamine activation in the nucleus accumbens. Late observations revealed that placebo-induced activation of both opioid and dopaminergic systems in several brain regions, including the nucleus accumbens, was associated with the anticipation of benefits and perceived effectiveness of the placebo. In contrast, nocebo responses were linked to reduced activity in these same systems. These findings highlight that placebo and nocebo effects produce opposite neurobiological responses within dopaminergic and endogenous opioid pathways.

11.5.3 Behavioural Conditioning

Classical conditioning involves cognitive components derived from previous therapeutic experiences. Thus, learning and anticipation are intertwined in the manifestation of the effect of placebo. Furthermore, learning is a fundamental mechanism in placebo responsiveness. Recent studies have shown that patients with chronic headaches, who regularly take medications for the same, may associate the pill's shape, colour, and taste with pain relief [20]. This conditioning means that a similar-looking sugar pill can also reduce pain. Numerous stimuli, including hospitals and healthcare professionals, can be similarly conditioned. Such an associative process, where a neutral stimulus (e.g., pill shape) becomes effective in symptom reduction through repeated pairing with an active principle, underlies many placebo effects. Studies have also shown that placebos administered after effective drugs elicit stronger responses than first-time placebos, highlighting the role of previous analgesic experiences in placebo efficacy [20,21].

11.5.4 Reinforced Expectations

Reinforced conditioning modulates placebo effect by strengthening the association between neutral stimuli and therapeutic outcomes, thereby enhancing the patient's expectations rather than creating an unconscious Pavlovian response. This process involves pairing a neutral stimulus, such as the colour, taste, or shape of a pill, with an active treatment that produces a desired effect. Recent studies have shown that when subjects are conditioned with reduced pain stimulation alongside a placebo, their subsequent responses to the placebo are significantly stronger [22,23]. This indicates that the conditioning procedure amplifies the patient's expectation of benefit, which is critical for the placebo effect to manifest. Reinforced conditioning thereby integrates cognitive and physiological components, demonstrating that the impact of placebo is not an automatic outcome but a complex interplay of learned expectations and physiological mechanisms.

11.5.5 Social Learning

Social learning, where individuals learn from one another through observation and imitation, also plays a role in placebo effects. A recent study compared placebo-induced analgesia resulting from social observations, conditioning, and verbal suggestion [24]. Under social observation conditions, subjects observed a demonstrator exhibiting analgesic responses when pain was associated with a green light. During the conditioning condition, participants experienced reduced stimulus intensity with a green light. In the verbal suggestion condition, participants were told to expect benefits from the green light. Results showed that social observation induced significant placebo responses, comparable to conditioning and significantly greater than verbal suggestion alone, highlighting the power of social learning in placebo effects [24,25].

11.6 THE NEURAL CIRCUIT INVOLVED IN PLACEBO ANALGESIA

The placebo analgesic response involves a very complex neural network. The cerebral cortex initiates a descending pathway that modulates and reduces pain signal transmission. Also, various cortical areas, including the anterior cingulate cortex and the dorsolateral prefrontal cortex, have been found to activate in response to placebo administration [26]. This activation extends to the hypothalamus, periaqueductal grey, and rostroventromedial medulla, and finally reaches the spinal cord, inhibiting dorsal horn neurons [27,28]. The aforementioned pathway is believed to be opioidergic, as supported by several studies showing that opioid antagonists inhibit placebo analgesia and that μ-opioid receptor activation has been observed in vivo during placebo analgesia [27,29]. Another neuronal circuit involving the dopaminergic reward system, where dopaminergic neurons projecting from the area of ventral tegmental to the nucleus accumbens play a significant role in the placebo effect [30]. Both the aforementioned neuronal circuits are antagonized at several areas, which is the basis of hyperalgesia induced by nocebo. For instance, a cholecystokinin-ergic (CCK-ergic) system inhibits the opioidergic circuit within the rostroventromedial medulla and reduced activity of μ-opioids and D2–D3 dopamine receptors in the nucleus accumbens dampens the dopaminergic reward system [23,30].

11.7 GENETICS AND PLACEBO

Recent studies have shown that specific genetic variants may enhance placebo responsiveness. However, limited genetic studies have been performed, warranting further research in order to validate and expand these findings. Understanding these predictors could significantly impact clinical trial designs and the customization of therapies for individuals.

11.8 PLACEBO IN CLINICAL TRIALS

Placebos are fundamental in modern clinical trials, serving as a benchmark for evaluating the effectiveness of new treatments. Since their widespread adoption post-World War II, placebo-controlled trials have become the gold standard for the evaluation of new treatments. These trials, conducted under double-blind conditions, provide the best evidence for assessing whether a treatment genuinely offers therapeutic benefits beyond psychological effects. It has been consistently observed that a significant proportion of patients in placebo groups experience dramatic improvements in their condition, as highlighted by Henry Beecher's influential proto-meta-analysis indicating a placebo response rate of approximately 35%. This underscores the importance of placebos in distinguishing true treatment effects from placebo effects, thereby ensuring the credibility and reliability of clinical trial outcomes.

11.9 ETHICS OF PLACEBO-CONTROLLED TRIALS

According to the Declaration of Helsinki: "In any medical study, every patient including those of control group, if any should be assured of the best proven diagnostic and therapeutic methods and no patient should suffer from unnecessary pain" [31]. In clinical trials where effective treatments already exist for a condition, employing a placebo control group is considered unethical as it denies patients access to known effective therapies. These trials seek to ascertain whether new drugs offer improved efficacy or safety compared to established treatments, rather than withholding proven care from participants.

11.10 METHODS TO ASSESS PLACEBO RESPONSE

Over the past few decades, several alternative approaches to the traditional double-blind placebo-controlled randomized clinical trial (RCT) have been suggested. Broadly, these designs fall into two categories. One category adapts experimental designs to allow more accurate estimation of placebo effects. The other category aims to reduce or eliminate placebo responses during data collection, thereby simplifying the inference of treatment effects. In this chapter, we will discuss a few designs that will provide a precise estimation of placebo effects, which include the following:

11.9.1 No-treatment-control arm
11.9.2 Balanced Placebo Design
11.9.3 Enrichment designs
11.9.4 Placebo lead-in phases
11.9.5 Sequential parallel comparison design
11.9.6 Enriched enrolment with randomized withdrawal design
11.9.7 Two-way enriched design

11.10.1 No-Treatment-Control Arm

According to the definition of placebo, the responses which are observed in subjects who received placebo are considered perceived placebo effect. This encompasses the impact of receiving a simulated treatment, such as an inert pill or injection, with other non-specific effects. In order to isolate the true placebo effect, these non-specific effects should be separated from the total observed responses. However, quantifying these non-specific effects in standard randomized clinical trials (RCTs) is challenging. One strategy to disentangle the placebo effect involves a no-treatment control (NTC) arm, where participants receive neither placebo nor an active treatment. The NTC serves as a control for the placebo intervention, like how the placebo controls the active treatment. Randomization ensures that non-specific influences are evenly distributed across all groups, allowing the placebo effects to be estimated by analysing the differences in responses between the NTC and placebo groups. However, there are serious ethical issues with this design as one group is deprived of any treatment.

11.10.2 Balanced Placebo Design (BPD)

The issues in standard RCTs, where participants know the chances of them receiving a placebo, have prompted researchers to design studies that manipulate expectations by altering information provided to participants. The Balanced Placebo Design (BPD) achieves this by providing incorrect information to half of the participants about their treatment. Subjects are randomly allocated to either placebo or active treatment, with half receiving correct information and half receiving false information. This design allows for a more accurate quantification of the placebo effect and enables testing the assumption of additivity between treatment and placebo effects [32]. However, using active placebos, which mimic side effects of the active treatment, is impractical in clinical trials due to availability issues [33]. The most important drawback of this design is that the participants are informed about the treatment they receive, which violates the principle of perfect blinding. Moreover, certain participants may distrust the truthfulness of information provided. On the other hand, participants receiving active treatment but told they are receiving a placebo may be less compliant, thus reducing the true treatment effect [33].

11.10.3 Enrichment Designs

Enrichment designs help to decrease the effect of placebo and thereby enhance the effect of treatment by randomizing only a selected subset of the initial sample enrolled in the study. This approach often results in larger effect sizes and allows inclusion of smaller sample sizes. A few enrichment designs are described as follows:

11.10.4 Placebo Lead-in Phases

This is one of the most commonly used enrichment designs, where a single-blind placebo lead-in phase is included. In this design, all the participants initially receive a placebo prior to randomization into either placebo or active treatment during the study. This phase aims to detect and remove individuals who respond to placebo from the study to enhance the precision of treatment effect. Even though this design is very effective in reducing placebo responders in the study, lead-in phases are time-consuming and costly. Also, their efficacy is debated in various studies.

11.10.5 Sequential Parallel Comparison Design (SPCD)

The sequential parallel comparison design comprises two stages. During the initial stage, subjects are randomly allocated to active treatment or placebo group, after which placebo responders are detected based on their observed responses and subsequently excluded from the study. In the second stage, non-responders to placebo are re-randomized to either active treatment or placebo. This design allows the treatment effect to be calculated within a refined sample, offering a more precise estimate by excluding placebo responders [34].

11.10.6 Enriched Enrolment with Randomized Withdrawal Design (EERW)

The Enriched Enrolment Randomized Withdrawal (EERW) design includes all participants beginning with a single-blind active treatment phase. Following this initial phase, participants who respond to treatment are randomized to either placebo group or the active treatment group in the next stage. Recent studies have shown that the subjects who initially respond positively to the active treatment are more likely to lose this benefit when switched to placebo. Therefore, this design is believed to maximize participant outcome and more closely replicate clinical practice, as all participants can benefit from the active treatment [35].

11.10.7 Two-Way Enriched Design

This design allows all the participants to be initially randomized in either the placebo group or active treatment group. In the next stage, responders to the active treatment are re-randomized to continue the treatment or receive placebo, enabling assessment of sustained efficacy. Similarly, participants who have shown negligible or no response to placebo in the first phase are re-randomized in the second phase to receive either active treatment or placebo. This design integrates the strengths of both the SPCD and the EERW design and therefore offers valuable insights into multiple dimensions of treatment and placebo effects, covering both short- and long-term efficacy. However, this design is too time-consuming and costly, which limits its practical use [36].

11.11 NOCEBO

The effect of nocebo represents the exact opposite of the effect of placebo, where unfavourable expectations or beliefs about a treatment cause harmful or adverse effects in patients, even when the patient receives an inert substance or sham treatment. This phenomenon demonstrates the powerful influence of psychological factors on physical health. The nocebo effect can induce symptoms such as pain, nausea, or fatigue solely due to the anticipation of negative effects. A nocebo effect can be induced by pairing an inactive treatment with negative verbal suggestions implying symptoms worsening, such as increased pain. In a recent study, healthy volunteers were told to expect painful sensations before being exposed to either touch stimuli or weak electrical shocks. These suggestions transformed tactile stimuli into pain and low-intensity pain into high-intensity pain, demonstrating that nocebo suggestions can produce hyperalgesia and allodynia (innocuous stimulation of pain response) [37]. The expectations of unfavourable outcomes can thus amplify pain by activating several regions of the brain, like the anterior cingulate cortex, prefrontal cortex, insula, and hippocampus, during pain anticipation. This highlights the critical need to carefully manage patient communication and expectations in clinical practice, as the effects of nocebo can significantly influence treatment outcomes and patient well-being.

REFERENCES

1. Aronson J. Please, please me. BMJ. 1999: 318:716.
2. Finniss DG, Kaptchuk TJ, Miller F, Benedetti F. Biological, clinical, and ethical advances of placebo effects. Lancet. 2010; 375: 686–695.
3. Tilburt JC, Emanuel EJ, Kaptchuk TJ, Curlin FA, Miller FG. Prescribing "placebo treatments": Results of national survey of US internists and rheumatologists. BMJ. 2008; 23: 337.
4. Carvalho C, Caetano JM, Cunha L, Rebouta P, Kaptchuk TJ, Kirsch I. Open-label placebo treatment in chronic low back pain: A randomized controlled trial. Pain. 2016; 157: 2766–2772.
5. Pardo-Cabello AJ, Manzano-Gamero V, Puche-Cañas E. Placebo: A brief updated review. Naunyn-Schmiedeberg's Archives of Pharmacology. 2022; 395: 1343–1356.
6. Kaptchuk TJ, Hemond CC, Miller FG. Placebos in chronic pain: Evidence, theory, ethics, and use in clinical practice. BMJ. 2020; 20: 370.
7. Mitsikostas DD, Blease C, Carlino E, Colloca L, Geers et al. European Headache Federation. European Headache Federation recommendations for placebo and nocebo terminology. J Headache Pain. 2020; 21: 117.
8. Price DD, Milling LS, Kirsch I, Duff A, Montgomery GH, Nicholls SS. Analysis of factors that contribute to the magnitude of placebo analgesia in an experimental paradigm. Pain. 1999; 83: 147–156.
9. Kirsch I, Sapirstein G. Listening to Prozac but hearing placebo: A meta-analysis of antidepressant medication. Prevention & Treatment. 1998;1(2):2a.
10. Enck P, Benedetti F, Schedlowski M. New insights into the placebo and nocebo responses. Neuron. 2008 July 31; 59(2): 195–206.
11. Price DD, Finniss DG, Benedetti F. A comprehensive review of the placebo effect: Recent advances and current thought. Annu Rev Psychol. 2008; 59: 565–590.
12. Benedetti F, Arduino C, Amanzio M. Somatotopic activation of opioid systems by target-directed expectations of analgesia. J Neurosci. 1999; 19: 3639–3648.
13. Kirsch I. Response expectancy as a determinant of experience and behavior. Am Psychol. 1985; 40: 1189–1202.
14. Vase L, Robinson ME, Verne GN, Price DD. The contributions of suggestion, desire, and expectation to placebo effects in irritable bowel syndrome patients: An empirical investigation. Pain. 2003; 105: 17–25.
15. Voudouris NJ, Peck CL, Coleman G. Conditioned response models of placebo phenomena: Further support. Pain. 1989; 38: 109–116.
16. Voudouris NJ, Peck CL, Coleman G. The role of conditioning and verbal expectancy in the placebo response. Pain. 1990; 43: 121–128.
17. Tobler PN, Fiorillo CD, Schultz W. Adaptive coding of reward value by dopamine neurons. Science. 2005; 307: 1642–1645.
18. Schultz W. Behavioural theories and the neurophysiology of reward. Ann Rev Psychol. 2006; 57: 87–115.
19. de la Fuente-Fernandez R, Ruth TJ, Sossi V, Schulzer M, Calne DB, Stoessl AJ. Expectation and dopamine release: Mechanisms of the placebo effect in Parkinson's disease. Science. 2001; 293: 1164–1166.
20. Colloca L, Benedetti F. Placebos and painkillers: Is mind as real as matter? Nat Rev Neurosci. 2005; 6: 545–552.
21. Colloca L, Benedetti F. How prior experience shapes placebo analgesia. Pain. 2006; 124: 126–133.
22. Benedetti F, Amanzio M, Vighetti S, Asteggiano G. The biochemical and neuroendocrine bases of the hyperalgesic nocebo effect. J Neurosci. 2006; 26: 12014–12022.
23. Benedetti F, Arduino C, Costa S, Vighetti S, Tarenzi L, Rainero I, et al. Loss of expectation-related mechanisms in Alzheimer's disease makes analgesic therapies less effective. Pain. 2006; 121: 133–144.
24. Colloca L, Benedetti F. Placebo analgesia induced by social observational learning. Pain. 2009; 144: 28–34.
25. Bootzin RR, Caspi O. Explanatory mechanisms for placebo effects: Cognition, personality and social learning. The science of the placebo: Toward an interdisciplinary research agenda. 2002: 108–132.

26. Wager TD, Billing JK, Smith EE, Sokolik A, Casey KL, Davidson RJ, et al. Placebo–induced changes in fMRI in the anticipation and experience of pain. Science. 2004; 303: 1162–1166.
27. Eippert F, Bingel U, Schoell ED, Yacubian J, Klinger R, Lorenz J, et al. Activation of the opioidergic descending pain control system underlies placebo analgesia. Neuron. 2009; 63: 533–543.
28. Eippert F, Finsterbusch J, Bingel U, Bu¨ chel C. Direct evidence for spinal cord involvement in placebo analgesia. Science. 2009; 326: 404.
29. Wager TD, Scott DJ, Zubieta JK. Placebo effects on human m–opioid activity during pain. Proc Nat Acad Sci. 2007; 104: 11056–11061.
30. Scott DJ, Stohler CS, Egnatuk CM, Wang H, Koeppe RA, et al. Placebo and nocebo effects are defined by opposite opioid and dopaminergic responses. Arch Gen Psychiatry. 2008; 65: 1225–1226.
31. Simon R. Are placebo-controlled clinical trials ethical? Editorial Ann Intern Med. 2000; 133: 474–475.
32. Kirsch I and Weixel LJ. Double-blind versus deceptive administration of a placebo. Behav Neurosci 1988; 102: 319–323.
33. Enck P, Klosterhalfen S, Zipfel S. Novel study designs to investigate the placebo response. BMC Med Res Methodol. 2011; 11: 90.
34. Fava M, Evins AE, Dorer DJ, et al. The problem of the placebo response in clinical trials for psychiatric disorders: Culprits, possible remedies, and a novel study design approach. Psychother Psychosom. 2003; 72: 115–127.
35. McQuay HJ, Derry S, Moore AR, et al. Enriched enrolment with randomised withdrawal (EERW): Time for a new look at clinical trial design in chronic pain. Pain. 2008; 135: 217–220.
36. Ivanova A and Tamura RN. A two-way enriched clinical trial design: Combining advantages of placebo lead-in and randomized withdrawal. Stat Methods Med Res. 2015; 24: 871–890.
37. Colloca L, Sigaudo M, Benedetti F. The role of learning in nocebo and placebo effects. Pain. 2008; 136: 211–218.

12 Role of Pharmacovigilance in Clinical Research

Kapish Bisht and Manoj Sharma
Global Pharmacovigilance Department Win-Medicare Pvt. Ltd

12.1 INTRODUCTION

Drug safety monitoring or pharmacovigilance has been used for considerably longer than 150 years. *The Lancet* findings published in 1893 reported the first recognized framework for the documentation and reporting of suspected adverse drug reactions (ADRs).[1] These findings were based on the reports of anesthesia-related mortality from doctors in Britain and their colonies that were published in *The Lancet*. This eventually triggered the concept of monitoring of drug safety among the medical community and later on beginning of the concept of "pharmacovigilance."

Pharmacovigilance, a word of French origin, refers to the discipline focused on identification, evaluation, and prevention of adverse effects of medicines. The term combines the Greek *pharmakon*, which means a drug or remedy, and the Latin *vigilans*, which means being careful or watchful[2]. According to the U.K. MHRA (Medicines and Healthcare Products Regulatory Agency), it is referred to as "a technical term used for identifying and addressing risk/benefit issues related to approved medicines in clinical settings, as well as for effectively disseminating of this knowledge to ensure their safe and effective utilization"[3]. World Health Organization (WHO) describes pharmacovigilance as "the science and activities related to the detection, assessment, understanding and prevention of adverse effects or any other drug related problem"[4].

12.2 CLINICAL TRIALS: ASPECTS OF SAFETY MONITORING

Clinical trials are voluntary research studies conducted in human beings to answer specific questions about the safety and/or effectiveness of drugs, vaccines, medical devices, and other therapies, or new ways of using existing treatments. During the drug development process (clinical trials phase I to III), pharmacovigilance (Figure 12.1) includes monitoring and evaluation of all adverse events with or without a causal relationship to the investigational medicinal product (IMP)*. The basic framework for pharmacovigilance during the clinical development process is presented in Figure 12.1.

Pharmacovigilance has a role during clinical development, in view of the number of drugs that have been withdrawn or have had warnings added to their labels due to hepatotoxicity. In the case of troglitazone (an antidiabetic drug, voluntarily withdrawn from the market by the licence holder in 2000), it was reported that 1.95% of patients treated with troglitazone in clinical trials developed elevations of aminotransferases that were greater than three times the upper limit of normal. A similar finding was noted in 0.6% of placebo-treated patients, so the increase seen in the active-treatment groups seems quite modest.[5]

For the past 35 years, there have been continued instances of drug recalls (removal of prescription or over-the-counter medication from the market). This includes the recall of valdecoxib (Bextra) and rofecoxib (VIOXX) from the worldwide market because of the increased risk of cardiovascular events.

 DOI: 10.1201/9781003533085-12

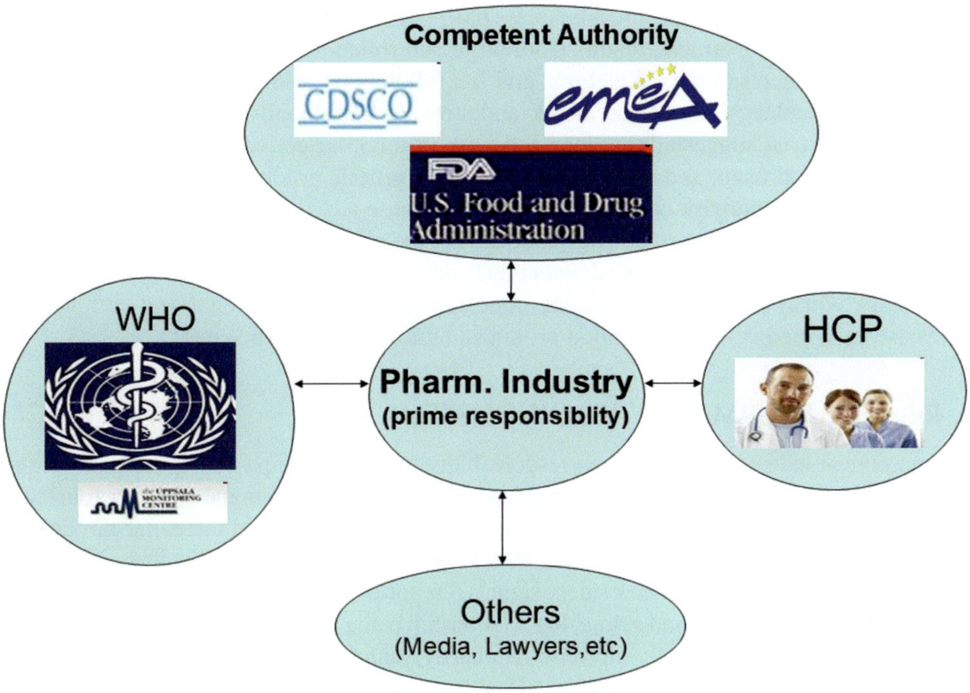

FIGURE 12.1 Pharmacovigilance framework during clinical development.

The other recalls posted on the website of the USFDA[6] include:

- voluntary nationwide recall of all accusure® insulin syringes.
- worldwide voluntary field removal of the original version of the 6F neuron 070 delivery catheter.

For details on other recalls made in the past 5 years, readers may visit the website http://www.fda.gov/Safety/Recalls.

Other precautionary statements (black box warning) or public health advisories due to the discovery of potential hazards during their use include:

- new safety information (severe, life-threatening, and in some cases fatal hepatotoxicity, including fulminant and cholestatic hepatitis, hepatic necrosis, and hepatic failure) added to the "WARNINGS and Boxed Warning for VIRAMUNE."
- new warning for Strattera, a drug approved for attention deficit hyperactivity disorder (ADHD) in adults and children. The labeling is being updated with a bolded warning about the potential for severe liver injury.
- public health advisory describing revisions to the WARNINGS, DOSAGE AND ADMINISTRATION, CLINICAL PHARMACOLOGY, and PRECAUTIONS sections of the labeling of Crestor (rosuvastatin calcium).
- public health advisory concerning the use of non-steroidal anti-inflammatory drug products (NSAIDs), including those known as COX-2 selective agents.
- recommendations of EMEA for the use of nimesulide[7].

Most of the aforementioned recalls and advisories have been issued on the basis of results from controlled clinical trials. For example, results from large controlled clinical trials[8–11] have shown that the COX-2 selective agents (Vioxx, Celebrex, and Bextra) may be associated with an increased risk of serious cardiovascular events (heart attack and stroke). Additionally, preliminary results from a long-term clinical trial suggested that long-term use of a non-selective NSAID, naproxen, which was sold as Aleve, Naprosyn, and other trade names and generic products, may be associated with an increased cardiovascular risk compared to placebo. These advisories and recalls form the basis for understanding the role of pharmacovigilance during the clinical trial process (clinical research), especially at a time when continuous advancement and introduction of new treatment approaches worldwide have widened pharmacovigilance concerns to include traditional and complementary medicines, herbals, medical devices, blood products, biologicals, and vaccines.

12.3 ROLE OF PHARMACEUTICAL INDUSTRY

The pharmaceutical industry has the prime responsibility toward the improvement of patient care (or clinical trial subjects) and safety related to the use of medicines, investigational products (during clinical trial) from the start of drug development (clinical research process) and thereafter throughout the lifetime of the drug. Pharmaceutical companies develop novel monitoring systems that are efficient for their contribution to the detection of new safety signals ("reported information on a possible causal association between an adverse event and a drug, the relationship being unclear or incompletely documented previously"). Other agencies—viz., competent (regulatory) authorities (US FDA, EMEA, UK MHRA, TGA, Health Canada, MCCA), WHO (World Health Organization collaborating center for international drug monitoring (in Uppsala), and CIOMS (Council for International Organization of Medical Sciences)—play an advisory role in harmonization of pharmacovigilance practices for the improvement of patient care and drug safety. Erice Declaration[12] on communicating drug safety has improved communication and exchange of information between the industry, regulatory authorities, and the public.

12.4 DRUG DEVELOPMENT PROCESS

For the introduction of a drug or any therapeutic or biological compound for the first time in the country for human use (which is also called the registration process), a process called clinical trial process, which is regulated by the specific regulatory guidelines (e.g., ICH GCP, USFDA guidelines), has to be undertaken. WHO defines clinical trial process as "for the purposes of registration, a clinical trial is any research study that prospectively assigns human participants or groups of humans to one or more health-related interventions to evaluate the effects on health outcomes." Clinical trials may also be referred to as interventional trials.[13] Clinical Trials Directive (2001/20/EC) defines clinical trial as "any investigation in human subjects intended to discover or verify the clinical, pharmacological and/or other pharmacodynamic effects of one or more investigational medicinal product(s), and/or to identify any adverse reactions to one or more investigational medicinal product(s) and/or to study absorption, distribution, metabolism and excretion of one or more investigational medicinal product(s) with the object of ascertaining its (their) safety and/or efficacy."[14]

- **Drug Recalls:** Recalls are actions taken by a firm to remove a product from the market. Recalls may be conducted on a firm's own initiative, by FDA request, or by FDA order under statutory authority. These can be categorized in following types:
  - **Class I recall:** A situation in which there is a reasonable probability that the use of or exposure to a violative product will cause serious adverse health consequences or death.
  - **Class II recall:** A situation in which use of or exposure to a violative product may cause temporary or medically reversible adverse health consequences or where the probability of serious adverse health consequences is remote.

- **Class III recall:** A situation in which use of or exposure to a violative product is not likely to cause adverse health consequences.
- **Market withdrawal:** Occurs when a product has a minor violation that would not be subject to FDA legal action. The firm removes the product from the market or corrects the violation. For example, a product removed from the market due to tampering, without evidence of manufacturing or distribution problems, would be a market withdrawal.
- **Medical device safety alert:** Issued in situations where a medical device may present an unreasonable risk of substantial harm. In some cases, these situations are also considered recalls.

- ***Investigational medicinal product***

> A pharmaceutical form of an active ingredient or placebo being tested or used as a reference in a clinical trial, including a product with a marketing authorization when used or assembled (formulated or packaged) in a way different from the approved form, or when used for an unapproved indication, or when used to gain further information about an approved use. [ICH E6]

Pharmaceutical companies or the drug companies with robust research and development (R&D) facilities continuously analyze thousands of compounds to choose the compounds of therapeutic value (Figure 12.2). This usually takes six to seven years of preclinical testing (a first stage of drug development involving synthesis and purification testing in the lab and animal testing) during which thousands of compounds are tested before entering into the second stage that requires filing of an IND (investigational new drug application) to the appropriate regulatory authority, which is also termed as FDA (Food and Drug Administration, e.g., US FDA in USA). If the IND is approved by the FDA and by an Institutional Review Board, the manufacturer may begin the first phase of development. The IND stage consists of three phases.

Phase I: In this phase, healthy individuals are recruited to determine the drug's basic pharmacokinetic properties and safety profile in humans.

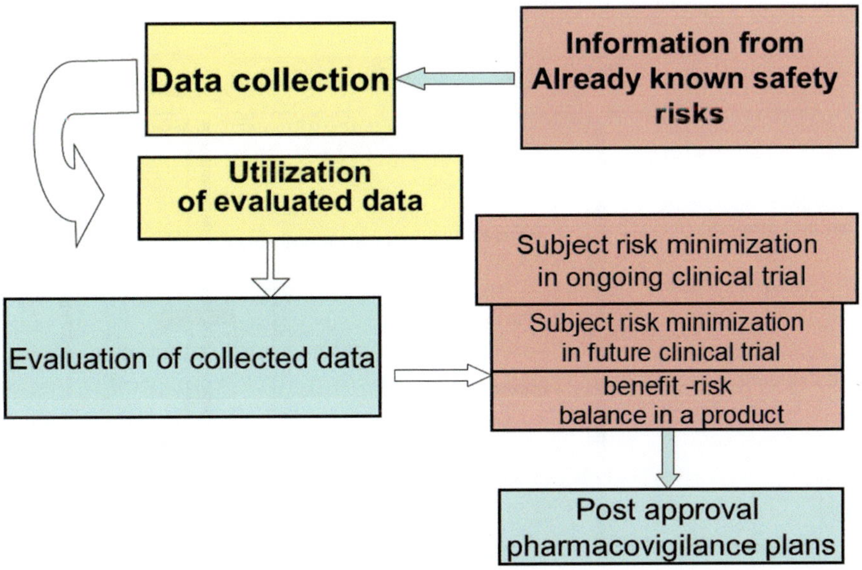

FIGURE 12.2 Drug development process and pharmacovigilance.

Phase II: During this phase, the drug is administered to the patients for the first time in the indication for which it is meant.

Phase III: The preliminary evidence gathered in Phase II that a drug is safe and effective for use in the intended indication and recipient population is confirmed in Phase III.

After the completion of Phase III, the manufacturer or the pharmaceutical company files or submits a New Drug Application (NDA) to the FDA for review of the efficacy, safety, and tolerability data generated during Phase I to Phase III. NDA review typically lasts for one to two years, thereby bringing total drug development and approval (that is, the IND and NDA stages) to approximately nine years. During the NDA stage, the FDA consults advisory committees made of experts from the different scientific disciplines (clinical pharmacologist, biostatistician, field expert, viz., cardiologist/endocrinologist/oncologist/rheumatologist) to obtain a broader range of advice on drug safety, effectiveness, and labeling. Once approved, the drug is marketed with FDA-regulated labeling, often called a therapeutic indication. During marketing of the drug in "real-world" clinical practice, where decisions of the prescribers do not follow strict eligibility criteria specified during subject enrollment in controlled clinical trials, the FDA gathers safety information on a continuous basis as the drug is used and adverse events are reported.

Clinical trial process, as discussed earlier, involves many stakeholders (Figure 12.3), viz., sponsors, regulators (government agencies), investigators, monitors, ethics committees or Institutional Review Boards (IRBs), participants, and a myriad of other public and private entities, as discussed earlier in this chapter, whose involvement greatly affects the clinical research process. During the conduct of clinical trials, it becomes imperative to assess the safety and tolerability profile of investigational new drugs (INDs), so the responsibility for monitoring the safety (a pharmacovigilance process) of study subjects during clinical trials is shared between trial sponsors, researchers, ethics committees, and drug regulators. In lieu of its pharmacovigilance role in clinical trials, the sponsor has the obligation to carry out various risk management activities during the clinical trial

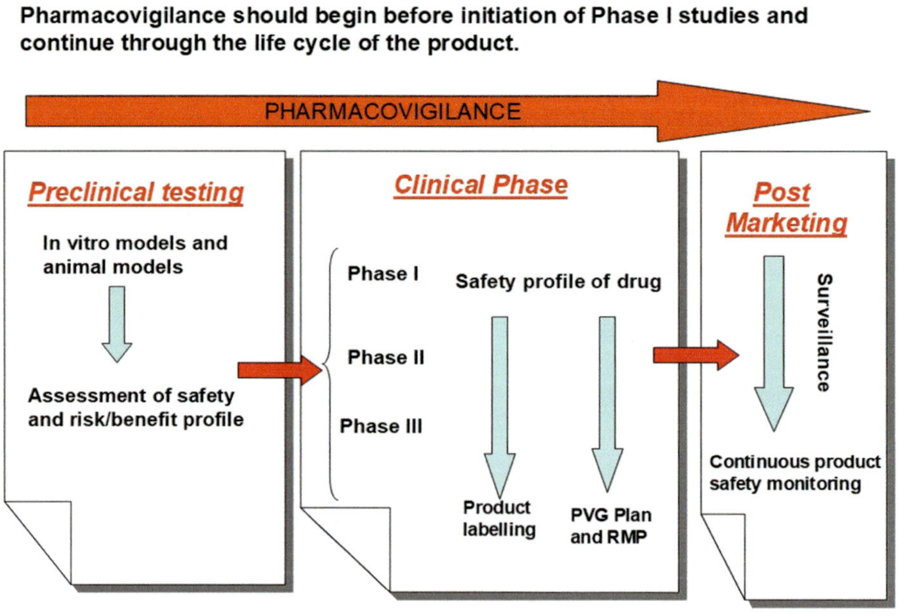

FIGURE 12.3 Stakeholders in pharmacovigilance.

process. These risk management activities include modifications in protocol due to safety or efficacy concerns (e.g., dosage changes, changes in study inclusion criteria, intensification of monitoring), restrictions in study population or indications; changes to the informed consent document relating to safety issues, formulation changes for safety reasons, addition of a special reporting requirement, issuance of a communication to investigators or healthcare professionals, and plans for new safety trials.

Here, it should be noted that since contract research organizations (CROs) and/or site management organizations (SMOs) are contracted by the sponsor to perform one or more of a sponsor's trial-related duties and functions, the pharmacovigilance roles and responsibilities as defined for sponsors for clinical trials will be applicable to them as well. To carry out some or all of the other functions, a sponsor has to execute specific legal "agreements" and "arrangements" with the other stakeholders as defined earlier in order to ensure safety for the subjects participating in the clinical trial. As part of the delegation of responsibilities as defined in the contractual agreement, a sponsor may transfer any or all of the pharmacovigilance tasks and functions to another person(s) or organization, but the ultimate responsibility for the fulfillment of all pharmacovigilance obligations and the quality and integrity of these pharmacovigilance functions always resides with the marketing authorization holder. It becomes imperative for the sponsor of the clinical trial to ensure that detailed and clear documented contractual arrangements for meeting pharmacovigilance obligations between the sponsor and the other stakeholders are in place. The contracted person(s) or organization should implement quality assurance and quality control and agree to be audited by or on behalf of the sponsor.

Now, for the understanding of the role of pharmacovigilance in clinical research, the roles and responsibilities of various stakeholders have been presented next:

12.5 SPONSOR: PHARMACOVIGILANCE RESPONSIBILITY

As per ICH-GCP (ICH E6), a sponsor is "an individual, company, institution, or organization which takes responsibility for the initiation, management, and/or financing of a clinical trial."[15]

For a sponsor, it becomes essential to use and adopt pharmacovigilance procedures to monitor adverse reactions occurring in clinical trials to ensure the immediate termination of any clinical trial in which there is an unacceptable level of risk. The sponsor has the prime responsibility to ensure the safety evaluation of the investigational medicinal products on a continuous basis (ongoing safety evaluation). In order to ensure ongoing safety evaluation, the sponsor is required to not only evaluate the safety of IMP when the trial finishes but also continuously assess any problems when both serious and non-serious ADRs are reported. As per regulations, the sponsor is responsible for the immediate notification of findings from the clinical trials that could adversely affect the health of subjects or if the findings could create an impact on the further conduct of the trial. For such findings, the sponsor has the prime responsibility of notifying all concerned investigator(s), the ethics committee, and competent authorities (regulatory authorities). In Europe, a sponsor has to notify the concerned investigator(s), the ethics committee, and competent authorities (regulatory authorities) of each concerned member state in order to ensure that the findings could alter the competent authority's authorization to continue the trial in accordance with Directive 2001/20/EC [14].

From the sponsor's perspective, its pharmacovigilance role in clinical research commences at the first stage during preparation of various essential documents, viz., protocol, investigator brochure, and case report forms (CRF). In the next stage, during the commencement of the clinical trial, the sponsor or its designated representatives report the occurrence of adverse events in a clinical trial as per the applicable regulatory guidelines and other company-specific standard operating procedures or as per specifications mentioned in the "pharmacovigilance section of the protocol." The importance of the incorporation of a pharmacovigilance section or safety section in the essential documents is discussed next.

12.6 PROTOCOL: PHARMACOVIGILANCE AND SAFETY REPORTING SECTION

ICH E6 defines protocol as "a document that describes the objective(s), design, methodology, statistical considerations, and organization of a trial. The protocol usually also gives the background and rationale for the trial, but these could be provided in other protocol referenced documents."[15]

Experts in the regulatory bodies and members of the ethics committees critically review and examine each and every section of the protocol and place much emphasis on the "pharmacovigilance and safety reporting section" of the protocol, as this remains a key section in guiding the proper recording and reporting of safety issues occurring in a clinical trial to ensure the safety of study subjects. The basic rules for what does or does not need to be recorded in the CRF or reported to the sponsor are usually mentioned in the protocol.

Following guidance should be provided in the "pharmacovigilance and safety reporting" section of the protocol.

- A definition of the adverse event (AE)/serious adverse event or reaction (SAE/SAR).
- A definition of the expectedness and unexpectedness of adverse event or reaction (AE).
- Specifications of the safety parameters to be studied as per the protocol, along with methods and timings for recording and analyzing.
- Standards for expedited reporting with reporting time frames.
- Declaration from the principal investigator (PI) that the PI will ask the study subjects during each scheduled visit or unscheduled visit (if any) about the experience of any events or hospitalizations, disability, or incapacity since their previous visit.
- The study subjects shall be provided with a contact address or telephone number of the PI or of any research personnel designated by PI to expedite the reporting of adverse events.
- In case of the occurrence of a serious adverse event in a blinded clinical trial, the management for blinded therapy cases should be given in detail, with clear responsibilities for breaking the blinding of code. During the conduct of a clinical trial, maintenance of blinding is advantageous till the final study analysis. However, in circumstances where a serious adverse reaction is judged to be reported in an expedited manner, it is advocated that the sponsor should break the blind for that specific patient only.
- A clear statement for adverse drug reactions that are not deemed to be reported to the sponsor unless they are considered to be occurring at a greater frequency or with greater severity than might be expected, as defined in the summary product characteristic (SmPC) or any other reference safety information.
- For example: in case of a licensed medicine or the approved pharmaceutical product, this might include a list of known ADRs as present or documented in the SmPC. A copy of SmPC or any other reference safety information should be added as an appendix to the protocol with an accompanying statement in the "Pharmacovigilance and Safety Reporting" section of the protocol as follows:

  > Adverse drug reactions listed under "undesirable effects" section in the SmPC are not deemed to be reported to the sponsor unless they are considered to be occurring at a greater frequency or with greater severity than might be expected, as defined in the summary product characteristics. (SmPC)

- A statement for serious adverse events that may not be deemed to be recorded and reported as per expedited reporting requirements should be clearly mentioned. For example, deaths due to disease in a study where death is a primary endpoint, as in the case of death from stroke in a stroke trial. Another example includes the case of hospitalization for an event that is an endpoint as a myocardial infarction, an AIDS event, or a cancer recurrence.
- In regard to therapeutic failures and defining the adverse events, it should be explicitly mentioned in the protocol that if the disease under investigation worsens during a clinical

trial, it will be considered as an AE or not. In some cases, if the disease entity under investigation worsens during a clinical trial. Then, it is not considered an AE; rather, it is considered a disease progression. The progressed disease, however, may cause a new symptom, which may be considered a new AE. For example, if a patient's pancreatic cancer spreads during a trial, and the new metastases result in increased pain, the worsened pancreatic cancer detected by restaging CT would not be considered an AE. The new pain may be reported as an AE, and in such cases the investigator should provide an attribution indicating that the pain is unlikely to be a result of the study therapy.

- Rather, we consider that as disease progression. The progressed disease, however, may cause a new symptom, which may be considered a new AE. So, for example, if a patient's pancreatic cancer spreads during a trial, and the new metastases result in increased pain. The worsened pancreatic cancer detected by restaging CT will *not* be considered an AE. However, the new pain may be reported as an AE. The investigator should provide an attribution that indicates the pain is unlikely to be the result of the study therapy.
- A statement regarding confirmation of reporting to the sponsor in case of the occurrence of a pregnancy or a follow-up till outcome in a female participant or in the female partner of a male participant should be provided. This is important for the drugs where there is a paucity of safety information concerning foetal exposure and development.
- A risk assessment statement should be provided in the protocol.
- Recording and reporting of post-study events that occurred after the patient had completed a clinical study (including any protocol-required post-treatment follow-up) should be clearly mentioned.
- The name and contact details of the sponsor's pharmacovigilance representative, who in most of the cases is qualified personnel for pharmacovigilance (QPPV), should be included for the purposes of reporting of SAE/SARs/SUSARs.

The risk assessment statement in the protocol ensures that an appropriate deliberation has been imparted by clinical investigators to potential safety issues in clinical trials that apply to investigational medicinal products/comparator products/non-investigational medicinal products (products that are not the entity for investigation such as rescue medication provided for preventive, diagnostic or therapeutic reasons to ensure that adequate medical care is provided for the subject participating in clinical trial).

Previous knowledge about the benefit/risk profile (frequency and severity of the adverse drug reaction) of the investigational medicinal product plays an important role in risk assessment. The risk is usually less in clinical trials that involve the licenced or marketed drugs that have been used or prescribed in a large number of patients and whose patient characteristics in whom the drug has been prescribed resemble those of clinical trial subjects. In such instances, it becomes appropriate that the investigators record known adverse drug reactions in the CRF but not report them to the sponsor unless they occur with unexpected frequency or severity.

In case of licensed drugs that are designated "black triangle" by the drug regulators, it is necessary that the sponsor should explicitly specify in the protocol that investigators need to report all SAEs to the sponsor and that unexpected events be considered potential SUSARs.

For investigational medicinal products tested in preliminary phases, viz., Phase I and II studies ("first-in-man"), where there is no information on the safety profile, the sponsor should explicitly mention that the investigators will record all adverse events in the CRF and will notify the sponsor of the adverse events that qualify the criteria for "seriousness."

12.7 INVESTIGATOR BROCHURE (IB)

As per ICH GCP, "Investigators Brochure" (IB) is a compilation of the clinical and non-clinical data on the investigational product(s) that are relevant to the study of the product(s) in human subject's.[15] As an essential document, it contributes to pharmacovigilance by not only providing investigators and other trial-related staff with the information that enhances their awareness of the justification for dosage, dosage frequency/interval, methods of administration but also outlining safety monitoring processes. In clinical research, expedited reporting is made on the basis of "expectedness" and "unexpectedness" of the serious adverse reaction. A key goal of expedited reporting during clinical trials is to keep regulatory bodies, principal investigator or investigator (s), IRBs, and other stakeholders aware of significant new findings on serious reactions, so the investigator brochure serves as a vital document for determining "expectedness" or "unexpectedness" of the adverse drug reaction. "Expected adverse drug reaction" refers to a response whose type of intensity aligns with the information provided in the relevant source documents. "Unexpected adverse drug reaction" is one whose severity or nature is inconsistent, accompanied by details contained in those source documents. An investigator brochure prepared and furnished as per the ICH guidelines by the sponsor serves as the primary source document for a medicinal product that has not received marketing approval in a given country. Like the "undesirable effects" section of the SmPC, where the adverse drug reactions are listed for the marketed product, the summary of adverse drug reactions is tabulated in the investigator brochure for the investigational product. The summarized data on adverse drug reaction severity and frequency in the investigator brochure acts as the source of reference for assessing the expectedness or unexpectedness of adverse reactions.

As per section 7.3.6 of ICH GCP,

> The IB should provide a description of the possible risks and adverse drug reactions to be anticipated on the basis of prior experiences with the product under investigation and with related products. A description should also be provided of the precautions or special monitoring to be done as part of the investigational use of the product(s).

12.8 CASE REPORT FORM (CRF)

A case report form is "a printed, optical, or electronic document designed to record all of the protocol required information to be reported to the sponsor on each trial subject."[15] As part of the clinical trial procedure, every adverse event identified or reported throughout trial visits must be recorded, unless the protocol provides specific exemptions (Table 12.1). The study protocol serves as a detailed framework for routine data collection, specifying the identification, management, reporting, and documentation of adverse events in the case report form. Within the context of pharmacovigilance, non-serious adverse events are also documented and reported if they hold importance to the monitoring of safety in a clinical trial or are regarded as essential to the assessment of a drug's safety (Table 12.2). Predictable adverse reactions are also recorded if they are mentioned in the protocol as factors that guide decisions regarding dosage adjustment. In addition to recording other data elements, for example, treatment regimen compliance, significant laboratory and diagnostic findings, medical history, and physical examination results, safety data are reported in case report forms using questionnaires for adverse drug events and a comprehensive symptom checklist organized by system organ class. As the identification of adverse reactions in clinical trials demands a thorough and systematic assessment of participants at all stages of exposure to the investigational product, quality control procedures are undertaken to maintain the integrity and accuracy of the findings. As per ICH-GCP, quality assurance is defined as "all those planned and systematic actions that are established to ensure that the trial is performed and the data are generated, documented (recorded), and reported in compliance with Good Clinical Practice (GCP) and the applicable regulatory requirement(s)."[15] The sponsor must ensure the implementation of effective quality assurance and quality control systems documented through SOPs to verify that the conduct of the clinical trial and the management of safety data align with the protocol, GCP principles, and all applicable regulatory requirements.

TABLE 12.1
Adverse Event Page in Case Report Form

ADVERSE EVENT FORM				
Is there any Adverse event experienced by the subject? *(If yes, kindly complete the adverse event form)*			Yes ❑ No ❑	
Adverse Event Description			**Adverse Event Number** [__I__]	
Is this an initial report of follow up report? *(Kindly tick which ever is applicable)*			Initial Report ❑ Follow up report ❑	
Date of onset (DD/MM/YY)		[__I__]-[__I__]-[__I__]		
Severity	Mild ❑	**Moderate** ❑	**Severe** ❑	**Life threatening** ❑
Mild = No interference with usual activities; Moderate = Significant interference with usual activities; Severe = Prevents usual activities Life threatening = Endangering life/risk of death				
Frequency	Isolated ❑	Intermittent ❑	Continuous ❑	Not Applicable ❑
Study Medication Adjustment		**None** ❑	**Dose modified/interrupted** ❑	**Discontinued** ❑
***Relationship to Study Medication**	**Certain** ❑	**Probable/Likely** ❑	**Possible** ❑	
	Unlikely ❑	**Conditional/ Unclassified** ❑	**Unassessible/Unclassifiable** ❑	
* *To confirm the possible relationship of the study treatment to the suspected reaction, please go through the standard description of above-mentioned terms (viz. certain, probable/likely, possible, unlikely, conditional/unclassified, unassessible/unclassifiable) on page no. X of CRF named 'Instructions to fill AE/Intercurrent illness Form and SAE form'.*				
Outcome	**Resolved with no sequelae** ❑ **Resolved with sequelae** ❑ **Specify**______		*Date of Resolution* [__I__]-[__I__]-[__I__]	
	Unresolved/ongoing at final contact ❑		**Death** ❑	**Unknown** ❑

Based on CIOMS VII, "an adverse event of special interest (serious or non-serious) is one of scientific and medical concern specific to the sponsor's product or program, for which ongoing monitoring and rapid communication by the investigator to the sponsor could be appropriate." Such an event might require further investigation in order to characterize and understand it. Depending on the nature of the event, rapid communication by the trial sponsor to other parties (e.g., regulators) might also be warranted.

12.9 SAFETY UPDATE REPORT

During the drug development process (clinical development) of an investigational medicinal product, regular assessment of safety findings becomes vital, which is essential for the continuous evaluation of potential risks to participants. Currently, in several countries or regions, drug regulatory authorities (Food and Drug Administration) mandate sponsors to provide periodic reports or development safety update reports (DSUR) to them, along with other involved parties or stakeholders (e.g., ethics committees) at regular intervals or defined timelines. These reports primarily outline the safety characteristics of an experimental product and actions undertaken to manage safety problems, such as early termination of the trial, ongoing status, adding a follow-up visit for the patient to assess safety. ICH E2F[16] guidelines on development safety update report (DSUR) ensure uniformity in yearly clinical trial safety reporting across ICH regions, enhancing the overall safety assurance for clinical trial subjects. As per the guidelines, the primary objectives of a DSUR are as follows:[16]

TABLE 12.2
Serious Adverse Event Page in Case Report Form

1. Patient Details		
Patient initial: [__I__I__]	Hospital/OPD record number (if any): [__I__I__I__I__I__]	
Age: [__I__] yrs	and/or	Date of Birth: [__I__]-[__I__]-[__I__]
Male ❑	Female ❑	(if female) Confirmed Pregnancy: Yes ❑ No ❑ Test not done ❑ If 'Yes' then weeks of gestation: [__I__] weeks

2. Suspected Drug(s)					
Generic name with dosage form and strength	Indication	Daily dose and regimen (specify units)	Route	Duration of Therapy	
				Starting date and time	Stop date and time

3. Other Treatments (prescription or nonprescription medications/non-drug therapy)					
Generic name with dosage Form and Strength/name of therapy	Indication	Daily dose and regimen (specify units)	Route	Duration of Therapy	
				Starting date and time	Stop date and time

4. Details of the Suspected Adverse Drug Reaction(s)/Description		
'Specific Diagnosis' for the reaction/event:	Associated Signs & Symptoms (if any):	
Full description of the reaction/event along with body site/system involved:		
Intensity/severity of reaction: Mild ❑ Moderate ❑ Severe ❑ Life threatening ❑		
Mild = No interference with usual activities; Moderate = Significant interference with usual activities; Severe = Prevents usual activities		
Criteria for reporting the event as an SAE- the adverse event resulted in (please tick as applicable): ❑ Death ❑ A life threatening experience ❑ Inpatient hospitalization or prolongation of existing hospitalization ❑ A persistent or significant disability/incapacity ❑ A congenital anomaly/birth defect ❑ A condition that required intervention to prevent permanent impairment or damage		
Start date and time [__I__]-[__I__]-[__I__] [__I__]:[__I__] hrs	Stop date and time [__I__]-[__I__]-[__I__] [__I__]:[__I__] hrs	Ongoing at final contact ❑
'Dechallenge and Rechallenge' done: Yes ❑ No ❑ If 'Yes' please provide details:		
Setting: Hospital ❑ Nursing ❑ Home ❑ Clinic ❑ Outpatient ❑ Others ❑__________		

5. Outcome
Resolved with no sequelae ❑ Resolved with sequelae ❑ Unresolved at final contact ❑ Death ❑ Unknown ❑
Results of specific tests/investigations/treatments that may have been conducted/given (if any):
In case of death (please mention cause of death)
Possible relationship of the study treatment to the suspected reaction: **unrelated** ❑ **Unlikely** ❑ **Possible** ❑ **Probable** ❑ **Likely** ❑
Post-mortem/autopsy done: **Yes** ❑ **No** ❑ If 'Yes', findings (if any):
Any other relevant information to facilitate the assessment of the case:

6. Details about the Investigator	
Name:	Profession (speciality):
Address:	Telephone No:
Date of reporting the event to the Licensing Authority: [__I__]-[__I__]-[__I__]	Date of reporting the event to the Ethics Committee overseeing the site: [__I__]-[__I__]-[__I__]

To provide a concise overview about current understanding of the product's known and potential risks, along with measures implemented for their management.

1. To identify and describe any new emerging safety concerns that may influence the protection and well-being of clinical trial participants.
2. To evaluate whether the safety information collected by the sponsor during the reporting period is consistent with the previously established safety profile of the investigational product.
3. To present an updated summary of the progress and current situation of the ongoing clinical research and overall development program.

A DSUR must be submitted once every year to the regulatory authority as long as the clinical trial with the investigational product is ongoing or until it is suitable for reporting in the purview of local safety requirements.[16] For periodic submission of safety related to an experimental product, an executive summary outlining the essential findings of the safety update report should be provided to the ethics committee, institutional review boards, or investigators. This should function as a "stand-alone" document suitable for submission to ethics committees and other relevant stakeholders, as mandated by local regulations. The executive summary of this report should include the following details:

- An introduction
- Information regarding experimental drug (such as its class, indications, dosage, route of administration, and mode of action)
- An estimated total exposure from clinical trial
- Number of countries (if any) in which medicinal product is authorized
- Overall safety assessment summary
- A summary or overall list of important identified and potential risks
- Action taken and proposed for safety reasons, including considerable changes to IB
- Conclusion

The executive summary must contain detailed lists of serious adverse reactions (specific terms used to classify them as serious) as warranted. In the line listing, the following data elements should be present: study ID (protocol number), case ID/subject number, country, age, gender, serious ADR, date of onset, time of onset, suspect drug, daily dose, route of administration, formulation, dates of treatment, treatment duration, outcome, and remarks. When presenting safety data from a clinical trial, it becomes essential that the report encompass adverse reactions of special interest in the line listings and adverse events of special interest in summary tables. The justification or criteria to identify the specific events should be documented.

Specific adverse events that are integral, that is, linked to efficacy endpoints, and documented in the protocol as "exempt" from data collection or inclusion in the safety database may be excluded from summary tabulations and line listings; however, the reason for these exclusions must be documented in the reports (e.g., deaths reported in congestive heart failure studies where overall mortality serves as the primary efficacy measure or disease in oncology trials).[16]

Here it should be noted that the primary goal of the DSUR is the presentation of information collected from clinical studies of investigational medicinal products, including biologicals, regardless of their marketing authorization status, along with information such as safety data and listings of serious adverse reactions, which may also be described in Periodic Safety Update Reports (PSURs) for approved products involved in ongoing clinical trials. In a DSUR, the safety data from all ongoing and completed clinical trials conducted by the sponsor during the reporting period must include:[16]

- clinical investigation (Phase I—III), such as human pharmacology, therapeutic exploratory, and therapeutic confirmatory trials (Phase I—III), conducted with an investigational drug irrespective of having marketing approval;

- clinical trials involving marketed drugs used for approved therapeutic indications (Phase IV or therapeutic use trials);
- additional therapeutic applications of investigational drug; and
- comparability studies designed to evaluate and justify manufacturing process modifications of pharmaceutical products.

Here it must be noted that other findings (e.g., clinical trial performed by a co-development partner under licensing agreement), safety data of clinical trials, significant safety findings from non-clinical trials, or necessary safety update from non-interventional studies or safety issues reported with the compassionate use should be included in the report if they have potential implications for the welfare safety of clinical trial participants.

Details regarding comparators are included solely when it has significance for participants' safety; otherwise, the investigational drug(s) should be the main focus of a safety update report. This report should be brief and comprehensive enough to reassure regulatory authorities that the sponsor is appropriately assessing and monitoring the safety profile of investigational product. Initial reporting of any newly identified safety concern should not be part of this document, because expedited reporting should have been used to notify regulatory authorities about them.

In the situations when drug development program or a clinical study is executed or conducted in mutual collaboration involving public enterprises (hospitals, academia, research institutions) or private institutions/business partners (contract research organization/site management organization) or another party, then a contractual agreement should (as discussed previously in the beginning of this chapter) be placed there by defining the responsibilities for submission as well as preparation of safety update report. This requirement also applies when responsibilities of preparation of the safety update report are delegated by the sponsor to an external party, for example, a contract research organization or an organization specialized in drug safety management aspects.

In special situations, for example, in cases where the sponsor has entered into a co-development or licensing collaboration with one or more partners, or where several partners jointly sponsor clinical studies of the investigational product, then a coordinated arrangement should be established to prepare a unified safety update report. In order for one sponsor to publish only one safety update report on behalf of every partner, written agreements need to be put in place that specify the method in which safety data will be distributed. Additionally, different sponsors can make an agreement for the preparation of a separate safety update report on a similar investigational product under the situations that differ in routes of administration, indications, or composition. For this, a rationale for the preparation of a separate development safety update report should be provided in each report.

In case of clinical studies including a fixed-dose combination product, a single safety update report should be prepared.[16]

Information on safety obtained during the period of reporting for the preparation of the safety update report is assessed based on "reference safety information." As discussed earlier, the "investigator brochure" acts as the "reference safety information." The Investigator's Brochure (IB) is initially of the reporting interval used as the "reference safety information" for the safety update report of an experimental drug, regardless of whether that drug has received marketing approval. The safety information (adverse event) received over the duration of clinical trial is compared with the "reference safety information" (IB). While preparing the report, the version number and date of the generation of IB are required to be mentioned in the report. It should be noted that the sponsor must include a copy of the updated IB along with the safety update report if it has been revised during the reporting period and the updated version has not previously been submitted to the competent authority. In situations where an IB is not required by local regulatory such as when noncommercial sponsors conduct a clinical trial using a marketed product, the relevant local product label may serve as the "reference safety information" (e.g., the Summary of Product Characteristics (SmPC) in the EU, the Japanese Package Insert in Japan, or the US Package Insert in the United States).[16]

Throughout the reporting period, the safety update report must include a concise summary of important safety observations that arise (if any) from market exposure of the investigational drug in any country. This becomes significant when the findings result in revisions to the product labeling or modifications to the risk management plan. A summary should be provided for significant safety observations from non-clinical *in vitro* and *in vivo* studies initiated or finalized during the period of reporting, including those on immunotoxicity, reproduction, and carcinogenicity. The effect of such studies' findings regarding the clinical safety of the investigational product must be reported in the safety update report.

In case of clinical trials conducted with innovative therapeutic products (e.g., tissue-engineered products, cell therapy products, and gene therapy), subjects are followed even when the trials are completed. In such cases, information from longitudinal assessment of subjects should be presented in the safety update report.

As a part of pharmacovigilance activities during clinical trials, it is deemed necessary that a sponsor make a periodic review of worldwide scientific literature for any emerging safety data that could arise during the conduct of clinical trial. For this, reviews are generally made into specific sites, viz *PubMed* (http://www.ncbi.nlm.nih.gov/pubmed/), Scopus (http://info.scopus.com/), or another database, for example, Cochrane database. Any updated safety information from animal/laboratory studies, clinical studies, or any new safety information on drugs of the same class that has been published during the period of reporting is incorporated in the safety update report. During the reporting period, if changes are introduced pertaining to the development and/or formulation design of an investigational medicinal product, then any significant safety concerns arising from such alterations are also mentioned in the safety update report. Reports of inadequate efficacy must be documented in the safety update report for clinical trials with vaccines or clinical trials where the investigational product is evaluating therapies to treat serious or life-threatening illnesses. In case of vaccine failure, the reporting becomes important as it may suggest emerging signals of decreased immunogenicity among a proportion of vaccinees, along with possible waning immunity or strain replacement.[16–17]

During the drug development process, it is the prime responsibility of the sponsor to continuously evaluate the potential risks that may develop with the usage of the investigational product in clinical trial subjects. For evaluation of risks in clinical trials, any significant variations in the type and severity of adverse drug reactions from previously identified reactions and identification of risk factors should be considered. For example, increase in the incidence of expected adverse reaction classified as very common (≥10%), common (≥ 1% and < 10%), uncommon or infrequent (≥ 0.1% and < 1%); increase in severity (to moderate or to severe); and changes in outcome and issues related to risk factors are considered for risk evaluation. These issues allow for consideration of further preventive measures in subjects. For evaluation, an emphasis should be given on signs, symptoms, and evidence (based on the laboratory values) of previously and newly identified clinically significant hepatic and renal toxicity, bone marrow toxicity, immunogenicity and hypersensitive reactions, CVS effects, CNS toxicity, and reactive metabolites.

Under Article 17 of Directive 2001/20/EC of the European Parliament concerning the coordination relating to the harmonization of member state laws, regulations, and administrative provisions for the application of Good Clinical Practice during clinical trials involving medicinal products for human use:

1. (a) It is the responsibility of the sponsor to record and report all relevant details regarding suspected serious unexpected adverse reactions that result in death or life-threatening conditions. These reports should be submitted without delay to the competent authorities of all concerned member states and to the ethics committee, and in any case, no later than seven days after the sponsor becomes aware of the case, with relevant follow-up information provided within the subsequent eight days.

(b) The sponsor must ensure that any other suspected serious unexpected adverse reactions are promptly communicated to the concerned competent authorities and ethics committee, within a period of not exceeding 15 days from the initial awareness of such information.
(c) It is the responsibility of each member state to ensure that all reports of suspected unexpected serious adverse reactions to an investigational medicinal product are duly documented and reported.
(d) The sponsor must inform all investigators.

2. Throughout the course of the clinical trial, the sponsor must provide the member states where the trial is conducted and the corresponding ethics committee with a summary listing of all suspected serious adverse reactions observed during that period, along with an evaluation of subjects' safety on an annual basis.[14]

12.10 PHARMACOVIGILANCE RESPONSIBILITY OF INVESTIGATOR

As per ICH E6, an investigator is defined as "an individual who is responsible for the conduct of the clinical trial at a trial site. When a clinical trial is conducted by a team of individuals at a trial site, the investigator who leads the team is designated as the Principal Investigator."

Article 2 of Directive 2001/20/EC of the European Parliament describes an investigator as

> a doctor or a person following a profession agreed in the Member State for investigations because of the scientific background and the experience in patient care it requires. The investigator is responsible for the conduct of a clinical trial at a trial site. If a trial is conducted by a team of individuals at a trial site, the investigator is the leader responsible for the team and may be called the principal investigator.[14]

A clinical trial investigator ensures that participants will receive appropriate healthcare treatment for any adverse reactions, including notable deviations in laboratory parameters, throughout trial conduct. To confirm the safety of participants and address an immediate risk during the clinical trial, an investigator can initiate a deviation or modifications from the preapproved protocol without prior approval/favorable considerations from the IRB/IEC. The amended protocol, along with the implemented changes or deviation must be forwarded to:

(a) the IRB/IEC for review approval/favorable opinion,
(b) the sponsor for agreement and, if required,
(c) the regulatory authorities.

Directive 2001/20/EC of the European Parliament sets out the principles for applying Good Clinical Practice in clinical trials conducted with medicinal products for human use[14] explicitly describes in its *Article 16* about the pharmacovigilance role of investigator related regarding the submission of adverse events. This directive states the following:

1. Investigator must report all serious adverse events to the sponsor, except for those explicitly exempted from immediate reporting as outlined in the protocol or investigator's brochure. The initial notification should be followed by comprehensive written documentation. Both the initial and follow-up reports should identify subjects using unique code numbers.
2. As per the reporting timelines specified in the protocol, all adverse events and/or laboratory abnormalities deemed essential for safety assessment must be reported to the sponsor.
3. In case a subject's death is reported, the investigator is required to provide any supporting details requested by the sponsor and the ethics committee.
4. All adverse events reported by the investigator(s) to the sponsor must be thoroughly documented. If requested, this information will be sent to the member states where the clinical trial is being carried out.

The investigator's pharmacovigilance responsibilities extend to the management of blinded therapy cases in blinded clinical trials, where investigator(s), monitor, subject(s), and, in certain instances, data analyst(s) remain unaware of the treatment assignment(s). For example, in cases, double blinded trials occurrence of serious adverse events requires a decision of breaking of the code for a particular patient to ensure patient safety. Methods of breaking the blinded codes are predefined in the clinical trial protocol. If the investigator unblinds a subject's treatment, the sponsor is expected to be informed and made aware of the treatment assignment for that particular patient.

Although maintaining the blind for all participants until the completion of the final study analysis is advantageous, it should be noted that, from the pharmacovigilance and reporting purposes, the maintenance of blinding has many disadvantages that outweigh the advantages. Some of the key disadvantages have been described next:

- By retaining the blind, there is always unnecessary filling of cases related to the placebo and comparator (usually a marketed product).
- Once the blind is opened, typically several weeks or months after regulatory reporting, the sponsor should ensure that company and regulatory databases are updated accordingly.
- It's not appropriate to notify the relevant parties (CRO, IRB) of the new information that has been updated in a blinded fashion in Investigator's Brochure, especially in case of new and potentially serious adverse events related to investigational medicinal products.

It should be noted that unblinding of a single patient has no considerable implication on the analysis of the complete clinical investigation data.

The incorporation of the Clinical Directive 2001/20/EC into national law established uniform procedures for adverse event reporting and documentation in clinical trials throughout Europe. It has been made statutory or compulsory that all serious unexpected suspected adverse reactions (SUSAR) arising from clinical trials must be reported to the ethics committee (IRB) and competent authorities within 7 days in case of death or life-threatening adverse reactions and within 15 days for all other cases. The goal of this directive is to discover and focus on SUSAR for the study analysis of safety signals. This allows the pharmaceutical industry (Manufacturing Authorization Holder) to conduct an annual review and make necessary revisions (Directive 2001/28/EC) of the product information (Investigator Brochure or Summary of Product Characteristics (SmPC). Additionally, when ADRs arise from concomitant medication used in clinical trials, and the sponsor is not the marketing authorization holder (MAH), such reactions must be reported directly either to the relevant competent authorities (regulatory authorities) or to the MAH of the concomitant medication to ensure regulatory compliance and timely reporting of serious cases within 15 days.[18]

12.11 PHARMACOVIGILANCE RESPONSIBILITY OF INDEPENDENT ETHICS COMMITTEE (IEC/INSTITUTIONAL REVIEW BOARD (IRB)

ICH E6 defines an ethics committee as an

> independent body (a review board or a committee, institutional, regional, national or supranational), constituted of medical professionals and non-medical members, whose responsibility is to ensure the protection of the rights, safety and well-being of human subjects involved in a trial and to provide public assurance of that protection, by, among other things, reviewing and approving/providing favorable opinion on, the trial protocol, the suitability of the investigator(s), facilities, and the methods and material to be used in obtaining and documenting informed consent of the trial subjects.

To fulfill its responsibilities toward the protection of rights, safety, and well-being of the participants, an IRB/IEC reviews essential documents, viz., trial protocol(s)/amendment(s), written informed consent form(s) (and consent form updates), Investigator's Brochure (IB), and current safety data on the investigational drug.

IRB/IEC must be timely notified for:

- all serious and unexpected adverse drug reactions (ADRs),
- every modification or deviation in the protocol to remove potential risk to the trial subjects,
- all relevant changes that raise the risks to participants and/or protocol modifications that affect the conduct of trial, and
- any updated data that could have a negative impact on the conduct of the trial or safety of subjects.

12.12 MANAGEMENT OF CASE SAFETY REPORTS DURING THE CONDUCT OF CLINICAL TRIALS

As stated earlier in this chapter, standard operating procedures are implemented by the sponsor to ensure necessary quality standards for data collection or recording, evaluation, validation, reporting, and archiving of the adverse drug reaction-related information. To implement pharmacovigilance responsibilities in clinical research, the sponsor must document a detailed record of all adverse events communicated by the investigator during the course of the clinical trial. Sponsor must thoroughly analyze each individual case safety report (ICSR) that the investigator provides in order to determine its seriousness, causality, and expectedness. For causality analysis, either the WHO causality assessment scale[19] or Naranjo's probability scale (NPS) is utilized.[20] In a clinical trial, an investigator makes an assessment on the adverse event since he/she has the opportunity to see the subject reporting the adverse event. From the sponsors' perspective, all the adverse events must be evaluated to enable a comprehensive understanding of their nature and frequency, both across individual trial sites (in a multicentric trial) and through pooled analyses of data from all participating centers. This helps the sponsor to provide additional information in comparison to that received by the individual investigator. This provides the rationale for conducting a causality assessment by both the investigator and the sponsor. In case a significant safety issue has been identified by the sponsor either on the receipt of an individual case safety report (ICSR) or through review of aggregated data (pooled analyses), as stated earlier, the sponsor must promptly communicate this information to all investigators. It should be noted that the sponsor cannot override the causality assessment provided by the investigator for the investigational product. In such situations sponsor may include remarks ("sponsors section" on comments in the ADR report) to document the disagreement. The report should be submitted with both investigator's and sponsor's opinion.

12.13 RISK INFORMATION DURING CLINICAL TRIALS

Risk assessment for a product involves making an assessment of any questions regarding safety, as well as existing risk information, which is evaluated in contrast to the product's established advantage. A product may be less acceptable if it has demonstrated fewer benefits and higher levels of risk. For elucidating maximum information from clinical trials, the sponsor should give careful consideration to the overall design of the safety evaluation.

During the preapproval phase, databases do not have sufficient population size to identify every safety issue that could arise after the product is marketed for use in the general population. Henceforth, it is unrealistic to assume that every possible risk related to a product can be identified, even from large clinical development programs. It is likely that during drug development, more serious adverse events will be identified with a larger and more extensive preapproval database. A number of factors influence the optimal size of the safety database required to support a new product:

- Whether the database is similar to available treatment or represents a new treatment
- Whether the other therapies are available and whether those therapies are safe in comparison to the newly developed product

- The targeted patient population and therapeutic indication
- The expected treatment duration

During preclinical or human clinical pharmacology studies, a large safety database might be necessary when risk signals are detected that require additional clinical evidence to clarify their nature and magnitude. In case of fatal diseases having no alternative adequate treatments, safety databases are often smaller compared to the products targeting conditions that do not lead to death or cause major, permanent disability. End-of-phase I meetings serve as an opportunity to discuss and finalize the design of Phase II trials for drugs targeting life-threatening or seriously debilitating illnesses, according to 21 CFR 312.82(b), "with the goal that such testing will be adequate to provide sufficient data on the drug's safety and effectiveness to support a decision on its approvability for marketing."

The ICH and FDA typically recommend that for investigational products targeted for long-term use in non-fatal diseases, approximately 1500 subjects should be exposed to the drug. Of these, 300 to 600 participants should receive treatment for at least 6 months, and about 100 participants should be treated for 1 year. This applies to therapies involving continuous use for 6 months or more, or to those given intermittently where the total treatment duration equals or exceeds 6 months.[20] Single-dose administration or brief exposure rarely results in significant adverse events such as hepatotoxicity and hematologic events. Therefore, only subjects who have received the product in multiple dose studies should be included in the 1500 subjects for chronic use products, according to the FDA's ICH guidance E1A.

According to the E1A guidance, there are specific situations where a safety database larger than 1500 patients may be considered appropriate. These circumstances include the following:

1. Where there is potential risk in which medicinal product may induce delayed-onset adverse reactions
2. When there is concern regarding time-dependent increases in the frequency or severity of adverse events
3. When there is a requirement to determine the rate of occurrence of an anticipated, rare adverse events, such as serious reactions observed with comparable medicinal products.

Apart from the considerations mentioned in E1A, the following circumstances may also require expansion of the safety database:

1. The treatment is aimed at individuals without active disease (e.g., a product developed for chemoprevention or a prophylactic vaccination).
2. A safe and effective therapeutic alternative to the investigational product is currently available in the market.

12.14 CONSIDERATIONS FOR RISK ASSESSMENT

12.14.1 Risk Assessment during Clinical Trials

Risk assessment strategies can be adapted as per the following situations:

- If a product has dose-related toxicities or is intended for chronic use (especially having a prolonged half-life). Examining the suitability of a reduced or less frequent maintenance dosing regimen in such cases.
- When a titration schedule is proposed within the dosing regimen, specific research studies should be conducted to establish the most appropriate titration method and to evaluate its influence on both efficacy and safety outcomes.

- If a drug has the potential to have adverse effects that patients are unlikely to identify or report without extra attention, additional clinical testing or targeted safety assessment should be undertaken. For example, sponsors include assessment of cognitive function, motor performance, and mood when developing a new drug with known CNS effects (particularly sedating properties). Similarly, new antidepressants should be assessed for their effects on sexual functions, as many agents in this class are known to have significant effects. Employing specific safety questionnaires or validated psychometric or other tools is frequently crucial for such evaluations because routine adverse event monitoring and safety assessments often fail to capture such effects.
- Special safety concerns should be taken into consideration if a product is intended for investigations in pediatric patients. Specific evaluations should include potential effects on growth and neurocognitive development in infants and young children, as well as safety of excipients and considerations related to universal immunization or school entry requirements.
- In situations where prior safety data suggested an unexpected or noteworthy issue, sponsor may consider storing blood samples or other biological materials obtained from participants in Phase III studies for subsequent evaluation.

12.14.2 Medication Errors during Clinical Trials

Medication errors refer to any error occurring during the prescribing, dispensing, or administration of a medicinal product, regardless of whether the error results in harm or adverse outcomes.[21] Medication errors may arise during any phase of the drug use process. Clinical trials have identified certain medication errors, particularly those related to parenteral formulations, prior to product marketing. Evaluating the potential for medication errors prior to product approval helps in minimizing their future occurrence. Medication errors may arise from the product's intrinsic characteristics or from unintended factors such as the proposed proprietary or established name, labeling elements (including container, carton, patient/consumer labeling, or professional package insert), and packaging design. Additionally, errors in dilution or administration techniques during clinical trial may result in non-optimal dosing. Such observations should be examined thoroughly as potential indicators of susceptibility to dosing errors, warranting possible modifications to its labeling, packaging, or overall design. If no medication errors are detected during trials, careful considerations should still be given to the design of the product, its packaging, and any device used for administration or deliver as these factors may influence safe use post-marketing. For example, packing is crucial when developing a concentrated product that needs to be further diluted before being administered intravenously. Placing the product in a prefilled syringe format could result in direct bolus administration without the required dilution, which may significantly elevate safety risks for patients. Likewise, the consequences of a device's mechanical failure should be considered during the development of a product intended for administration or delivered through a device. Any such incidents must be documented, reported, and reviewed to determine corrective actions, such as redesigning the device or revising usage instructions.

12.15 CONCLUSION

The scope of pharmacovigilance and the emphasis on understanding the safety issues during drug development process have broadened with the ongoing advancement and emergence of new treatment approaches facilitated by clinical trials involving traditional and complementary medicines, herbals, medical devices, blood products, biologicals, and vaccines. Safety data reporting outcomes in clinical trials should maintain the same level of quality and precision as that of efficacy data reporting outcomes. Safety update reports should detail the frequency and nature of adverse events in each treatment group, including the number of subjects discontinued or withdrawn from the trial.

REFERENCES

1. Ruth HS. Anesthesia study commissions. J Am Med Asso 1945; 127 (9): 514–517.
2. Stephen J, Evans W. Pharmacovigilance: A science or fielding emergencies? *Statist Med* 2000; 19: 3199–3209.
3. http://www.mhra.gov.uk/Glossary/. Accessed on September 25, 2009.
4. http://apps.who.int/medicinedocs/en/d/Js4893e/9.html. Accessed on September 25, 2009.
5. Lin Y-L, Chern H-D, Chu M-L. Hepatotoxicity in the review of clinical safety data. *DIA* 2003; 37 (2): 155–158.6. http://www.fda.gov/safety/recalls/. Accessed on November 2009.
7. Press Release. European Medicines Agency Recommends Restricted Use Nimesulide-Containing Medicinal Products. Doc. Ref. EMEA/430988/2007, September 21, 2007.
8. Geba GP, Weaver AL, Polis AB, Dixon ME, Schnitzer TJ, Vioxx, Acetaminophen, Celecoxib Trial (VACT) group: Efficacy of rofecoxib, celecoxib, and acetaminophen in osteoarthritis of the knee. *JAMA* 2002; 287: 64–71.
9. Bombardier C, Laine L, Reicin A, Shapiro D, Burgos-Vargas R, Davis B, et al. Comparison of upper gastrointestinal toxicity of rofecoxib and naproxen in patients with rheumatoid arthritis. *N Engl J Med* 2000; 343: 1520–1528.
10. Schnitzer TJ, Burmester GR, Mysler E, Hochberg MC, Doherty M, Ehrsam E, et al. Comparison of lumiracoxib with naproxen and ibuprofen in the therapeutic arthritis research and gastrointestinal event trial (TARGET), reduction in ulcer complications: Randomised controlled trial. *Lancet* 2004; 364: 665–674.
11. Mamdani M, Juurlink DN, Lee DS, et al. Cyclo-oxygenase-2 inhibitors versus non-selective non-steroidal anti-inflammatory drugs and congestive heart failure outcomes in elderly patients: A population-based cohort study. *Lancet* 2004; 363: 1751–1756.
12. http://www.prescrire.org/docus/ericeEn.pdf. Accessed on November 2009.
13. http://www.who.int/ictrp/en/. Accessed on September 25, 2009.
14. Directive 2001/20/EC of the European Parliament and of the Council of 4 April 2001.
15. ICH Harmonised Tripartite Guideline Guideline for Good Clinical Practice E6(R1) Current *Step 4* version dated 10 June 1996.
16. International Conference on Harmonization of Technical Requirements for Registration of Pharmaceuticals for Human Use. Development Safety Update Report (E2F). Current *Step 2* version dated 5 June 2008.
17. Volume 9A of the Rules Governing Medicinal Products in the European Union: Pharmacovigilance for Medicinal Products for Human Use, September 2008.
18. Panos Tsintis P, La Mache E. CIOMS and ICH initiatives in pharmacovigilance and risk management overview and implications European agency for the evaluation of medicinal products. *London, United Kingdom Drug Safety* 2004; 27 (8): 509–517.
19. http://www.who-umc.org/. Accessed on November 25, 2009.
20. ICH Harmonised Tripartite Guideline. The extent of population exposure to assess clinical safety for drugs intended for long-term treatment of non-life-threatening conditions E1. *Status: Step* 1994; 4.
21. Williams DJP. Medication errors. *J R Coll Physicians Edinb* 2007; 37 (4): 343–346.

13 Statistical Considerations in Clinical Research

Ruchika Sharma[1], *and Anoop Kumar*[2]
[1]Delhi Pharmaceutical Sciences and Research University (DPSRU), New Delhi, India
[2]Department of Pharmacology, Delhi Institute of Pharmaceutical Sciences and Research (DIPSAR), Delhi Pharmaceutical Sciences and Research University (DPSRU), New Delhi, India

13.1 INTRODUCTION

In clinical trials, statistics play a crucial role. The range of statistical challenges includes trial design and protocol development, data management, data analysis, trial outcomes reporting, and data monitoring and conduct during an ongoing experiment. It can be challenging for non-statisticians to comprehend statistical concepts. To maintain the integrity of a trial, however, it is critical that clinicians working on clinical trials comprehend basic statistical concepts (Daniel & Cross, 2018). When reading medical publications, it's also critical to have a basic understanding of biostatistics and study design.

13.2 BASIC CONCEPTS (ARMITAGE ET AL., 2008)

- **Data:** Numbers, or data, are the foundation of statistics. While multiple numbers are referred to as data, a single number is called a datum.
- **Statistics:** Gathering, organizing, analyzing, and summarizing data. Data sources include surveys, experiments, and records.
- **Biostatistics**: Information analyzed comes from medicine and the biological sciences.
- **Variable:** Traits that have varying values in various people, locations, or objects. For instance, heart rate, blood sugar, diastolic blood pressure, etc.
- **Quantitative variable:** Provides details on the amount.
- **Qualitative Variables:** A lot of traits can only be divided into.
- **Random Variable:** Impossible to forecast with precision beforehand. For instance, we are unable to precisely forecast a child's height at birth.
- **Discrete Random Variable:** Needs to be a whole number, like 0, 1, 2, or 3. No number like 1.5, 2.9, or 3.3 can represent the number of admissions on a certain day. Any value can be assigned to the continuous random variable. The different measures that can be taken of people, such as height, weight, and skull circumference, are examples of continuous variables.
- **Population:** The greatest group of things in which we are interested at a given moment. A sample is a subset of the population, measurement is the process of allocating numbers to things or occurrences in accordance with a set of guidelines, and nominal scale is the lowest measurement scale. It entails "naming" observations or grouping them into a number of mutually exclusive and all-encompassing categories.

DOI: 10.1201/9781003533085-13

- **Ordinal Scale:** Observations are considered to be measured on an ordinal scale if they may be ranked based on a criterion in addition to being distinct from one category to another. It is possible to classify patients as unimproved, improved, and much improved.
- **Interval Scale:** The interval scale is more advanced than the nominal or ordinal scales since it allows one to order measurements and determine the separation between any two measurements. The process by which we make conclusions about a population from the data in a sample taken from that population is known as statistical inference.

13.3 DESCRIPTIVE STATISTICS (HOLLANDER ET AL., 2013)

- **Mean:** The mean is impacted by every value in a set of data since every single value is used to calculate the mean. Therefore, extreme values affect the mean and can sometimes distort it to the point where it is no longer a useful indicator of central tendency.
- **Median:** The median is the number that splits a finite set of values into two equal portions so that the number of values that fall below or correspond to the median is equal to the number of values that exceed or correspond to the median. The median, or middle value when all the values are sorted by magnitude, will be determined if the number of values is odd. When the number of numbers is even, there isn't a single middle value. Instead, there are two middle values. In this case, the median is taken to be the mean of these two middle values after all values have been sorted by magnitude.
- **Mode:** The value that appears the most frequently in a set of values is called the mode. There is no mode if every value is different; nonetheless, a collection of values may have multiple modes.

13.4 MEASUREMENT OF DISPERSION

Insights regarding the level of variation within a particular data set. There is no dispersion when all the values are the same; data dispersion occurs when they are not.

- **Range:** This is the variation between a collection of observations' maximum and smallest value. The range's utility is restricted. It is an inadequate measure of dispersion because it considers just two variables. Using the range has the primary benefit of being easy to calculate.
- **Variance:** A set of observations has less dispersion when its values are closer to their mean than when they are widely dispersed. Given this, measuring dispersion in relation to the scatter of the values about their mean would make natural sense. The variance is where such a measure is realized and the average squared difference between each value and the chosen mean (Dey & Mulekar, 2018).
- **Degree of Freedom:** n-1 represents the sample
- **Standard Deviation:** The variance is an inappropriate measure of dispersion when we wish to express this concept in terms of the original units because it represents squared units. The degree of dispersion in original units can be computed by taking the square root of the variance. This yields the standard deviation.
- **Coefficient of Variation**

  As a gauge of variance within a particular set of data, the standard deviation is helpful. However, comparing the two standard deviations can produce inaccurate findings when attempting to evaluate the dispersion in two sets of data. It's possible that the two variables in question have different units of measurement. For instance, we would want to know if serum cholesterol levels, which are expressed in milligrams per 100 milliliters, are more variable than body weight, which is expressed in pounds, for a particular population.

Moreover, the two means may differ significantly even though the same unit of measurement is applied. When the weight standard deviations of first graders and high school freshmen are compared, it may be seen that the latter standard deviation is quantitatively greater than the former. This is not because the dispersion is greater, but rather because the weights themselves are larger. In such circumstances, a measure of relative variance, not absolute variation, is required. The coefficient of variation contains such a metric. Since the mean and standard deviations are expressed in the same unit, we find that the unit of measurement cancels out when computing the coefficient of variation. Therefore, our measurement is independent of the unit of measurement.

13.5 SAMPLE SIZE CALCULATION

A crucial stage in carrying out a clinical study is estimating the sample size. To guarantee that research time, staff effort, and expenses are not lost, the sample size must be carefully considered. It frequently happens that a study's small sample size prevents it from detecting even significant treatment effects. This crucial aspect of clinical study preparation is addressed with the assistance of a biostatistician. Clinical investigators can use relatively simple calculations to estimate the proper sample size for conventional study designs in the absence of a biostatistician.

A few study design elements and the stated statistical assumptions typically determine the right sample size. These consist of the intended statistical power, significance threshold, predicted measurement variability, and the smallest meaningful observable difference (effect size).

Since proving the efficacy and safety of the drug products being studied is the main goal of the majority of clinical trials, determining the sample size at the planning stage is crucial to guaranteeing that there are enough participants to provide an accurate and trustworthy evaluation of the drug products with a certain level of statistical assurance. In reality, hypotheses about the study drug's scientific or medical issues are typically developed in accordance with the main goals of the research. In order to verify that the test results are correct and dependable with a specific level of statistical assurance, the hypotheses are next assessed using suitable statistical tests within a legitimate study design.

It should be emphasized that determining a proper sample size requires the use of appropriate statistical tests for hypotheses that accurately reflect the study objectives within a legitimate study design. It is consequently recommended that the assumptions be clearly indicated when calculating the sample size. For each of the previously described hypotheses, a distinct sample size is necessary to achieve a specific level of statistical assurance.

Estimation/determination, justification, correction, and re-estimation are the basic categories into which sample size calculation fits. Sample size estimation/determination is the process of computing the required sample size to attain a specified level of statistical accuracy and dependability, such as 80% power. In contrast, sample size justification seeks to give statistical evidence for a chosen sample size, which is often restricted due to cost restrictions and/or unique medical reasons. Most clinical trials have to correct for confounders or dropouts in order to have enough evaluable persons for a reliable statistical assessment of the study medication.

Sample size adjustment is the term for this kind of sample size computation. Interim analyses, whether planned or unplanned, may be helpful in many clinical trials as they are being conducted. For clinical studies that include planned or unplanned interim analyses, the sample size should be changed to account for an overall type I error rate at the nominal significance level. To determine whether the chosen sample size is sufficient to achieve the needed power at the end of the trial, sample size re-estimation based on cumulative information gathered up to a certain time point during interim analyses is also required. Depending on whether the sample size re-estimation or interim analysis will add bias into the clinical evaluation of participants after the time point at which it is performed, the process can be blinded or unblinded.

13.6 TYPICAL STATISTICAL ISSUES IN CLINICAL RESEARCH

Common statistical issues in clinical trials include inaccurate p-value interpretation, the need to display confidence intervals, the intent-to-treat principle, missing data, multiplicity, subgroup analyses, association versus causation, proper trial result reporting, probability and Bayesian statistics, clinician-statistician interaction, and the importance of effective communication.

13.7 STATISTICAL POWER

The type II mistake is associated with clinical trial statistical power. The findings in a clinical study either support HA (right judgment) or do not support HA (type II error) if the underlying truth is that the HA is true. Clinical trials with a prospective design should have a type II error of ≤0.20, which is equivalent to at least 80% statistical power.

13.7.1 One-Sided and Two-Sided Hypothesis Tests

One-sided and two-sided hypothesis tests are also possible. If a researcher wants to see if there is a difference between treatments A and B, a two-sided hypothesis test is acceptable. A one-sided hypothesis test can be used to determine whether an experimental treatment (A) is superior to the control arm therapy (B). Given that the A is evenly distributed across the two possible statistically significant differences in a two-sided test, a 0.05 test yields 0.025 a for A being better than B and 0.025 a for B being better than A. Because all of the data in a 1-sided test go to the single potential statistically significant difference, a 0.05 test, as seen in the previous example, has a 0.05 false positive rate. Therefore, with a one-sided test of the same level as a two-sided test, the false positive rate is greater. Therefore, an alpha of 0.025 is typically used for a 1-sided test in definitive phase III trials; nevertheless, a 1-sided test with an alpha of 0.05 is very uncommon, especially in trials targeting more uncommon cancers (Razali & Wah, 2011).

13.7.2 Stratification and Blinding

Reducing bias in clinical trials is the main goal of statisticians in order to minimize any factors that can complicate the interpretation of treatment effects in studies. Two related difficulties are the use of stratification criteria and whether patients and physicians will remain unaware of the patient's treatment. While randomization helps balance factors between treatment arms that may influence the trial's endpoints, stratification ensures balance for elements known to be associated with the primary outcome. Blinding occurs when neither the patient nor the physician is aware of the treatment being administered during a clinical trial. It goes without saying that biases may arise when the patient and/or physician are aware of the treatment being provided.

Depending on the specific outcome under evaluation, these biases could vary. However, blinding in every randomized clinical trial is not always realistic or even logistically possible. "Sham" radiation therapy or surgery would be necessary for the non-treatment arm of trials that randomly assigned participants to receive either radiation or surgery. In a drug trial, when a patient may be taking a tablet, it is more practical to have identical pills for the active medicine and the placebo.

Additional logistical issues arise in trials where the medication is administered intravenously. Rules for unblinding must be established. Generally speaking, unblinding should only be carried out if the information is required to treat the patient for an urgent problem before the patient fails the primary endpoint. Guidelines for unblinding patients after they fail the primary endpoint should also be taken into account. For example, in the case of a PFS primary endpoint, will patients in the control arm who progress be switched to the experimental treatment, and if so, how will this affect an OS secondary endpoint? Depending on a number of logistical, resource, and occasionally legal requirements, the decision to blind or not is made trial by trial.

Blinding or masking is used in clinical experiments to lessen the likelihood of both conscious and unconscious bias in the execution and interpretation of the experiment. The potential influence of treatment knowledge on subject assignment and selection techniques, post-treatment care, treatment attitudes, end-point evaluation, withdrawal management, data exclusion from analysis, and other procedures may be the cause of this bias. Preventing therapy identification until all potential biases have been eliminated is the primary goal.

In a double-blind experiment, neither the participant nor any of the sponsor or investigator personnel participating in the clinical evaluation or treatment of the participants is aware of the treatment they received. Anyone who determines subject eligibility, assesses protocol compliance, or evaluates endpoints falls under this category. Throughout the experiment, this degree of blinding is maintained, and the relevant staff will only be unblinded once the data has been cleaned to a satisfactory standard. The sponsor should have sufficient standard operating procedures in place to prevent the improper distribution of treatment codes if any of the staff members who are not involved in the subjects' clinical evaluation or treatment must be unblinded to the code.

In a single-blind experiment, the participant is unaware of the therapy, but the researcher and/or his team are, or vice versa. In an open-label experiment, everyone is aware of the treatment's identification. The best method is the double-blind trial. This necessitates that the blind be kept in a suitable state throughout the experiment and that the treatments to be administered cannot be differentiated (by appearance, taste, etc.) either before or during administration.

The following factors may make it difficult to achieve the double-blind ideal: the treatments may be entirely different, such as medication therapy and surgery; two drugs may have different formulations, and while using capsules may make them indistinguishable, altering the formulation may also alter the pharmacokinetic and/or pharmacodynamic properties, necessitating the establishment of bioequivalence between the formulations; and the daily schedule of administration of two treatments may differ. In these situations, a "double-dummy" technique is one method of creating double-blind conditions. This method may occasionally compel an administration plan that is sufficiently out of the ordinary to negatively affect the individuals' motivation and compliance. However, a lot of work should be done to get beyond these obstacles.

The apparent treatment-induced effects may impair the double-blind character of some clinical trials. In these situations, blinding investigators and pertinent sponsor personnel to specific test results may enhance blinding. Trials where distinct or particular treatment effects may result in unblinding individual patients should take into account similar strategies for reducing bias in open-label trials.

The single-blind option should be taken into consideration if a double-blind study is not practical. In certain situations, it is only ethically or practically feasible to conduct an open-label trial. Additional flexibility is offered by single-blind and open-label trials; nevertheless, it is crucial that the choice to enroll the subject should be made before the researcher is aware of the randomized treatment. The use of a centralized randomization technique, like telephone randomization, to assign randomized treatment should be taken into account for these trials.

Medical personnel who do not treat the participants and who are blind to therapy should also perform clinical evaluations. Every attempt should be taken to minimize the several known causes of bias in single-blind or open-label trials, and the primary variables should be as objective as feasible. The protocol should provide an explanation of the rationale behind the chosen level of blinding as well as the measures taken to reduce bias in other ways. For instance, while cleaning the database before releasing it for analysis, the sponsor should have sufficient standard operating procedures in place to guarantee that access to the treatment code is suitably controlled.

13.7.3 Randomization

In a clinical trial, randomization adds a purposeful element of chance to the subjects' treatment assignments. It offers a solid statistical foundation for the quantitative assessment of the evidence pertaining to treatment effects during further examination of the trial data. Additionally, it frequently results in treatment groups with comparable distributions of known and unknown prognostic variables. Randomization, when used in conjunction with blinding, helps prevent any bias in subject allocation and selection that may result from the predictability of treatment assignments.

A clinical trial's randomization schedule documents how individuals are randomized to treatments at random. In its most basic form, it is a list of treatments in sequential order, or codes that correspond to subject numbers. Though the logistics of some trials, such as those involving a screening stage, may complicate matters, the specific pre-planned assignment of treatment, or treatment sequence, to the subject should be obvious. Creating randomization schedules will require different ways depending on the trial design. The randomization procedure should be repeatable if necessary.

In multicenter research, randomization procedures should be centralized. There should be a random scheme specific to each center, such as stratification by center or the distribution of multiple whole blocks to each center. To promote fair distribution within strata, stratification based on major prognostic markers evaluated at baseline may generally be useful at times; small trials may gain more from this.

Using more than two or three stratification factors is rarely necessary and is less effective in achieving balance, as well as being logistically challenging. Adopting a dynamic allocation technique may help achieve balance across many stratification criteria at the same time, assuming that the remaining trial protocols can be modified to suit such an approach. Randomized stratification factors should be considered later in the investigation.

Dynamic allocation is a different process where a subject's treatment is assigned based on the current balance of treatments that have been assigned, as well as the subject's stratum and the balance within that stratum in a stratified trial. Every treatment allocation should have a suitable amount of randomization, and deterministic dynamic allocation processes should be avoided. The trial's double-blind status should be maintained at all costs. For instance, access to the treatment code can be limited to a central trial office, which typically controls the dynamic allocation over the phone.

This in turn creates access into the experiment and allows for further eligibility criterion checks, both of which are beneficial in some kinds of multicenter trials. It is then possible to follow the standard procedure of pre-packaging and labeling drug supplies for double-blind trials, but the sequence in which they are used is no longer sequential. The central trial office staff should be kept in the dark about the treatment code by using the proper computer algorithms. When thinking about dynamic allocation, it is important to carefully assess the logistics' complexity and any effects on the analysis.

13.8 TRIAL DESIGN CONSIDERATIONS

13.8.1 Parallel Group Design

The parallel group design, in which participants are randomly assigned to one of two or more arms, each with a different treatment, is the most common clinical trial type for confirmatory trials. These treatments will consist of one or more doses of the investigational substance along with one or more control treatments, like an active comparator or a placebo. Compared to most other designs, this one has simpler underlying assumptions. Covariates, repeated measurements over time, interactions between design parameters, protocol violations, dropouts, and withdrawals are a few examples of extra trial aspects that could make analysis and interpretation more difficult, as is the case with other designs (Valentinuzzi et al., 2004).

13.8.2 Crossover Design

Each participant in the crossover design serves as his own control for treatment comparisons since he is randomly assigned to a series of two or more treatments. This straightforward technique is appealing mainly because it, occasionally to a significant degree, lowers the number of individuals and assessments required to reach a given power. In the most basic 2×2 crossover design, each participant receives two treatments in a random order over the course of two consecutive treatment sessions, frequently interspersed by a washout interval. Comparing n(>2) treatments over n periods, with each subject receiving all n treatments, is the most popular extension of this (Armitage et al., 2008).

There are several variations, including designs where a subset of n(>2) treatments are given to each subject or designs where treatments are repeated within a subject. Numerous issues with crossover designs have the potential to render their findings erroneous. Carryover, or the lingering effects of treatments in later treatment periods, is the main challenge. Direct treatment comparisons will be skewed in an additive model due to unequal carryover. The proper contrast is "between subject," hence the test for either of these effects lacks power. Additionally, the carryover effect in the 2×2 design cannot be statistically separated from the interaction between treatment and period. Although less severe in higher-level designs, this issue cannot be completely disregarded (Valentinuzzi et al., 2004).

Therefore, it's crucial to avoid carryover while using the crossover design. The easiest way to accomplish this is to apply the design selectively and carefully, based on sufficient understanding of the disease area and the novel drug. The condition being studied ought to be steady and chronic. During the course of treatment, the medication's pertinent effects should fully manifest. For the pharmacological action to be fully reversible, the washout times should be long enough. Prior knowledge and data should be used to demonstrate that these conditions are likely to be met before the trial begins.

In crossover studies, there are other issues that require careful consideration. The most prominent of them are the difficulties in interpreting and analyzing data that result from subject loss. Additionally, the possibility of carryover makes it challenging to assign the proper treatment to adverse outcomes that transpire during later treatment periods. ICH E4 describes these and other difficulties. Generally speaking, the crossover design should only be used in circumstances where it is anticipated that there would be minimal subject losses from the study (Moore et al., 2005).

The 2×2 crossover design is commonly used to demonstrate bioequivalence between two versions of a drug. If the wash-out time between the two periods is sufficient, carryover effects on the relevant pharmacokinetic variable are unlikely in this particular application in healthy volunteers. On the basis of the data collected, it is nevertheless crucial to verify this assumption during analysis, for instance, by proving that no drug is detectable at the beginning of each session (Serdar et al., 2021).

13.8.3 Factorial Designs

A factorial design uses different combinations of treatments to evaluate two or more treatments at the same time. The most basic example is the 2×2 factorial design, where participants are assigned at random to one of four potential pairings of two treatments, let's say A and B. These are neither A nor B, both A and B, B alone, and A alone. This approach is frequently employed specifically to investigate how A and B interact. If the sample size was determined using the test for main effects, the statistical test of interaction might not have the power to identify an interaction. When using this design to examine the combined effects of A and B, this consideration is crucial, especially if the treatments are anticipated to be given in tandem (Serdar et al., 2021).

Establishing the dose-response characteristics of concurrently using treatments C and D is another crucial application of the factorial design, particularly in cases when the effectiveness of each monotherapy has been demonstrated at a particular dose in earlier studies. An equivalent number, n, of doses of D is chosen, along with a number, m, of doses of C, typically containing a zero dose (placebo). Each of the m×n treatment groups in the whole scheme receives a unique mix of dosages of C and D.

An acceptable combination of C and D doses for clinical use may then be determined with the aid of the response surface estimate that is produced. By comparing the effectiveness of the two treatments with the same number of people as would be needed to compare the effectiveness of either treatment alone, the 2×2 design may occasionally be utilized to maximize the usage of clinical trial participants. For very large mortality trials, this approach has proven quite useful (Valentinuzzi et al., 2004; Serdar et al., 2021).

The efficacy and validity of this strategy depend on the fact that treatments A and B do not interact with one another in order for their effects on the major efficacy variables to follow an additive model. Therefore, whether or not A adds to the effect of B, its effect is essentially the same. When it comes to the crossover trial, facts and past knowledge should be used to show that this condition is likely to be met prior to the start of the experiment.

13.8.4 Analysis

"A number that needs to be <0.05 so the trial can be published in a good journal" is not the solution. Simply defined, a P number represents the probability that, if the Ho is true, the data will produce a result that is as extreme as or more extreme than the observed result. In general, if the hypothesis is correct, a smaller p value indicates that the observed events are unlikely to have occurred.

13.9 COEFFICIENT OF DETERMINATION

The computer will produce a result known as the coefficient of determination, or R2, after regression analysis is completed. Usually given as a percentage, this indicates how much of the data's variability can be explained by the regression line.

Consequently, it provides a measure of the regression line's fit to the data (R2 value 0 to 1). Greater values show that the data points and regression line fit each other more closely (Casella & Berger, 2021).

- **Confirmation Interval**
  Interval of confidence = Point estimate± Skewness and critical value × S.E.
  Mode > median > positive (right)-mean
  (left)-negative mean<median
  When data is skewed, use the median with the IQR.
  Important Gaussian Curve Features
  The curve's left and right sides are mirror images.
  The mean, median, and mode are all at the middle.
  The standard deviation
  The mean is within ±1SD of 68% of the data.
  95% fall between 2SD and the mean.
  99.7% of them fall within 3SD of the average</median

13.10 CONCLUSION

In conclusion, statistical techniques are essential to clinical research. Currently, a wide range of statistical techniques are accessible to handle various data circumstances. A thorough understanding of the study design and data collection is necessary for the proper application of these strategies. Clinical research producers and consumers need to have a basic understanding of prevalent statistical approaches and how they differ and are similar.

REFERENCES

Armitage P, Berry G, Matthews JNS. Statistical methods in medical research. Chichester: John Wiley & Sons, 2008

Casella G, Berger RL. Statistical inference. Belmont, CA: Cengage Learning, 2021

Daniel WW, Cross CL. Biostatistics: A foundation for analysis in the health sciences. Chichester: Wiley, 2018

Dey R, Mulekar MS. Effect size as a measure of difference between two populations. In: Alhajj R, Rokne J. (eds) Encyclopedia of social network analysis and mining. New York: Springer, 2018. pp.715–26

Hollander M, Wolfe DA, Chicken E. Nonparametric statistical methods. Chichester: John Wiley & Sons, 2013

Moore DS, Dawson LG, McCabe GP. Introduction to the practice of statistics excel manual with macros. London: Macmillan, 2005

Razali NM, Wah YB. Power comparisons of Shapiro-Wilk, Kolmogorov-Smirnov, Lilliefors and Anderson-Darling tests. J Stat Model Anal 2011;2:21–33

Serdar CC, Cihan M, Yücel D, Serdar MA. Sample size, power and effect size revisited: Simplified and practical approaches in pre-clinical, clinical and laboratory studies. Biochem Med 2021;31:27–53

Valentinuzzi ME, Friedman LM, Furberg CD, DeMets DL. Fundamentals of clinical trials. 3rd ed. Cham: Springer, 2004

14 Emerging Trends and Innovations in Clinical Research

Haya Majid[1] *and Raman Sehgal*[2]
[1]Department of Translational and Clinical Research, School of Chemical and Life Sciences, Jamia Hamdard, New Delhi, India
[2] Department of Clinical Research, Medanta-The Medicity, Gurugram, Haryana, India

14.1 INTRODUCTION

Clinical research is evolving at an unprecedented pace, driven by advances in technology, data science, and a deeper understanding of human biology. As the demand for more efficient, patient-centric, and innovative approaches grows, the traditional models of clinical trials are being redefined. Emerging trends and innovations in clinical research are reshaping how studies are designed, conducted, and analyzed, with a profound impact on the speed, accuracy, and efficacy of developing new therapies (Kandi and Vadakedath 2023).

In recent years, this field has witnessed a paradigm shift toward digital transformation, personalized medicine, and data-driven decision-making. Decentralized clinical trials (DCTs) are gaining traction, utilizing digital tools to conduct studies remotely, enhancing patient engagement, and broadening participant diversity. Concurrently, artificial intelligence (AI) and machine learning (ML) are revolutionizing every stage of the research process, from identifying potential participants to optimizing trial designs and analyzing complex datasets (McComb, Bies, and Ramanathan 2022; Aghamiri, Amin, and Helikar 2022).

Moreover, real-world evidence (RWE) and real-world data (RWD) are becoming essential components of clinical research, offering insights into how treatments perform in broader, more diverse populations beyond the controlled environment of traditional clinical trials. Wearable devices, electronic health records (EHRs), and mobile health applications enable continuous monitoring and real-time data collection, providing a richer, more comprehensive understanding of patient outcomes. Additionally, the emergence of precision medicine and genomic research is transforming therapeutic development by tailoring treatments to the genetic profiles and molecular characteristics of individual patients. Innovations in biomarkers, genomics, and bioinformatics are enabling more targeted therapies, improving efficacy, and reducing adverse effects (Inokuchi et al. 2022; Evans 2016).

As the clinical research ecosystem becomes more interconnected and data-driven, regulatory frameworks are also evolving to accommodate new methodologies and technologies. Collaborative models involving academia, industry, regulators, and patients are fostering a more agile and adaptive approach to clinical research, ensuring that innovative therapies reach patients faster while maintaining rigorous safety and efficacy standards. This chapter explores the key trends and innovations driving the future of clinical research, highlighting the opportunities and challenges in adopting new approaches. By understanding these developments, stakeholders can better navigate the complexities of clinical research and contribute to the advancement of medical science in the 21st century (Figure 14.1).

DOI: 10.1201/9781003533085-14

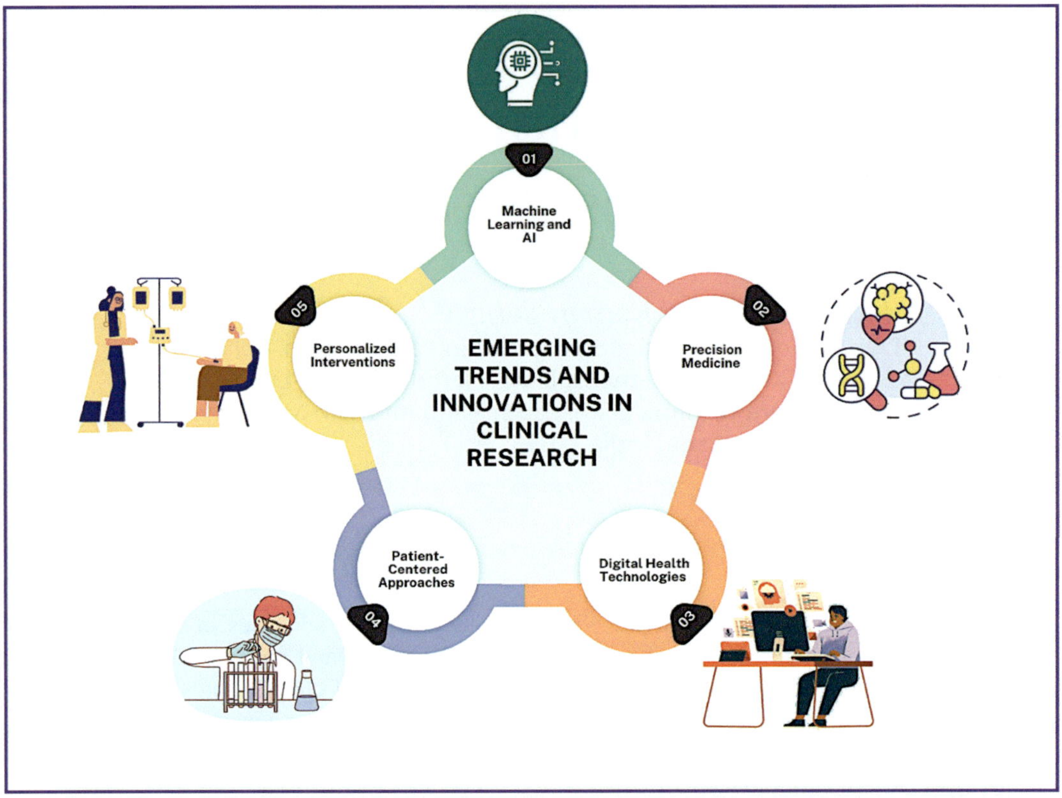

FIGURE 14.1 Emerging trends and innovations in clinical research.

14.2 PRECISION MEDICINE AND PERSONALIZED INTERVENTIONS

Precision medicine or personalized medicine represents a transformative approach to healthcare that takes into account genetic, environmental, and lifestyle heterogeneity across individuals to develop tailored therapeutic strategies. Unlike the traditional "one-size-fits-all" model, which assumes that a standard treatment will work uniformly across a population, precision medicine aims to identify the most effective treatments for specific patient subgroups according to their distinct molecular and genetic characteristics. This paradigm shift is driven by the growing recognition that diseases, even those with the same clinical diagnosis, can manifest differently in different patients due to underlying biological differences. Precision medicine seeks to understand these differences at a molecular level and use this information to guide clinical decision-making.

14.2.1 History of Precision Medicine

14.2.1.1 Origins of Precision Medicine: Early Insights and Concepts

Precision medicine, while seemingly modern, can trace its roots back over a century. The earliest inklings of what would later evolve into precision medicine began in the 19th and early 20th centuries when scientists and physicians began to recognize that individuals often responded in contrast to the same therapies. This was specifically evident in observations related to infectious diseases, where the same pathogen could cause mild symptoms in one person and severe illness or death in another. At this time, however, there was limited comprehension of the basic biological factors driving these variations, and medicine largely relied on empirical observations rather than tailored approaches.

The formal foundation of precision medicine was laid in the early 20th century with the burgeoning field of pharmacogenetics, which sought to understand how genetic differences influence medication reactions of patients. In 1902, British physician Archibald Garrod made a landmark contribution to this field with his study of alkaptonuria, a rare metabolic disorder. Garrod suggested that the condition was the result of a "chemical individuality" due to an inborn error of metabolism, which was among the first suggestions that genetic factors could influence how people metabolize certain substances. This idea was revolutionary at the time and foreshadowed the future direction of precision medicine.

14.2.1.2 Mid-20th Century: The Rise of Genetics and Pharmacogenomics

The mid-20th century marked significant progress in the understanding of genetics, which would become a cornerstone of precision medicine. The discovery of the structure of DNA by James Watson and Francis Crick in 1953 provided a critical framework for understanding how genetic information is encoded and passed on, setting the stage for future advances in molecular biology and genetics. In the ensuing decades, research into genetic inheritance, gene function, and gene-environment interactions deepened the understanding of the biological basis for individual differences in health and disease.

By the 1960s and 1970s, the term "pharmacogenetics" began to gain prominence, focusing specifically on the study of how genetic variations influence drug metabolism and efficacy. Researchers began identifying specific genetic polymorphisms that affected how individuals metabolize common drugs, such as the role of the enzyme glucose-6-phosphate dehydrogenase (G6PD) in sensitivity to certain antimalarial medications. These discoveries highlighted the potential to tailor drug therapy based on an individual's genetic profile, a foundational concept for precision medicine.

14.2.1.3 The Late 20th Century: Molecular Biology and Genomics Revolution

The latter part of the 20th century saw explosive growth in molecular biology and genomics, fueled by advances in DNA sequencing technologies and bioinformatics. The development of polymerase chain reaction (PCR) technology in the 1980s allowed for rapid amplification and analysis of DNA, making it easier to study genetic variations associated with diseases and drug responses. During this period, researchers discovered numerous genetic markers linked to specific diseases, such as cystic fibrosis, Huntington's disease, and certain forms of cancer, providing critical insights into the genetic underpinnings of human health.

The 1990s brought the advent of the Human Genome Project (HGP), a massive international research effort launched in 1990 with the goal of mapping the entire human genome. Completed in 2003, the HGP was a monumental achievement that marked the beginning of the genomic era, providing a reference map of the 3 billion DNA base pairs that make up the human genome. The HGP paved the way for identifying genes associated with a wide range of diseases and enabled researchers to understand how genetic variations contribute to individual differences in disease susceptibility, progression, and response to treatment.

In parallel, advances in computational biology and the development of powerful bioinformatics tools facilitated the analysis of large-scale genomic data. This capability was crucial for the identification of genetic mutations and polymorphisms that could serve as biomarkers for disease risk, prognosis, and treatment response, laying the groundwork for the personalized approaches that define precision medicine today.

14.2.1.4 The Early 21st Century: Precision Medicine Takes Shape

The early 21st century marked a period of rapid acceleration in the field of precision medicine. Building on the foundational work of the Human Genome Project, scientists began to explore the implications of genomics for clinical practice more deeply. Key to this era was the development of next-generation sequencing (NGS) technologies, which dramatically reduced the cost and time required to sequence DNA, making it feasible to apply genomic analysis in clinical settings. NGS technologies enabled large-scale studies, such as genome-wide association studies (GWAS), which have identified numerous genetic variants associated with complex diseases, including diabetes, heart disease, and various cancers.

The concept of "personalized medicine" began to emerge more prominently during this time, with a focus on using genetic information to guide treatment decisions. Oncology quickly became a key area for the application of personalized approaches, with the discovery of specific genetic mutations in tumors, such as the HER2 gene in breast cancer and the BRAF mutation in melanoma. These discoveries led to the development of targeted therapies, such as trastuzumab for HER2-positive breast cancer and vemurafenib for BRAF-mutant melanoma, which significantly improved outcomes for specific patient subgroups and demonstrated the potential of precision medicine to transform clinical care.

In 2003, the term "precision medicine" gained broader recognition when the National Academy of Sciences published a report titled "Toward Precision Medicine: Building a Knowledge Network for Biomedical Research and a New Taxonomy of Disease." This report highlighted the need to move beyond traditional disease classifications based on symptoms and pathology toward a more nuanced understanding of diseases based on molecular and genetic characteristics.

14.2.1.5 The 2010s: Formalizing Precision Medicine Initiatives

The 2010s witnessed significant institutional support for precision medicine, particularly in the United States. In 2015, President Barack Obama announced the Precision Medicine Initiative (PMI) during his State of the Union Address, launching a national effort to advance precision medicine research and implementation. The PMI aimed to leverage advances in genomics, big data, and health information technology to develop more personalized approaches to disease prevention, diagnosis, and treatment. The initiative emphasized the gathering and evaluation of vast amounts of health data from diverse populations to uncover the genetic, environmental, and lifestyle factors contributing to disease.

Concurrent with the PMI, numerous other countries and institutions launched similar efforts to advance precision medicine. For instance, the United Kingdom's 100,000 Genomes Project intended to sequence the genetic material of 100,000 people suffering from malignancy and uncommon disorders, integrating genomic data with clinical information to drive research and improve patient care. Other initiatives, such as the European Union's Horizon 2020 program and China's National Precision Medicine Strategy, underscored the global commitment to advancing precision medicine as a critical component of future healthcare systems.

14.2.1.6 The Present and Future of Precision Medicine

Today, precision medicine is increasingly becoming a reality in clinical practice, driven by continued advancements in genomics, molecular biology, and data science. The integration of genomic data with EHRs, the use of AI and machine learning (ML) to analyze complex datasets, and the development of novel biomarkers for disease risk and treatment response are expanding the scope and impact of precision medicine. In addition to oncology, precision medicine is making inroads into other fields, such as cardiovascular disease, neurology, infectious diseases, and pharmacogenomics, offering new opportunities to enhance the results for patients and reduce healthcare costs.

The future of precision medicine is likely to involve even greater integration of multi-omics data (including genomics, proteomics, metabolomics, and microbiomics) to provide a more comprehensive understanding of disease mechanisms and treatment responses. Advances in gene editing technologies, such as CRISPR-Cas9, hold promise for not only diagnosing but also curing genetic disorders by directly correcting disease-causing mutations. Moreover, the expansion of biobanks, coupled with advances in data sharing and collaborative research, will continue to drive the discovery of new biomarkers and therapeutic targets.

The foundation of precision medicine lies in advances in genomics, molecular biology, and bioinformatics. Rapid developments in next-generation sequencing (NGS) technologies have made it possible to sequence an individual's entire genome quickly and cost-effectively, providing an elaborate map of genetic mutations, variations, and expressions. This information can reveal critical insights into the mechanisms underlying various diseases, such as cancer, cardiovascular disorders, and neurological conditions, allowing clinicians to design more targeted and effective treatments. For example, in oncology, precision medicine has led to the identification of specific genetic mutations, such as the HER2 gene in breast cancer or the EGFR mutation in lung cancer, which can be targeted by specific drugs, resulting in improved patient outcomes and reduced side effects.

14.2.2 Personalized Interventions: Tailoring Treatment to the Individual

Personalized interventions, an extension of precision medicine, focus on tailoring treatment plans to an individual's unique genetic, molecular, and phenotypic profile. The goal of personalized interventions is to optimize therapeutic effectiveness while reducing negative consequences, thereby enhancing overall patient care and quality of life. This individualized approach involves a comprehensive assessment of multiple factors, including a patient's genetic makeup, lifestyle, environment, and even their microbiome—the complex ecosystem of microorganisms living within the body.

For instance, pharmacogenomics, a key component of personalized medicine, studies how genetic variations affect response to drugs. These variations can influence drug metabolism, efficacy, and toxicity, leading to significant differences in how patients respond to the same medication. By analyzing a patient's genetic profile, medical professionals can predict their response to certain medications, enabling them to choose the most effective treatment with the least risk of side effects. This approach is particularly valuable in managing conditions like depression, epilepsy, cardiovascular diseases, and cancer, where significant variability in drug response exists among patients.

Additionally, personalized interventions often involve the use of biomarkers—measurable indicators of biological processes, diseases, or responses to treatment. Biomarkers can help stratify patients into subgroups that have a greater probability of gaining advantages through specific therapies, thereby enhancing the precision of treatment. For example, in oncology, the use of PD-L1 expression as a biomarker helps identify patients who are more likely to respond to immunotherapies targeting the PD-1/PD L1 pathway. Similarly, in cardiovascular medicine, biomarkers like LDL cholesterol levels, C-reactive protein (CRP), and genetic markers like PCSK9 mutations are used to personalize treatment approaches for conditions like hypercholesterolemia and atherosclerosis.

14.2.3 Technological Advances Driving Precision Medicine and Personalized Interventions

Several technological advances are accelerating the adoption of precision medicine and personalized interventions in clinical practice. Genomic technologies, such as CRISPR-Cas9 for gene editing, have opened new avenues for developing targeted therapies, particularly for genetic disorders where specific mutations are known to cause disease. CRISPR enables precise modifications to the genome, potentially correcting disease-causing mutations or altering gene expression to prevent disease progression. This technology holds promise for treating conditions like cystic fibrosis, sickle cell anemia, and certain types of cancers, where specific genetic mutations play a pivotal role.

In addition to genomic technologies, advancements in bioinformatics and computational biology are crucial for processing and interpreting the vast amounts of data generated by proteomic, genomic, and metabolomic studies. Machine learning algorithms and AI tools are being employed to analyze complex datasets, identify novel biomarkers, and predict patient responses to therapies. These resources allow researchers to discover previously hidden patterns in large datasets, facilitating the development of new diagnostic tools and therapeutic strategies that are more tailored to individual patient needs.

Wearable devices and digital health tools also play a significant role in advancing personalized interventions. These devices enable continuous monitoring of physiological parameters, such as heart rate, glucose levels, and activity levels, providing real-time data that are able to personalize treatment plans. For example, in managing chronic conditions like diabetes, continuous glucose monitors (CGMs) provide detailed insights into an individual's glucose patterns, allowing for more precise insulin dosing and lifestyle recommendations. Similarly, in cardiology, wearable ECG monitors can detect arrhythmias or changes in heart rate variability, enabling timely interventions and personalized adjustments to treatment regimens.

14.3 CHALLENGES AND OPPORTUNITIES IN IMPLEMENTING PRECISION MEDICINE

While precision medicine and personalized interventions hold immense promise, their implementation doesn't come without difficulties. One of the primary obstacles is the need for robust, standardized methods for data collection, storage, and analysis. The vast amount of data generated by genomic and other high-throughput technologies requires secure, interoperable systems to ensure data privacy, accuracy, and accessibility. Moreover, integrating these diverse datasets—from genomic and clinical data to patient-reported outcomes and environmental exposures—into a cohesive framework that can be applied to clinical judgement is a complex task that requires interdisciplinary collaboration.

Another significant challenge is ensuring fair access to precise medical care. The cost of genomic testing, advanced diagnostics, and targeted therapies can be prohibitive for many patients, raising concerns about health disparities. To fully achieve precision medicine's capabilities, it is crucial to develop cost-effective technologies and expand access to underserved populations. Initiatives like population-based genomic studies and efforts to include diverse patient groups in clinical trials are steps in the right direction, aiming to create a more inclusive foundation for precision medicine (publica and 2019 2024; M. Kosorok, its, and 2019 2024; Lobitz et al. 2024; Bylstra et al. 2021; K. B. Johnson et al. 2021; Ginsburg and Phillips 2018; Ashley 2016; M. R. Kosorok and Laber 2019).

14.4 DIGITAL HEALTH TECHNOLOGIES IN CLINICAL RESEARCH

Digital health technologies are revolutionizing the field of clinical research by providing innovative tools and platforms that enhance the efficiency, accuracy, and inclusivity of clinical trials. These technologies encompass a wide range of digital tools, including electronic health records (EHRs), wearable devices, telemedicine, mobile health (mHealth) applications, and digital platforms for data collection and analysis. By integrating these technologies into clinical research, researchers can conduct studies more efficiently, recruit and retain diverse patient populations, collect real-time data, and monitor participants remotely. This shift toward digital solutions is making clinical research more patient-centric, accessible, and adaptable, paving the way for new advancements in medical science (Figure 14.2).

14.4.1 Electronic Health Records (EHRs) and Digital Data Repositories

EHRs are digital versions of patients' medical histories, including information on medications, immunization dates, diagnoses, allergies, treatment plans, laboratory test results, and radiology images. EHRs play a crucial role in clinical research by providing a rich source of real-world data (RWD) that can be used to identify eligible participants, monitor patient safety, and observe new interventions.

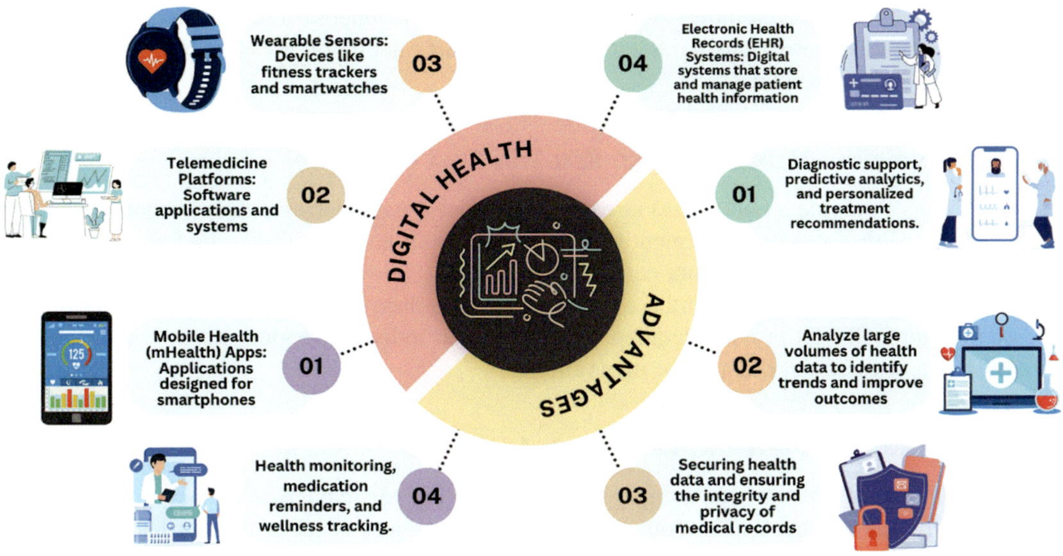

FIGURE 14.2 Digital health technology and advantages.

14.4.2 Enhancing Participant Recruitment and Screening

One of the significant challenges in clinical trials is recruiting and screening eligible participants. EHRs can streamline this process by providing access to vast amounts of patient data, enabling researchers to identify potential participants who meet specific eligibility criteria. For example, using algorithms to query EHR databases, researchers can quickly find patients with certain medical conditions, genetic markers, or medication histories, significantly reducing the cost and time associated with manual recruitment methods.

14.5 MONITORING PATIENT SAFETY AND OUTCOMES

EHRs enable continuous monitoring of patient safety and outcomes throughout a clinical trial. Researchers can access up-to-date patient information, detect adverse events promptly, and ensure timely interventions if necessary. Additionally, EHRs provide a longitudinal view of patient health, allowing researchers to assess the long-term effects of treatments and understand disease progression over time.

14.5.1 Improving Data Quality and Reducing Redundancy

EHRs improve the quality and accuracy of data collected during clinical trials by reducing the need for manual data entry and minimizing transcription errors. Data can be automatically extracted from EHR systems, ensuring consistency and reducing redundancy. Furthermore, EHRs facilitate data standardization across multiple sites and studies, enabling more straightforward comparison and integration of data from different sources.

14.5.2 Wearable Devices and Sensors

Wearable devices and sensors have become powerful tools in clinical research, enabling the continuous, non-invasive collection of physiological and behavioral data from study participants. These devices include smartwatches, fitness trackers, ECG monitors, glucose monitors, and implantable sensors that can measure various parameters, such as heart rate, blood pressure, physical activity, sleep patterns, and glucose levels.

14.5.3 Continuous Monitoring and Real-Time Data Collection

Wearable devices provide a continuous stream of real-time data, offering a deeper comprehension of a patient's health status and treatment response. For instance, in clinical trials for cardiovascular diseases, wearable ECG monitors can detect arrhythmias or changes in heart rate variability, allowing for early detection of potential adverse events. Similarly, in diabetes research, continuous glucose monitors (CGMs) provide detailed insights into an individual's glucose patterns, enabling more precise assessment of therapeutic interventions.

14.5.4 Enhancing Patient Engagement and Adherence

Wearables encourage greater patient engagement by allowing participants to actively monitor their health and provide feedback. The convenience of these devices reduces the burden on participants, as they no longer need to make frequent visits to clinical sites for monitoring. This increased engagement can lead to higher adherence rates and more accurate data collection, improving the overall quality of the trial.

14.5.5 Remote Patient Monitoring and Decentralized Trials

Wearable devices are integral to the shift toward decentralized clinical trials (DCTs), where participants can be monitored remotely without the need for frequent site visits. Remote monitoring allows researchers to collect data from participants in their natural environments, providing a more accurate representation of how treatments perform in real-world settings. This approach is particularly beneficial in studies involving vulnerable populations, such as the elderly or those with mobility issues, who may find it challenging to travel to clinical sites.

14.5.6 Mobile Health (mHealth) Applications

Mobile health (mHealth) applications are smartphone-based tools designed to support health monitoring, patient engagement, data collection, and communication in clinical research. These apps are increasingly being used in clinical trials to improve participant experience, streamline data collection, and enhance study efficiency.

14.5.7 Improving Data Collection and Participant Reporting

mHealth apps allow participants to enter data directly, such as daily symptoms, medication adherence, or lifestyle behaviors, which can be instantly transmitted to researchers. This direct data entry minimizes errors associated with manual transcription and recall bias, resulting in more accurate and reliable data. For example, in clinical trials for chronic pain management, mHealth apps is able to gather patient-reported outcomes (PROs) on pain levels, medication use, and side effects, providing valuable insights into treatment efficacy.

14.5.8 Facilitating Communication and Follow-Up

mHealth apps facilitate real-time communication between participants and researchers, improving study coordination and follow-up. Participants can receive reminders for medication intake, upcoming appointments, or data entry tasks, helping to maintain adherence and compliance. Moreover, mHealth apps can provide educational content and support tools to empower participants, fostering a sense of involvement and ownership in the research process.

14.5.9 Enabling Remote Consent and Enrollment

The use of mHealth apps simplifies the process of obtaining informed consent by providing digital platforms for electronic consent (eConsent). Participants can review study information, ask questions, and provide consent remotely, reducing the need for in-person visits and enhancing study accessibility. Digital consent forms can be tailored to improve understanding and engagement, using multimedia elements such as videos, animations, and interactive quizzes to clarify complex information.

14.5.10 Telemedicine and Virtual Visits

Telemedicine involves the use of digital communication tools, such as video conferencing, to conduct remote consultations, assessments, and follow-ups with clinical trial participants. The incorporation of telemedicine into clinical research is significantly expanding the reach and flexibility of trials, especially in geographically diverse or underserved populations.

14.6 EXPANDING ACCESS AND DIVERSITY IN CLINICAL TRIALS

Telemedicine eliminates geographical barriers, allowing participants from remote or underserved areas to participate in clinical trials without needing to cover large distances to clinical sites. This expanded access can enhance the diversity of trial populations, making study findings more generalizable to broader patient groups. For example, telemedicine has been widely used in COVID-19 vaccine trials to enroll participants from diverse locations, contributing to more comprehensive data on vaccine efficacy across different demographics.

14.6.1 Reducing Costs and Burden on Participants

By minimizing the need for in-person visits, telemedicine reduces costs associated with transportation, accommodation, and time off work, which can be significant barriers to participation. This reduction in burden can increase participant retention and decrease dropout rates, ultimately enhancing the efficiency and success of clinical trials.

14.6.2 Facilitating Real-Time Data Collection and Monitoring

Telemedicine enables real-time data collection and monitoring, allowing researchers to conduct virtual assessments, monitor adherence, and address any concerns promptly. For example, in mental health trials, telemedicine platforms can be used for remote psychological assessments, therapy sessions, and monitoring of treatment adherence, providing timely support to participants and ensuring data quality.

14.6.3 Digital Platforms for Data Integration and Analysis

Digital platforms designed for data integration and analysis are revolutionizing how clinical trial data is managed, shared, and analyzed. These platforms enable the aggregation of diverse datasets from multiple sources, including EHRs, wearables, mHealth apps, and telemedicine tools, into a unified, interoperable system.

14.6.4 Enhancing Data Management and Interoperability

Digital platforms offer advanced tools for data management, ensuring data is standardized, de-identified, and stored securely. This interoperability is crucial for multicenter trials, where data must be integrated from various locations and sources. Cloud-based platforms enable real-time data sharing and collaboration among researchers, fostering a more agile and adaptive approach to clinical research.

14.6.5 Facilitating Advanced Data Analytics and AI Integration

These platforms are equipped with advanced analytical tools, including AI and machine learning algorithms, which can analyze large datasets to optimize trial designs, identify patterns, and predict outcomes. For instance, predictive modeling can help identify patient subgroups most likely to gain from a specific treatment, while machine learning can automate data cleaning, reducing the cost and time associated with manual data curation.

14.6.6 Ensuring Regulatory Compliance and Data Security

Digital platforms must comply with regulatory standards, such as GDPR in Europe and HIPAA in the United States, to ensure data privacy and security. These platforms often include built-in features for audit trails, data encryption, and access controls, ensuring that data is handled in a manner that meets regulatory requirements and protects patient confidentiality.

14.6.7 Challenges and Future Directions

While digital health technologies offer immense potential to transform clinical research, their implementation has challenges. Key issues include security and privacy concerns, the need for robust infrastructure, and ensuring equitable access to digital tools. Data interoperability between different digital systems remains a significant challenge, as does the need for standardized guidelines for the application of technology in digital health within clinical trials.

Moreover, the adoption of digital technologies requires significant investment in training and capacity building for researchers, healthcare providers, and participants to ensure effective and ethical use. Addressing these challenges will be crucial to fully realizing the potential of digital health technologies in clinical research (Borges Do Nascimento et al. 2024; Scott et al. 2020; Kemp et al. 2024; Khan et al. 2017; Awad et al. 2024; Societies and 2014 2014; Lupton 2014).

14.7 PATIENT-CENTERED APPROACHES AND PARTICIPATORY RESEARCH MODELS

Patient-centered approaches and participatory research models represent a transformative shift in clinical research, emphasizing the involvement of patients as active partners rather than passive subjects. These approaches prioritize patients' experiences, values, and preferences, integrating their insights into every stage of the research process—from study design and implementation to data processing and distribution of results. The goal is to enhance the relevance, transparency, and effectiveness of clinical trials, ultimately improving health outcomes and ensuring that research findings are more applicable to real-world patient populations. By adopting patient-centered and participatory research models, researchers can develop studies that better reflect the needs and priorities of patients, reduce barriers to participation, and increase trust and engagement within communities. These models are especially crucial in addressing health disparities, as they provide a framework for more inclusive research that involves diverse patient populations and addresses their unique health challenges.

14.7.1 Defining Patient-Centered Approaches in Clinical Research

Patient-centered approaches in clinical research focus on the holistic involvement of patients throughout the research lifecycle. This means engaging patients not only as study subjects but as key stakeholders whose perspectives are vital in shaping the research agenda. These approaches align closely with the principles of shared decision-making, respect for patient autonomy, and recognition of individual preferences and values.

14.7.2 Engaging Patients in Study Design

In patient-centered research, patients are involved in the study design phase to ensure that the research questions are relevant to their needs and concerns. This involvement can take various forms, including patient advisory boards, focus groups, and surveys, where patients provide feedback on study objectives, protocols, and outcomes. By involving patients early in the design process, researchers can identify potential barriers to participation, such as complex procedures or frequent site visits, and make necessary adjustments to enhance patient engagement and retention. For instance, in studies involving chronic diseases like diabetes or cancer, patient input can help determine the most meaningful outcomes to measure, such as quality of life, pain levels, or treatment side effects. Traditional clinical trials often focus on clinical endpoints (e.g., blood sugar levels or tumor size), which may not fully capture the aspects of care that matter most to patients. By integrating patient perspectives, researchers can ensure that the chosen endpoints align more closely with patients' priorities, making the study outcomes more relevant and impactful.

14.7.3 Incorporating Patient-Reported Outcomes (PROs)

Patient-reported outcomes (PROs) are a key component of patient-centered research. PROs involve collecting data directly from patients about their symptoms, health status, quality of life, and treatment satisfaction, without interpretation by clinicians or researchers. These outcomes provide valuable insights into the patient's experience and help capture aspects of health that are not always evident through clinical measures.

For example, in clinical trials for chronic pain management, PROs may include patient-reported pain severity, duration, and interference with daily activities. By integrating these outcomes into the research, studies can offer a more comprehensive view of treatment effectiveness and ensure that the patient's voice is central to the evaluation process. PROs can also be used to monitor patient safety, detect adverse events, and make real-time adjustments to treatment plans.

14.7.4 Participatory Research Models: Engaging Patients as Co-Researchers

Participatory research models take patient-centered approaches a step further by actively involving patients and communities as co-researchers rather than just participants. These models are rooted in principles of empowerment, co-creation, and collaboration, emphasizing shared decision-making, mutual learning, and collective ownership of the research process.

14.7.5 Community-Based Participatory Research (CBPR)

Community-Based Participatory Research (CBPR) is a widely recognized participatory research model that involves researchers, organizational representatives, and community members in all phases of the research process. CBPR recognizes the community as a unit of identity and emphasizes the importance of building trust, sharing power, and addressing community-identified needs.

In CBPR, patients and community members are actively involved in formulating research questions, developing study protocols, collecting and analyzing data, and disseminating findings. This approach helps ensure that the research is culturally sensitive, ethically sound, and directly relevant to the community's needs. For example, in studies involving marginalized populations, such as indigenous communities or low-income urban residents, CBPR can help address historical mistrust and ensure that research outcomes are meaningful and beneficial to the community.

CBPR has been successfully applied in various areas, such as infectious disease research, mental health, and public health interventions. For instance, in HIV prevention research, CBPR has been used to develop culturally appropriate interventions tailored to specific community needs, enhancing their acceptability and effectiveness. By involving community members in designing and implementing interventions, researchers can leverage local knowledge and cultural practices to improve health outcomes and reduce disparities.

14.7.6 Patient and Public Involvement (PPI) in Research

Patient and Public Involvement (PPI) in research refers to the active involvement of patients, carers, and the public in the design, conduct, and dissemination of research. PPI is increasingly recognized as a standard practice in clinical research, with funding bodies and regulatory agencies requiring evidence of meaningful patient engagement.

PPI can take many forms, such as patient advisory panels, steering committees, or participatory workshops. The involvement of patients in these capacities ensures that research questions address real-world concerns, study materials are understandable and accessible, and dissemination strategies reach the intended audiences. For example, in rare disease research, involving patient advocacy groups can help identify patient priorities, improve recruitment strategies, and enhance the relevance of study findings to the patient community.

14.7.7 Co-Production of Research

Co-production is an emerging model within participatory research that involves patients and researchers working together as equal partners throughout the research process. Co-production goes beyond consultation and involves co-designing the study, co-creating interventions, co-analyzing data, and co-disseminating results. This approach is based on the principles of reciprocity, mutual respect, and shared decision-making, acknowledging the unique expertise and contributions that both patients and researchers bring to the table.

For instance, in mental health research, co-production can involve people with lived experience of mental health conditions collaborating with researchers to design interventions, develop measurement tools, and interpret findings. This collaboration helps ensure that the research is grounded in real-world experiences and addresses the nuances and complexities of mental health from the patient's perspective (McMillan et al. 2013; Lee et al. 2018; Bokhour et al. 2009; Buawangpong et al. 2020; Berry, Seiders, and Wilder 2003; Tran 2021).

14.8 BENEFITS OF PATIENT-CENTERED AND PARTICIPATORY RESEARCH MODELS

14.8.1 Improved Relevance and Impact of Research

By involving patients and communities in the research process, patient-centered and participatory models ensure that the research addresses the actual needs and priorities of those it intends to benefit. This relevance enhances the applicability and impact of research findings, leading to more effective treatments, interventions, and policies that reflect the real-world experiences of patients.

14.8.2 Enhanced Recruitment and Retention

Research shows that studies designed with patient input are more likely to achieve their recruitment and retention targets. Patient-centered approaches help identify and address potential barriers to participation, such as complex procedures, high travel costs, or lack of culturally appropriate materials. As a result, these studies tend to have higher participant engagement, lower dropout rates, and more diverse study populations, ultimately improving the generalizability of research findings.

14.8.3 Greater Trust and Transparency

Participatory research models foster trust and transparency between researchers and participants, particularly in communities that have historically been marginalized or exploited in research. By engaging patients and communities as partners, these models help build relationships based on respect, reciprocity, and mutual benefit. This trust is essential for moral research procedures and can improve the willingness of individuals and communities to participate in future studies.

14.9 CHALLENGES IN IMPLEMENTING PATIENT-CENTERED AND PARTICIPATORY MODELS

14.9.1 Balancing Power Dynamics

One of the key challenges in participatory research is managing power dynamics between researchers and patients or community members. Ensuring that all voices are heard, valued, and respected requires a commitment to equitable participation, transparency, and capacity building. Researchers need to share power, listen actively, and be open to incorporating patient and community feedback, even when it challenges established norms or practices.

14.9.2 Resource and Time Constraints

Implementing patient-centered and participatory approaches can be resource-intensive, requiring additional time, funding, and personnel to facilitate meaningful engagement. Building trust and fostering collaboration often requires sustained efforts, ongoing communication, and flexibility in adapting to the needs and schedules of patients and community members. These challenges may be particularly pronounced in under-resourced settings or studies with tight timelines (Berry, Seiders, and Wilder 2003).

14.9.3 Ensuring Representativeness and Diversity

While patient-centered and participatory models aim to enhance inclusivity, ensuring representativeness and diversity in patient and community involvement remains a challenge. Engaging a broad range of voices, including those from marginalized or underrepresented groups, requires targeted outreach, culturally competent practices, and strategies to address barriers to participation, such as language, literacy, and socioeconomic factors (L. B. Johnson and Smalley 2019; Lauver et al. 2002).

14.9.4 Future Directions and Opportunities

As the healthcare landscape evolves, there is growing recognition of the value of patient-centered and participatory research models. Future directions include developing standardized frameworks and best practices for meaningful patient engagement, leveraging digital tools and platforms to facilitate remote participation, and fostering partnerships between researchers, patients, and communities. Advances in digital health technologies, such as telemedicine, mobile health apps, and virtual communities, offer new opportunities for patient-centered and participatory research. These tools can help overcome geographical and logistical barriers, enable real-time communication, and enhance patient engagement in research. For example, virtual patient communities can provide platforms for patients to share their experiences, collaborate on research projects, and advocate for their needs and priorities (Lee et al. 2018).

14.10 CONCLUSION

The field of clinical research is experiencing a significant shift due to the emergence of novel ideas and trends that place an emphasis on patient-centeredness, technology integration, and customized methods. Digital health technologies, such as electronic health records (EHRs), wearable devices, mobile health (mHealth) applications, telemedicine, and advanced data platforms, are revolutionizing how clinical trials are planned, carried out, and evaluated. These tools enable real-time data collection, enhance participant engagement, reduce barriers to participation, and foster more efficient and adaptive study designs. Simultaneously, the rise of individualized treatments and precision medicine is shifting the focus toward treatments tailored to individual genetic, molecular, and phenotypic profiles. By leveraging advancements in genomics, bioinformatics, and digital health tools, personalized approaches offer the capacity to enhance patient results, decrease adverse effects, and make healthcare more effective and efficient. There is a growing commitment to patient-centered and participatory research models, which actively involve patients and communities as partners throughout the research process. These models emphasize shared decision-making, transparency, and mutual respect, ensuring that research is relevant, inclusive, and responsive to the real-world needs of diverse patient populations. While these advancements bring immense opportunities, they also present challenges, such as data privacy concerns, technological disparities, resource constraints, and the need for equitable access to new tools and methods. To overcome these obstacles, it is necessary to have interdisciplinary collaboration, regulatory adaptation, and sustained efforts to build trust and engagement with patients and communities.

REFERENCES

Aghamiri, Sara Sadat, Rada Amin, and Tomáš Helikar. 2022. "Recent Applications of Quantitative Systems Pharmacology and Machine Learning Models across Diseases." *Journal of Pharmacokinetics and Pharmacodynamics* 49 (1). J Pharmacokinet Pharmacodyn: 19–37. https://doi.org/10.1007/S10928-021-09790-9.

Ashley, Euan A. 2016. "Towards Precision Medicine." *Nature Reviews Genetics* 17 (9). Nature Publishing Group: 507–22. https://doi.org/10.1038/nrg.2016.86.

Awad, A., S.J. Trenfield, T.D. Pollard, . . . J.J. Ong—Advanced Drug Delivery, and undefined 2021. 2024. "Connected Healthcare: Improving Patient Care Using Digital Health Technologies." *Elsevier*. Accessed September 9. https://www.sciencedirect.com/science/article/pii/S0169409X21003513.

Berry, Leonard L., Kathleen Seiders, and Susan S. Wilder. 2003. "Innovations in Access to Care: A Patient-Centered Approach." *Annals of Internal Medicine* 139 (7). American College of Physicians: 568–74. https://doi.org/10.7326/0003-4819-139-7-200310070-00009.

Bokhour, Barbara G., Mary Jo Pugh, Jaya K. Rao, Ruzan Avetisyan, Dan R. Berlowitz, and Lewis E. Kazis. 2009. "Improving Methods for Measuring Quality of Care: A Patient-Centered Approach in Chronic Disease." *Medical Care Research and Review* 66 (2): 147–66. https://doi.org/10.1177/1077558708327174.

Borges Do Nascimento, Israel Júnior, Hebatullah Abdulazeem, Lenny Thinagaran Vasanthan, Edson Zangiacomi Martinez, Miriane Lucindo Zucoloto, Lasse Østengaard, Natasha Azzopardi-Muscat, Tomas Zapata, and David Novillo-Ortiz. 2024. "Barriers and Facilitators to Utilizing Digital Health Technologies by Healthcare Professionals." *Nature.Com*. Accessed September 9. https://doi.org/10.1038/s41746-023-00899-4.

Buawangpong, Nida, Kanokporn Pinyopornpanish, Wichuda Jiraporncharoen, Nisachol Dejkriengkraikul, Pakorn Sagulkoo, Chanapat Pateekhum, and Chaisiri Angkurawaranon. 2020. "Incorporating the Patient-Centered Approach into Clinical Practice Helps Improve Quality of Care in Cases of Hypertension: A Retrospective Cohort Study." *BMC Family Practice* 21 (1). BioMed Central Ltd. https://doi.org/10.1186/S12875-020-01183-0.

Bylstra, Yasmin, Weng Khong Lim, Sylvia Kam, Koei Wan Tham, R. Ryanne Wu, Jing Xian Teo, Sonia Davila, et al. 2021. "Family History Assessment Significantly Enhances Delivery of Precision Medicine in the Genomics Era." *Springer* 13 (1). BioMed Central Ltd. https://doi.org/10.1186/s13073-020-00819-1.

Evans, R. S. 2016. "Electronic Health Records: Then, Now, and in the Future." *Yearbook of Medical Informatics* 25 (S 01). Georg Thieme Verlag KG: S48–61. https://doi.org/10.15265/IYS-2016-S006/ID/JRS006-47/BIB.

Ginsburg, Geoffrey S., and Kathryn A. Phillips. 2018. "Precision Medicine: From Science to Value." *Health Affairs* 37 (5). Project HOPE: 694–701. https://doi.org/10.1377/HLTHAFF.2017.1624.

Inokuchi, Ryota, Yutaka Kondo, Kei Nishiyama, Friedemann Schad, and Anja Thronicke. 2022. "Real-World Evidence—Current Developments and Perspectives." *International Journal of Environmental Research and Public Health* 19 (16). Multidisciplinary Digital Publishing Institute: 10159. https://doi.org/10.3390/IJERPH191610159.

Johnson, Kevin B., Wei Qi Wei, Dilhan Weeraratne, Mark E. Frisse, Karl Misulis, Kyu Rhee, Juan Zhao, and Jane L. Snowdon. 2021. "Precision Medicine, AI, and the Future of Personalized Health Care." *Clinical and Translational Science* 14 (1). Blackwell Publishing Ltd: 86–93. https://doi.org/10.1111/CTS.12884.

Johnson, Lorraine B., and Jaye Bea Smalley. 2019. "Engaging the Patient: Patient-Centered Research." *Strategies for Team Science Success: Handbook of Evidence-Based Principles for Cross-Disciplinary Science and Practical Lessons Learned from Health Researchers*, January. Springer International Publishing, 135–47. https://doi.org/10.1007/978-3-030-20992-6_10.

Kandi, Venkataramana, and Sabitha Vadakedath. 2023. "Clinical Trials and Clinical Research: A Comprehensive Review." *Cureus* 15 (2). Cureus Inc. https://doi.org/10.7759/CUREUS.35077.

Kemp, E., J. Trigg, L. Beatty, . . . C. Christensen—Health Promotion, and undefined 2021. 2024. "Health Literacy, Digital Health Literacy and the Implementation of Digital Health Technologies in Cancer Care: The Need for a Strategic Approach." *Wiley Online Library*. Accessed September 9. https://onlinelibrary.wiley.com/doi/abs/10.1002/hpja.387.

Khan, Numan, Francoise A. Marvel, Jane Wang, and Seth S. Martin. 2017. "Digital Health Technologies to Promote Lifestyle Change and Adherence." *Current Treatment Options in Cardiovascular Medicine* 19 (8). Springer Healthcare. https://doi.org/10.1007/S11936-017-0560-4.

Kosorok, Michael R., and Eric B. Laber. 2019. "Precision Medicine." *Annual Review of Statistics and Its Application* 6. Annual Reviews Inc.: 263–86. https://doi.org/10.1146/ANNUREV-STATISTICS-030718-105251/CITE/REFWORKS.

Kosorok, Michael R., Eric B. Laber—Annual review of statistics and its, and undefined 2019. 2024. "Precision Medicine." *Annualreviews.Org*. Accessed September 9. https://www.annualreviews.org/content/journals/10.1146/annurev-statistics-030718-105251.

Lauver, Diane R., Sandra E. Ward, Susan M. Heidrich, Mary L. Keller, Barbara J. Bowers, Patricia Flatley Brennan, Karin T. Kirchhoff, and Thelma J. Wells. 2002. "Patient-Centered Interventions." *Research in Nursing and Health* 25 (4): 246–55. https://doi.org/10.1002/NUR.10044.

Lee, Joy L., Sydney M. Dy, Ayse P. Gurses, Julia M. Kim, Catalina Suarez-Cuervo, Zackary D. Berger, Rachel Brown, and Yan Xiao. 2018. "Towards a More Patient-Centered Approach to Medication Safety." *Journals.Sagepub.Com* 5 (2). SAGE Publications: 83–7. https://doi.org/10.1177/2374373517727532.

Lobitz, G., K. Armstrong, J. Concato, . . . B.H. Singer—Psychotherapy and, and undefined 2019. 2024. "The Biological and Biographical Basis of Precision Medicine." *Karger.Com*. Accessed September 9. https://karger.com/pps/article/88/6/333/283175.

Lupton, Deborah. 2014. "Critical Perspectives on Digital Health Technologies." *Sociology Compass* 8 (12). Wiley-Blackwell: 1344–59. https://doi.org/10.1111/SOC4.12226.

McComb, Mason, Robert Bies, and Murali Ramanathan. 2022. "Machine Learning in Pharmacometrics: Opportunities and Challenges." *British Journal of Clinical Pharmacology* 88 (4). John Wiley & Sons, Ltd: 1482–99. https://doi.org/10.1111/BCP.14801.

McMillan, Sara S., Elizabeth Kendall, Adem Sav, Michelle A. King, Jennifer A. Whitty, Fiona Kelly, and Amanda J. Wheeler. 2013. "Patient-Centered Approaches to Health Care: A Systematic Review of Randomized Controlled Trials." *Medical Care Research and Review* 70 (6): 567–96. https://doi.org/10.1177/1077558713496318.

publica, JAB Iriart—Cadernos de saúde, and undefined 2019. 2024. "Precision Medicine/Personalized Medicine: A Critical Analysis of Movements in the Transformation of Biomedicine in the Early 21st Century." *SciELO Brasil*. Accessed September 9. https://doi.org/10.1590/0102-311X00153118.

Scott, Benjamin K., Geoffrey T. Miller, Stephanie J. Fonda, Ronald E. Yeaw, James C. Gaudaen, Holly H. Pavliscsak, Matthew T. Quinn, and Jeremy C. Pamplin. 2020. "Advanced Digital Health Technologies for COVID-19 and Future Emergencies." *Telemedicine and E-Health* 26 (10). Mary Ann Liebert Inc.: 1226–33. https://doi.org/10.1089/TMJ.2020.0140.

Societies, D. Lupton, and undefined 2014. 2014. "Beyond Techno-Utopia: Critical Approaches to Digital Health Technologies." *Mdpi.Com* 4: 706–11. https://doi.org/10.3390/soc4040706.

Tran, Brandon Q. 2021. "Strategies for Effective Patient Care: Integrating Quality Communication with the Patient-Centered Approach." *Social and Personality Psychology Compass* 15 (1). Wiley-Blackwell. https://doi.org/10.1111/SPC3.12574.

Index

Note: Page numbers in *italics* indicate figures, and page numbers in **bold** indicate tables.

K

L

M

N

O

P

U

V

W